AF839506

Routledge Revivals

Speech Disorder in Nineteenth Century Britain

Originally published in 1980, this comprehensive study of stuttering in Britain in the nineteenth century was the first detailed examination of one speech problem as manifested in a particular time and place. It examines the problems posed by stuttering and illustrates how it became the linguistic handicap most responsible for laying the roots of professional speech therapy. The impediment was seen as a challenge to the physician in that the cure was tantalisingly elusive and the cause highly problematic. From these first attempts at treatment the profession of speech therapy developed. Many of the nineteenth century therapists were themselves stutterers who conquered their own impediment. As systematic management of speech defects emerged it matched the development of both humane mental health services and special education. It also demonstrated the community's response to disabled people which took the form of private philanthropy on the one hand and government legislation on the other.

Speech Disorder in Nineteenth Century Britain

The History of Stuttering

Denyse Rockey

ROUTLEDGE REVIVALS

Routledge
Taylor & Francis Group

First published in 1980 by Croom Helm Ltd

This edition first published in 2026 by Routledge
4 Park Square, Milton Park, Abingdon, Oxon, OX14 4RN
and by Routledge
605 Third Avenue, New York, NY 10158.

Routledge is an imprint of the Taylor & Francis Group, an informa business

© 1980 Denyse Rockey

All rights reserved. No part of this book may be reprinted or reproduced or utilised in any form or by any electronic, mechanical, or other means, now known or hereafter invented, including photocopying and recording, or in any information storage or retrieval system, without permission in writing from the publishers.

ISBN 13: 978-1-041-15919-3 (hbk)
ISBN 13: 978-1-003-68200-4 (ebk)
ISBN 13: 978-1-041-15950-6 (pbk)
Book DOI 10.4324/9781003682004

SPEECH DISORDER IN NINETEENTH CENTURY BRITAIN

The History of Stuttering

Denyse Rockey

CROOM HELM LONDON

© 1980 Denyse Rockey
Croom Helm Ltd, 2-10 St John's Road, London SW11

British Library Cataloguing in Publication Data

Rockey, Denyse
Speech disorder in nineteenth century Britain.
1. Speech, Disorder of – Great Britain – History – Sources
I. Title
616.8'55'00941 RC423

ISBN 0-85664-809-4

Typeset by Leaper & Gard Ltd, Bristol
printed and bound in Great Britain
by Billing and Sons Limited
Guildford, London, Oxford, Worcester

CONTENTS

To Edwina Bryson

LIST OF FIGURES AND TABLES

Figures

Tables

ABBREVIATIONS AND BIBLIOGRAPHICAL DETAILS

References which appear in the Bibliography are identified by the author's name only in the Notes, and qualified by the date where necessary. Anonymous notes are represented by a contracted title.

DNB indicates the *Dictionary of National Biography*. Standard abbreviations are used for journal articles. Full references can be found in the Bibliography.

Unless otherwise stated, Foster refers to J. Edgar Foster; Hunt to James Hunt; Wright to James Wright and Yearsley to James Yearsley.

Square brackets surrounding a date indicate that it was derived from a source other than the title page. Round brackets surrounding reference numbers indicate the full extent of the article, where this does not appear in the Bibliography.

ACKNOWLEDGEMENTS

I am most grateful to the Cambridgeshire Libraries for permission to use Finley's etching of Brampton Park and to the Bodleian Library, Oxford, for allowing me to reproduce advertisements from the John Johnson Collection, together with illustrations from Dieffenbach's *Memoir* and James Hunt's *Stammering and Stuttering*. Charles Phillips' surgical illustration appears by courtesy of the Wellcome Trustees. Permission to quote from copyright material has kindly been granted by Irvington Publishers, Inc., for a passage in M.E. Wingate's *Stuttering*; by Harper & Row for a passage in Claude Bernard's *An Introduction to Experimental Medicine*; and by Houghton Mifflin for a passage in C. Mackenzie's *Alexander Graham Bell*. Full bibliographic details are to be found in the references or bibliography.

PREFACE

This book is based on an Oxford University D. Phil. thesis entitled *Stuttering in Britain in the Nineteenth Century*. Though most of the source material was available in Oxford, my enquiries also led further afield and entailed the writing of innumerable letters. As space does not permit me to thank everyone by name, I shall content myself with mentioning only Mary Plackett, chief librarian of the Royal National Institute for the Deaf, London, who, along with the staff of the Bodleian and Radcliffe Science Libraries, Oxford, I troubled more than most.

Historical research was a discipline new to me and therefore I am particularly grateful for the encouragement, guidance and criticism I received from Mr Brian Farrell, Dr Brian Harrison and Dr Charles Webster, all of Corpus Christi College, who supervised my studies at various times. The choice could not have been more fortunate.

Mary Deane similarly gave generously of her time during the preparation of the manuscript, whilst my husband and brother provided other forms of practical assistance. Lastly, I must thank my parents, who supported me in ways too numerous to mention.

Wellcome Unit for the History of Medicine
Oxford

INTRODUCTION

For the historian of speech disorders, the nineteenth century holds special interest, for then the multiplicity of problems began to be differentiated, more closely evaluated and extensively treated. No longer was speech breakdown worth only passing comment in some medical or rhetorical treatise. Nor were the inarticulate to be stranded largely without help. Elocutionists moved beyond their traditional bounds, offering assistance to those whose speech was defective rather than unpolished and thus initiating what might loosely be called a profession of speech correction, albeit an unorganised one, with its members bound together by their occupation rather than by any institution or commonly shared views. Herein lay the potential for dissent, and, as the seventeenth century had seen the debate on deafness between Holder and Wallis, so the nineteenth century witnessed speculation and controversy over another type of verbal impediment.

In Britain, the period is conventionally bracketed by two figures whose stature and perspicacity were as notable as their mode of expression and interpretation were diverse. John Thelwall and John Wyllie each took a broad view, interesting themselves in the totality of speech problems, but while the former's approach was that of a layman with an affection for the English tongue, the latter analysed impediments with the eye of a modern physiologist. They were pioneers, cast in very different moulds. Thelwall, the political agitator, called upon rhetoric and enthusiasm to establish his new profession: Wyllie, university lecturer and physician, replaced missionary zeal with the dedication of a careful experimenter, and as a retiring bachelor, was well disposed for the task of collecting and synthesising contemporary knowledge on linguistic handicaps. Thelwall's *Letter to Henry Cline* of 1810 was the first book concerned solely with speech problems to be published in English; Wyllie's *The Disorders of Speech*, appearing 84 years later, may be regarded as the first British textbook on the subject, and in its day was considered the most comprehensive in any language. Finally, these men were landmarks in a special sense, for whereas Thelwall is arguably Britain's first 'speech therapist',[1] Wyllie's book has been taken as the date from which modern speech therapy actually started.[2]

This study ranges widely over its subject. The book falls into three sections. The first two chapters deal with patients and the professional response to them, the following three are concerned with causes and the final three with cures. Stuttering is important in the evolution of speech rehabilitation because, in Victorian Britain, the history of the two may almost be equated. It was the first complaint to provoke widespread interest. This was partly because it was considered particularly pernicious, but also because it lent itself to the sort of pseudo-scientific speculations that were so attractive. Other disorders could scarcely compete. Operative techniques for cleft palate were crude, and the prognosis consequently poor; serious developmental handicaps were barely recognised; vocal disorders were generally insufficiently disabling or challenging to make a significant impression; whilst language breakdown following brain injury stimulated theoretical rather than therapeutic interest, when it caught the medical imagination later in the century.

History is a new frontier in speech pathology. There are virtually no detailed inquiries into past attitudes to or the management of verbal handicaps, contributions to date being mainly limited to poorly documented chronologies or surveys so sweeping that they are unable to do justice to any question within their purview. The former have merely reviewed the literature, along the lines prefacing scientific treatises, but projected further back in time. To judge from their titles, some were ostensively general studies but, in actuality, stuttering was their real focus, which fact underscores its importance to earlier thinkers. The result is that such histories amount to little more than a catalogue of names, dates, professions and nationalities of the leading theorists and therapists, together with brief comment on their views. This format was adopted by James Hunt, in the last century, when he sketched ideas from antiquity to the late Renaissance, and also provided a review of those notions current in his own day.[3] Others followed suit, and continue to do so, often presenting fewer rather than more facts. An example is the survey in Samuel Potter's prize winning essay *Speech and Its Defects* (1882). Potter, who became a member of the Royal College of Physicians, London, published this in Philadelphia, America having become his home around 1864, when he emigrated from Ireland at the age of seventeen. His work, important in its time, was the source of other studies, some of which bear his stamp.[4] Since the turn of the twentieth century, there have been over a dozen such surveys in English from speech pathologists, some of which appear in the bibliography.[5] Notwithstanding their greater frame of reference, the educational historians Frampton and Rowell have been content with this approach.[6] While they rely on secondary sources, Pritchard ignores speech therapy before 1906 and limits his discussion to a brief account of the events of 1945, when local authorities were first obliged to educate verbally impaired children and the College of Speech Therapists, London, came into being.[7]

One weakness of these studies is the tendency to accept the words *stammer* and *stutter* at face value. By projecting our own vocabulary and conceptual framework onto the past we assume, first, that these words have not changed meaning and, secondly, that patients were diagnosed according to present criteria. Neither assumption is fully justified and hence publications so based are liable to be mistitled and lacking in critical insight. To avoid these confusions, I have used the term *stuttering*, currently favoured in America, for the disorder under discussion. This is not to suggest that *stuttering* is without ambiguity, but its connotations are generally less misleading than its older synonym. For present purposes, the definition by the College of Speech Therapists will suffice:

> Speech characterized by interruptions of its fluency by the repetition of sounds, syllables or phrases, and blocks, overt or disguised, often accompanied by concomitant movements and disruption of normal breathing rhythm. There may be avoidance reactions either of words or speech situations.[8]

The word *stammering* is used only in quotations or where the author's meaning is uncertain.

Another deficiency of the chronological method is that it has led to a certain patronising attitude to the past and corresponding self-complacency, despite the growing realisation that many modern notions are but old ideas in new clothing. This situation arises not only because speech correctionists and historians differ in orientation, but also because the former, anxious to establish their occupation as a profession and their discipline as a science, have been striving to rid themselves of outmoded ideas. With the growth of professional confidence, however, the present should be able to reflect upon the past without the fear of being engulfed by it.

By exploring the manifold intellectual and social influences upon them, Victorians may be seen in their own light, and thus some of their bizarre and apparently misguided thoughts and actions become less foolish. Of particular significance were social factors, not only in provoking stuttering, but also in dictating who would give and who receive treatment, and under what conditions. Furthermore, professional rivalries and prejudices could be as important in determining beliefs as any scientific finding. Unfortunately, neither space nor time has permitted a complete account of all the factors impinging upon a given idea or treatment, nor has it been possible to analyse the internal coherence of any one theory or personal contribution in detail. The aim has been to present the questions Victorians were asking, to indicate their avenues of enquiry, and to note the assumptions underlying their treatment. Regarding surgery, however, as some studies are available,[9] I have been content to restate the situation in Britain, introduce new material and comment on the diagnoses.

As circumstances may be highlighted through contrast, it is sometimes helpful to step outside the Victorian era, the stuttering problem, and Britain. In doing so, I may appear to have strayed beyond my brief in three ways. First, retrospective glances to earlier centuries assist in assessing the speed and direction of scientific progress and also serve to indicate sources of change. Hartley's associationism, for example, was said to have had more impact in the nineteenth century than in his own time. Modern concepts and experimental findings, by contrast, are helpful in bringing into focus the particularly puzzling features of the disorder, the distinctions that Victorians made, the conceptual framework under which they laboured and the ways this affected them for good or ill. This dialectic of past and present, however, is not intended as a yardstick whereby the one can be judged by the other, but as a tool by which the difficulties of Victorians, their aims and achievements, may be more readily discerned.

A second source of comparison is other handicaps. The development of services and techniques for helping the deaf, blind, insane, mentally retarded and even cripples have been well documented, and it is informative to contrast their circumstances with those of defective speakers. Reference is also made to a variety of speech disorders, both because differential diagnosis was problematical and because it is interesting to see how others fared *vis-à-vis* the stutterer.

Thirdly, I have made geographical excursions. Though the majority of practitioners were situated in London, and it is there that most books and articles appeared, it would be wrong to suggest that the new movement was primarily English, or was intellectually nurtured from this source. Many doctors had embarked upon their careers whilst Edinburgh still dominated the academic scene and some that were not native Scotsmen made it their business to spend time in the northern capital, which was also the home of notable elocutionists. Significant contributions likewise came from Ireland, with stutterers being able to find help, at various times, in Dublin and Belfast. But many ideas originated farther afield, and as it would be impossible to write a history of modern British speech therapy without reference to the United States, so any study of the last century must consider Continental attitudes. These became known through journal reports or books that were either written in English or translated, as well as by direct experience. Publications have been consulted also, which, though printed abroad, were either later editions of a work originating in this country and no longer readily available, or were based upon an idea having its root here. As regards Britain itself, ideas were widely scattered and reflected the proclivities of individuals rather than the thinking of particular regions or schools.

In number and length, Victorian publications far exceeded those of previous centuries. They are noteworthy either as technical or social documents, some being addressed to the professionally concerned, some to fellow sufferers, and some to the public. Many people reflected upon stuttering, but the most influential concepts came from elocutionists and medical men. However, as academic standing provided no certain guide to its understanding, and the insights of an observant layman might be as astute as any professional, all commentators deserve fair consideration. In addition to special treatises and articles in medical journals, stuttering featured in dictionaries, encyclopaedias, literary magazines, theses[10] and even novels. These, then, in the main provide the sources of reference. The material they contain ranges from highly personal accounts to embryonic statistics, from diverting anecdotes to factual case histories, from pamphlets offering words of cheer to more technical analyses. Much of the information is fragmentary and apparently written in ignorance of other contemporary enquiries, so the picture that emerges in the following pages results from the piecing together of many isolated facts, often inconsequential if taken alone. Thus, in trying to present these coherently, there is the risk of conveying a false sense of order in what was a very confused field.

It is disappointing that in an entrepreneurial age, with quacks supposedly lurking around every corner, so little ephemera has come to light. The advertisements I have found are all reasonable in their claims and language. Some appear in books, and indeed many publications were intended as much for publicity as for the dissemination of knowledge. From a modern standpoint, few have inherent merit and few are of historical importance in the sense of being turning points or exerting lasting influence. Indeed, most were soon forgotten. This has made the compilation of a bibliography difficult. In addition to the meagre works of substance, the best that could be done was to include a selection of writings giving the range and flavour of current ideas. Also listed are secondary sources from which some background material may be derived, but unfortunately in those areas most pertinent to my topic such histories are all too few – speech pathology before 1800[11] and after 1900, its development in Continental Europe during the period under investigation, the latter stages of the elocutionary movement, nineteenth century British linguistics and certain aspects of psychology. Hence, conclusions of a universal character must await further research. My findings stay closer to the study, which represents a small piece in the jigsaw of Victorian medical and social life.

Notes

1. Rockey (1977), pp. 83-4; Rockey (1979), pp. 156, 158-60.
2. George Sykes, 'The Growth and Development of Speech Therapy in Great Britain, 1894-1962' (St Andrew's Univ., Dundee, BA thesis in education, 1962), 1, p.5.
3. The most detailed account appears in Hunt's 7th edn (1870), pp. 13-192.
4. G. Klingbeil, 'The historical background of the modern speech clinic', *Journal of Speech Disorders*, 4 (1939), 115-31. Abstracted in *A Compendium of Research on Theory on Stuttering*, ed. Charles Diehl (Springfield, Illinois, Charles C. Thomas, 1958), pp. 5-13.
5. Appelt, pp. 1-4; Bluemel, vol. 1, ch. 7, esp. 277-8, vol. 2, pp. 25, 260-1; Department of Education and Science, pp. 4-9; Eldridge, p. 1 ff; Van Riper, pp. 285-8, 335-8; Wingate, pp. 129-41, 153-6; 279-93. Cf. Schoolfield, pp. 111-16.
6. Merle Frampton and Hugh Rowell (eds.), 'History' in *Education of the Handicapped* (London, G.G. Harrap & Co., Ltd, [1938]), vol. 1, 87-100.
7. Pritchard, pp. 212-13.
8. 'Terminology . . .', p. 39.
9. Burdin, pp. 43-64; L. Stevenson, pp. 527-54.
10. It is unfortunate that two MD theses in Glasgow appear not to have been published: J.T. Whittaker's 'Physiology of Stammering' (1876) and A.G. Park's 'Defects in Speech' (1892). I was unable to obtain copies of these before going to press.
11. Since completing this book Ynez Violé O'Neill's study has come to my notice: *Speech and Speech Disorders in Western Thought before 1600* (Westport, Conn., Greenwood Press, 1980).

Oh! tis a sore affliction, to restrain,
From mere necessity, the glowing thought;
To feel the fluent cateract of speech
Check'd by some wintry spell, and frozen up,
Just as it leapeth from the precipice!
To be the butt of wordy captious fools,
And see the sneering self-complacent smile
Of victory on their lips, when I might prove,
(But for some little word I dare not utter,)
That innate truth is not a specious lie;
To hear foul slander blast an honour'd name,
Yet breathe no fact to drive the fiend away;
To mark neglected virtue in the dust,
Yet have no word to pity or console;
To feel just indignation swell my breast,
Yet know the fountain of my wrath is seal'd;
To see my fellow-mortals hurrying on
Down the steep cliff of crime, down to perdition,
Yet have no voice to warn, – no voice to win!

'Tis to be mortified in every point,
Baffled at every turn of life, for want
Of that most common privilege of man,
The merest drug of gorged society,
Words, – windy words.

Martin Tupper, from his
The Stammerer's Complaint

1 EMERGENCE OF THE PROBLEM

Some idea of the general awareness of speech problems may be gained from the *Encyclopaedia Britannica*. In 1798, aphasia was confined to the vocabulary of sceptic philosophy, which defined it as silence arising from doubt; neither lisping nor stuttering were mentioned at all. The contrast with deafness and dumbness is striking. Between them, these subjects covered several columns in 1798 and by 1877 they filled over seventeen. Though stuttering was not included until 1860, when it commanded less than four columns, it should not be inferred that the problem was ignored before mid-century. Some scientifically oriented dictionaries had already taken note of it and a miscellany of people were engaged in describing its characteristics, as well as its personal and social ramifications.

These early writings succeeded in establishing basic information about the problem's existence, though its nature continued to be obscure. Symptomatology remained at a pre-scientific level with stutterers providing vivid accounts of their sufferings and tales being recounted of their bizarre behaviour. Even professionals adopted this line, preferring to stimulate the imagination than search for general principles of behaviour. A move towards objectivity had begun, however, with enquiries into the incidence and distribution of the impediment; and, amidst abundant guesswork, some genuine facts started to emerge.

Popular Impressions

The chameleon-like character of stuttering bewildered the sufferer, whilst provoking a certain fascination amongst bystanders. Why was it that, often for no apparent reason, speech would halt under circumstances and in a manner that varied greatly from person to person? Numerous illustrative accounts of stutterers' speech point to an implicit recognition that their vacillations could be examined from three points of view. Obvious fluctuations existed in the utterance itself, but there were also physiological and environmental changes that affected a person's ability to communicate. These phenomena, when portrayed through compelling anecdotes, could entertain the casual observer, but they taxed theorists who, obliged to take them seriously, had to find an explanation that could encompass them all.

A well recorded symptom was the stutterer's ability to sing, which perhaps inspired the French saying: 'Les bègues chantent toujours bien'.[1] Their skill received early recognition in this country through Allan Ramsay's *On Wit: The Tale of the Manting Lad* (1716).[2] The nineteenth-century equivalent of this tale was often recounted, and involved a ship's crew being saved from mutiny through attention being diverted at the crucial moment by a stutterer singing out the plight of a cook, who had fallen overboard with his bucket.[3] Stutterers were not always so fluent, however, for Cull had observed hesitation during singing on three occasions,[4] a symptom that one German colleague took as a poor prognosis.[5] It was also realised that whistling presented no difficulty and that stutterers often spoke well in an assumed voice, or foreign tongue.

More perplexing was the tendency for speech to become arrested at certain words or sounds, particularly consonants. One typical story concerned an officer who, on giving an order, stuck on *f-f-f*, until he thought to shout: 'D—n your eyes, you know what I mean – *shoot*'. Another person was unable to say 'a pint of porter', but could order 'two half pints of porter' with ease.[6] Considerable attention was also paid to the freeness of some speech, once the initial barrier had been overcome. This had been noted by Aristotle, but Victorians preferred Shakespeare's more colourful version:

> I pr'ythee, tell me, who is it? quickly, and speak apace.
> I would thou could'st stammer that thou might'st pour this concealed man out of thy mouth, as wine comes out of a narrow mouth'd bottle, either too much at once, or none at all.[7]

This phenomenon provoked much speculation, one writer quoting Swift's comment that those whose minds are filled with ideas, crowding to be expressed, are apt to hesitate, whereas those with one set of ideas may be likened to people at a church door, who file through quickly when it is almost empty.[8]

The effects of health, alcohol, tobacco and even the weather were likewise fully appreciated. Liquor was said to free the tongue, but there came a time when incoherency ensued and this intoxicated speech was sometimes called stammering. If it did not render the person completely dumb, strong emotion might also have a salutary effect, as Bathsheba was informed when paying her new employee, Andrew

Randle: ' 'A can cuss, mem, as well as you or I, but 'a can't speak a common speech to save his life.'[9] Further reports told of stutterers speaking well when swimming, asleep, blindfolded, masked or in certain company, some acquiring greater fluency amongst friends and others with strangers. Charles Dodgson, for example, was most at home with little girls.

Accompanying these overt symptoms was an inner turmoil and by the end of the century the most authoritative medical opinion was that 'the sum-total of unhappiness inflicted upon a people by this single defect is not much less than that produced by all other derangements of speech put together'.[10] Numerous harrowing accounts contributed to this opinion, many supplied by speech correctionists who had once stuttered themselves. Particular publicity, however, derived from two literary figures, one reputedly the most popular man in England at the time of his death, and the other 'lifted to a height of fame that has been exceeded by few writers, during their lifetime'.[11] For Charles Kingsley, stuttering was 'that fearful curse', seemingly afflicting him more than most, sapping his vitality and debarring him from witty converse.[12] To Martin Tupper, it was an affliction 'unnumbered amongst this world's sorrows' and one for which 'life hath no grief more galling'.[13] These lines were expressed in his best selling volume of poetry *Proverbial Philosophy* and they so caught the sentiment of the times that they were used to preface numerous treatises on stuttering. In the same vein was his *The Stammerer's Complaint*, and with such graphic portrayals of the disorder available few were moved to offer more scientific descriptions.

The fortunes of a stutterer could be conveyed convincingly in literary form. Those requiring holiday reading might enjoy *Stuttering Sam – the Whitest Sport of Santa Fe*,[14] whereas the more serious could turn to Lord Lytton's two volume novel of romance, honour and humility. In this story, a key part is played by George Morley, a man of intellect and theological learning, whose stuttering frustrated his ambition to enter the Church. After being helped to overcome his complaint, he is fortuitously enabled to repay his benefactor by speaking fluently on his behalf at a most timely moment.[15] Even more realistic episodes in the life of a stutterer were unfolded in *The Unspeakable*, a quasi-fictional narrative of events known to or experienced by its anonymous author.[16] The book, commended to every mother by Kingsley,[17] and widely reviewed, is filled with Dickensian characters. The hero, Charles Theodore Monckton, and his stepmother, nicknamed Brocade, could double for the young

Copperfield and Miss Murdstone. In the course of his youth, various unpleasant characters chastise the sensitive lad until he became an inveterate stutterer trailing from elocutionist to doctor and quack in search of help. As many of these individuals are only thinly disguised, the story provides an interesting slant on their activities.

In an obvious allusion to this book, Dickens suggests how it might be set to music as a tragi-comic opera.[18] The comic aspects of stuttering were most theatrical and were used in a romantic context in two Continental operas. Smetana portrayed Vasek as a simpleton in *The Bartered Bride*,[19] whilst in *Le Voyage en Chine*,[20] elocutionary lessons relieve the impediment of Monsieur Alidor de Rosenville to the delight of his future father-in-law. When put to the test, however, both men fail to get their tongues around *incombustibilité*.[21] Meanwhile, English speakers were entertained by Lord Dundreary, the inept fop with idiosyncratic gait, eyeglass and stutter, played by Sothern and bringing him fame and fortune. His speech impediment, in particular, was thought hugely funny and audiences each side of the Atlantic flocked to *Our American Cousin*, reputedly one of the biggest attractions known to the American stage.[22]

Of course, stutterers had been the butt of ridicule long before the nineteenth century. Tartaglia,[23] for instance, had become a theatrical institution through the Commedia dell'Arte. Originally, he was portrayed as an obstructive civil servant but he later took the form of some other elderly government official, who was enabled to make satirical comments on current affairs under the guise of his impediment.[24] Those with unfortunate characteristics were also ready objects for practical joking. One wit gave dinner parties and amused himself at the expense of his guests as they gradually realised what united them. Having entertained a group of squinters and another with long chins, he gathered some stutterers together, setting an amanuensis behind a screen to record their dialogue. The man's task was not arduous as no more than twenty words were spoken during the first course, and during the second, one guest took a quarter of an hour to say 'the Ducklins and Sparrow-grass were very good' and 'another took up the same time in declaring himself of the same Opinion'. The joke turned sour, however, when one of the guests took umbrage and issued his host a challenge.[25]

To the general public, then, the stutterer may have appeared a comical character or a bumbling fool, but those who knew him better often thought otherwise and they began to enquire more closely into factors that may have disposed him to misfortune.

Civilisation and Language

Though the founding of cities is generally considered a landmark in human progress, Rousseau had questioned the suitability of man for this civilised state, and the deplorable condition of much urban life provided impressive support for the argument. Those with more moderate views certainly interpreted such advance as a mixed blessing:

> It is not civilization, but the increasing want which it brings in its train . . . which set the mind in passive motion; . . . Civilization . . . carries the poison and the antidote in the same hand . . . If savages show such a happy exemption from insanity they are indebted for it, not merely to the want of civilization, but probably also to the indomitable energy of their corporeal vitality.[26]

Degeneracy in all its forms was a contentious issue in the nineteenth century and speech problems were associated with physical degeneracy and criminality. The weakened nervous system of Bohemian gypsies, partly attributed to intermarriage, also produced a proclivity to disorders like epilepsy and insanity, as well as stuttering.[27] However, it was not until the twentieth century that the impediment was expressly described as a functional disease of civilisation, due to the tendency for instinctive actions to be performed consciously. 'In the matter of speech', Jones asserted, 'this tends to produce stammering.'[28]

This was not idle speculation. During the nineteenth century, explorers had penetrated many unknown regions and one question they were asked was whether primitives stuttered. Facts were few and conflicting. The impediment was said to be common in West Africa, where it was fashionable.[29] Further details are contained in a letter to Hunt, in which Clarke suggested that some natives, with their well-developed imitative faculties, thought it prestigious to stutter, having observed certain Europeans doing so. He went on to surmise that when the complaint arose in later life it was through the natives' predilection for strong tobacco and alcohol. Hunt also drew attention to a French report of a so-called stuttering negro tribe, the Neambaga, whose speech was characterised by the insertion of the syllable, *shill*, into the middle of words. And he makes mention of the Hottentots, thought to have been so named by the Dutch, on account of their 'stuttering' speech. However, Amman, around 1700, was using *hottentotism* for a severe articulatory defect.[30]

Another traveller to Africa was a former patient of Abbotts, who had stuttered himself and was therefore a reliable witness. In the Cape he came across two or three stuttering tribesmen, but in each case, he reported 'the sufferer had been subjected more or less to the influences and enervating habits of civilised life'. In Central Africa, however, a Commander Cameron had found no trace of any impediments.[31]

In an attempt to clarify the issue, Cazalet wrote to Livingstone enquiring about his experiences in the African interior, and received the following reply, dated 11 February 1858:

> SIR, – I never met with a single case of Stammering in any part of Africa. I saw but one dumb man, and another partially so, and I heard of a third – a woman – but did not see her. Defects of hearing and speaking are extremely rare.
>
> I am, etc.,
> DAVID LIVINGSTONE
>
> If the case is as stated at Sierra Leone, it is very remarkable indeed.[32]

Cazalet also approached Sir James Brooke about Borneo, and learned that he could recall no instance either among these people or the Dyaks and Malays, but he pointed out that the latter, though living in a simple state, were hardly uncivilised.[33]

Negative findings also came from George Catlin, an American painter and ethnologist, whose work was well known in London. He had moved through some 150 tribes in North and South America, containing over two million people, and never once heard of a stutterer, idiot, lunatic or hunchback, though a few cases of deaf-mutism were reported. Nor was mortality high, except amongst those perverted by Western influences. Catlin castigated Europeans for their deplorable life-styles, particularly their pernicious habit of the 'hanging jaw' – a posture never found amongst Indian tribesmen. Evidently the tribal practice was to close infants' mouths after suckling, thus establishing healthy patterns for life.[34] Catlin's friend, William Abbotts, while agreeing that a drooping jaw was injurious to health and 'certainly increases the affection of stammering where it exists' did not think it engendered the disorder in all cases; indeed, totally diverse causes might be operative.[35] Nevertheless, he gave weight to these and the African reports, concluding that in 'a condition of savage simplicity, stammering and stuttering are next to unknown'.[36] Of course, as some perceived, much turned on the exposure of tribesmen to foreign influences, as well as the definition of 'primitive' and 'stuttering'.

A century after Catlin's explorations the North American Indians were visited anew, by a team which confirmed his findings but offered a different explanation, since they had found no word for stuttering in the native language. This fitted well with Johnson's diagnosogenic theory of the complaint and with Korzibski's semantic philosophy, to which he subscribed, the contention being that normal non-fluencies do not become stuttering until so called.[37] Since then, however, stuttering has been found among some Indian tribesmen,[38] as well as amongst Zulus and Bantus[39] and the debate continues.

Victorians found linguistic explanations more attractive than sociological ones. Henry McCormac of Belfast, one of the first British physicians to write on stuttering, could speak authoritatively. Not only was he widely travelled, but he had a prodigious command of some 20 languages.[40] In his opinion, primitive languages were evolving and hence their consonantal complement was incomplete, leaving them more melodic.[41] He made no effort to correlate this with stuttering though others were ready to suggest that Catlin's Indians were more fluent because of their musical language.[42] Support for this hypothesis came from Potter, who personally had found no stuttering amongst the vocalic sounding Pimos, in contrast with the Apaches and Maricopes of Arizona, whose language was harsh.[43] By extension, it could be argued that musically gifted people might be less apt to stutter, but the only comment on this point came from Abbotts who believed it to be rare amongst wind instrumentalists, a fact he attributed to their good breathing habits.[44]

Another linguistic parameter was rhythm, supposedly marked in primitive languages and varying in degree amongst the civilised. One report tells of frequent stuttering amongst the Mongolian inhabitants of China, where it was 'given the suggestive name of "kchi-ko" '.[45] But more attention was focused on the Cochin area of China on account of a French consul's son, whose case was investigated in 1839 by the French speech correctionist, Dr Marc Colombat. The lad, a Eurasian, grew up speaking two languages, but though stuttering in French, the local Chinese dialect tripped easily from his tongue, as it did for most of the population.[46] It was not so much the rhythmic intonation, however, nor precisely the similarity of Chinese words in sound or measure, that impressed Hunt, but the fact that they are monosyllabic, as are the tribal languages of some North American Indians where stuttering is absent.[47]

For every anecdote, there was usually another to controvert it. For instance, Sir George Braithwaite Broughton's stuttering left him when he spoke French,[48] as it did for Erasmus Darwin's eldest son,[49] yet for another man this was when the problem appeared.[50] Then there was the Frenchman who only experienced difficulty in English,[51] whilst one medical man could speak English better than either his native tongue or Persian.[52] From this, little could be deduced with safety but there was a feeling that even among European languages, melodiousness and the prevalence of stuttering were causally linked. English was not ranked on the hierarchical scale but presumably was considered more musical than German, a hard language apt to produce stutterers.[53] It compared unfavourably with the harmonious Italian tongue. The Spanish were also remarkably free from the disorder.[54] These languages had a vocalic emphasis approaching that of song, which might account for the ease with which they were articulated. No reasons were offered for the frequency of the complaint in Constantinople.[55]

Similarly, certain dialectal regions could be assumed to foster stuttering. Knighted for his work on statistics, Sir William Wilde, oto-laryngologist and father of the playwright, had cause for interest in the subject. As one of the 1851 Irish Census Commissioners, he was partly responsible for collecting the first statistical information on deaf-mutism in the British Isles.[56] His observations on other verbal impediments were less well founded. Stuttering was reputedly rare amongst the sonorous speakers of Mayo and Galway[57] and Wilde believed this true of Dublin, but not of Northern Ireland. Abbotts agreed, adding that Cornwall, Liverpool and Manchester were also bad areas.[58]

Hunt postulated that hesitation – the precursor to stuttering – might be more common in regions where two languages or dialects were juxtaposed, since the inhabitants had a firm grasp of neither. The meeting point of Gaelic and English, or Yorkshire and Lancashire, were two examples. For this reason, northerners might be more disposed to the complaint,[59] though this could be because their dialect was harsher.[60] Bearing in mind the population of the counties at that time, neither conjecture was confirmed by Hunt's map, the deficiencies of which he realised, but which he saw as a first step in the demographic study of stuttering (Figure 1.1, p. 38). Hunt also reproduced Chervin's military statistics, showing that in France, too, the south was more affected,[61] the cause here being attributed to poor educational standards rather than dialectal variations.[62] Education, however, could have less desirable effects and should be considered alongside the related questions of social status and intellectual ability.

Social Class and Intelligence

The maxim for social advancement in England, on a par with keeping a good wine cellar, was, according to Dickens: 'Be a fluent speaker.'[63] This was possibly of less consequence to the aristocracy, whose financial and social status was assured, but for an ambitious middle-class man, hesitant speech could frustrate his professional aspirations. Erasmus Darwin evidently considered it no hindrance to a young physician starting a practice, it might even have publicity value;[64] but few suggested that this held for the pulpit, bar, senate or army. True, stuttering did not prevent Kingsley from joining the Church – he could speak for God but not himself[65] – yet it must have been a factor in Dodgson's initial reluctance to take priest's orders. It certainly did debar Martin Tupper, as it had Charles Lamb. Tupper also failed to become an advocate or MP and in grave financial anxiety wrote to Gladstone, his close friend, asking him to find 'some situation requiring the pen rather than the tongue'.[66] And for entertainment he turned to chess, one means by which a sufferer 'can conquer in argument without the toil of speech'.[67]

Chess is no game for the dullard, yet the stuttering schoolboy was frequently bottom of the class through his inability to speak up, even when he knew the answers better than most.[68] It is easy to equate verbal agility with intellectual prowess, and Melville Bell censured educationalists for their false values:

> Quickness of utterance being the quality most prized by mistaken schoolmasters, the thoughtful boy, who is often shy, and who is generally of better part than the pert, guessing lads, that are always first with their answers, has no chance; and in his efforts to expedite his thoughts, he confuses them, or they come faster than his tongue can utter them, so that jumbling rapidity, inarticulate hurry, stuttering, or convulsive impediment, is very naturally created.[69]

Furthermore, merciless teasing by peers was compounded by the 'reign of terror' instituted by teachers. It was for such reasons that 'many eminent physicians' believed stuttering to be increasing greatly.[70] In Charles Monckton's school the impediment was not permitted,[71] but elsewhere there were other pressures. Cramming was the very negation of education,[72] and though by Beasley's time legislation existed to prevent bodily overworking of children, there was nothing to stop undue mental exertion, which benefited the child little, but served to demonstrate 'the proficiency of this or that scholastic establishment'.[73]

The public schools came in for particular censure. Before Dr Arnold's Rugby, their system had been one of 'anarchy tempered by despotism'.[74] But the system he established was little better, for a man whose philosophy was that 'the first, second, and third duty of a schoolmaster was to get rid of unpromising subjects' can hardly have been a sympathetic mentor to diffident pupils. However, though nearly every public school could 'furnish an example' of stuttering,[75] there is no reason to believe that the situation was any better in state schools, either here or abroad (Table 1.3, p. 37). In fact, these were places where the defect flourished to such an extent that they might be called 'Institutes for teaching Stammering',[76] and in Vienna, Coën advised that stuttering children should avoid 'public' schools.[77]

Stutterers had their own tales to tell. Despite the 'severity of the masters' and the 'tyranny of the monitors' at Christ's Hospital, Lamb did not ascribe his own speech impediment to this source.[78] Less fortunate was his schoolmate, Leigh Hunt, whose hesitancy caused the impatient Dr Boyer to knock out a tooth with the back of a Homer.[79] At Eton – where 'a boy suffers more injustice, and is taught more moral and physical corruption'[80] – problems also existed, since it was evidently necessary to have an elocutionist within its precincts expressly for correcting impediments.[81] Unfavourable mention was similarly made of Charterhouse – 'Slaughterhouse as Thackeray was wont to style it' – Martin Tupper's school. He was admitted at the age of eleven when it was run by a despotic headmaster who 'worked so upon an over-sensitive nature to force a boy beyond his powers, as to fix for many years the infirmity of stammering'.[82]

Victorians commonly equated sensitivity with intelligence, though the idea was not new, as Carlyle points out in one of his numerous letters to Emerson, concerning a mutual friend:

> James is a very good fellow . . . and . . . confirms an observation of mine, which indeed I find is hundreds of years old, that a stammering man is never a worthless one. Physiology can tell you why. It is an excess of delicacy, excess of sensibility to the presence of his fellow creature, that makes him stammer. Hammond l'Estrange says, 'Who ever heard of a stammering man that was a fool?' Really there is something in that.[83]

Beasley certainly believed stutterers to be intellectually superior, and that this was an acquisition obtained through the habit of thinking, reading and contemplation, into which they retreated after being cut off from social intercourse.[84] This appears to have been the predicament of the solitary and romantic George Darley, an able mathematician and poet, who describes his affliction as 'a hideous mask upon my mind which not only disfigures, but nearly suffocates it'.[85]

We also find suggestions that while stutterers may be intelligent and anxious to please their teachers, their problem may stem from impatience, or be found amongst stupid children unable to formulate ideas.[86] With the development of intelligence tests, the concept of idiocy has undergone revision and we would not be inclined to Thelwall's view that every stutterer and 'unconscious reiterator' is partially 'either idiotic, or deranged' because he is constantly doing the reverse of what he intends.[87]

Although there was no suggestion that girls were more intelligent than boys, they were considered more sensitive and this posed theoretical difficulties, as they were less apt to stutter (Tables 1.1 and 1.2, pp. 33, 35) despite their proclivity to other nervous disorders, like hysteria and chorea. Reference was not made to their schooling, but it was argued that they were freer from pressure and, as adults, untroubled by business worries. However, men's stronger constitution should compensate for these added stresses.[88] Young girls' facility with language was also noted, they were brought up more in society, conversed with greater ease, and were not so naturally timid about speech as boys.[89] In short, not only did girls think more quickly, and at an earlier age, but they had a finer organisation of the speech mechanism and a quicker apprehension, which enabled fluent and voluble articulation. These observations were in line with Rousseau's opinion that, compared with boys, the speech organs of girls are more supple and their nervous system more developed, giving them greater skill in the social graces and a richer inner life. This at once provided an explanation 'why stammering should be so rare, and other nervous affections so common, in females'.[90]

Many of these statements were merely personal impressions founded upon scanty evidence and reflecting prevailing mythologies. Intelligence and personality testing lay far in the future, as did sociological investigation. Certain other factors were, however, amenable to crude quantitative analysis.

Some Statistics

Statistics as a science was popularised by Gottfried Achenwall in the mid-eighteenth century, but its roots reached back to Hermann Conring a hundred years before. Germany led the way, but it was Pierre Louis, in 1825, who applied it to the reporting of disease. In Britain, the tradition of numbering the people began during the Puritan Revolution.[91] Fact gathering included mortality statistics, also a feature of Bisset Hawkins' *Elements of Medical Statistics* (1829), the first textbook in this country. Another innovation was census taking, during 1801, and fresh impetus was given to statistics by the typhus epidemics, erupting around 1832. In the following two years the Manchester and London Statistical Societies were formed and in 1837 the Registrar General's Office started recording births, marriages and deaths in accordance with the Registration Act passed the previous year. The main subjects for statistical endeavour were education, crime, trade, sanitation and the health of the armed forces.[92] Speech pathologists had no statistical expertise and their interest merely reflected contemporary trends. Neither for common diseases, nor stuttering, was any significant attempt made to correlate symptoms with a variety of possible causal factors. Regarding speech, the most suitable subjects for quantification were the frequency and distribution of problems, and only Mason looked further afield (Table 3.1, p. 79).

Continentals led the field on stuttering statistics, with the work of Otto and Colombat. Their figures and those of subsequent Europeans were quoted widely but incompletely in the English literature. Little information was provided on how the figures were acquired, and some secondary sources disagree or contain errors in computation. Moreover, certain estimates, from either side of the Channel, seem to be guesswork or hearsay, rather than the result of objective measurement. Statistical methods were not subject to critical analysis and so the crude percentages in the following tables are not strictly comparable. But despite these shortcomings, it is interesting that Victorian estimates are broadly in line with modern surveys. The latter show wide variations, an indication that the difficulty in obtaining adequate samples and determining criteria for abnormality has yet to be overcome.

One of the first features to impress investigators was the prevalence of males and throughout the century this point was noted, even if no data were provided. Estimates were usually based upon cases in treatment and the increase of females probably reflects social changes rather than a real increase in their numbers. The British learned that Itard, Rullier and Astrié, writing between 1817 and 1824, had seen no females, though they did not deny their existence. By 1830, Colombat put the figure at 4.66 per cent and subsequently this grew from about

12 per cent to 33 per cent with the experience of Klencke, Wyneken, Norden and Coën.[93] British statistics are recorded in Table 1.1; they show a rather lower proportion of females than recent modern studies, where the incidence ranges from 16 per cent to 33 per cent.[94] The exception is Blake's figure, supplied by Benjamin Ward Richardson and based upon the situation at the Jews' Free School in London's East End,[95] which if accurate, raises many questions.

Table 1.1: Percentage of Females in the Stuttering Population

1841	Cull	*Penny Cyclop.*, p. 434	13%
1841	J. Yearsley	*Stammering*, p. 21	5%
1843	J. Yearsley	*Lancet*, I, p. 246	7%
1843	Physician	*Treatise*, p. 14	5%
1853	A.M. Bell	*Observations*, p. 27	20%
1870	J. Hunt	*Stammering*, pp. 342-3	12-13.25%
1879	Shuldham	*Stammering*, p. 21	20%
1885	Mason	*Elocutionist*, 3, p. 11	11.8%
1890	Blake	*Lip Chorea*, p. 10	≑50%*J
1894	Abbotts	*Stammering*, p. 16	25%
1894	Wyllie	*Disorders*, p. 22	16.6-20%
1909	W. Yearsley	*Treatise*, p. 29	25%*

* Children
J Jews

Source: Derived from figures given by the above British authors. For full reference of books not listed in this chapter, see the bibliography.

The relationship between the sexes is further evident in Table 1.2, where the high number of young people undergoing treatment, both here and in one German practice, is also exposed. With Hunt and Klencke, the percentages are based upon 200 people or less, with Mason on approximately 650 people, attending their respective clinics over a number of years.[96] Adolescence and early adult life is the time when symptoms are worst, yet then social and professional pressures make fluency most desirable. Victorians recognised the correlation between age and the severity of stuttering, most agreeing that it usually began in early childhood, diminished by middle age and disappeared during decline. As treatment was far from satisfactory we may assume that after 30, people were either relieved of the complaint or so disheartened that they forsook the practitioner's office. Undoubtedly, however, advancing age brought on a decline and this prompted speculation. Yearsley, who knew of only one case between 60 and 70, and that possibly a vocal paresis, suggested that after the age of 25 the stutterer 'begins to acquire a cunning which serves him in evading the infirmity to a surprising extent'.[97] Relatively little was said about avoidance tactics, and the course of the disorder, but it was realised that evasion should not be equated with cure.[98]

Various interpretations were put on the absence of stuttering in the elderly. One concerned the voice. In childhood, intonation changes are marked, the pitch high, running into falsetto, and the loudness of speech frequently takes the form of a crescendo. The aging voice, although rarely manifesting a diminuendo, differs in being tremulous, of a slow, steady and uniform rate, punctuated by deliberate pauses, the accent coming through extensions of length, rather than stress. Since stutterers reputedly experienced greater difficulty with the diminuendo, short unextended syllables, narrow pitch changes, accent by stress, and a conversational as opposed to a falsetto tone, Cull thought he had one explanation for their paucity amongst the elderly. However, his argument is far from convincing, as their conversational tone and restricted pitch range would, by his reasoning, tend to perpetuate any problem they may have.[99] Further, the contention that stutterers are more fluent when the pitch intervals are wider, as in song or declamation, needs to be squared with their similar freedom when speaking in a monotone.

It was also said that stuttering diminished with age because an individual's character was more integrated,[100] by then he had acquired dignity, his thought processes were no longer hasty and he was not anxious to express new ideas.[101] Moreover, nervous sensibilities were blunted[102] and the passions held less sway.[103] A more gloomy analysis was given by the elder Poett, who believed that strain from the complaint caused organic disease, consigning stutterers 'to an early tomb'.[104] For Catlin, it was not the impediment that caused the premature demise; rather, both resulted from the hanging jaw and consequent bad breathing habits.[105] Tartaglia was, therefore, a parachronistic figure.

Other speculations concerned the onset of stuttering. Estimates ranged from upwards of three years[106] to about ten,[107] with McCormac arguing that it arose only after the speech powers had fully matured, that is, around the ages of seven or eight.[108] These estimates are rather

Table 1.2: Percentage of Stutterers According to Age in Three Practices

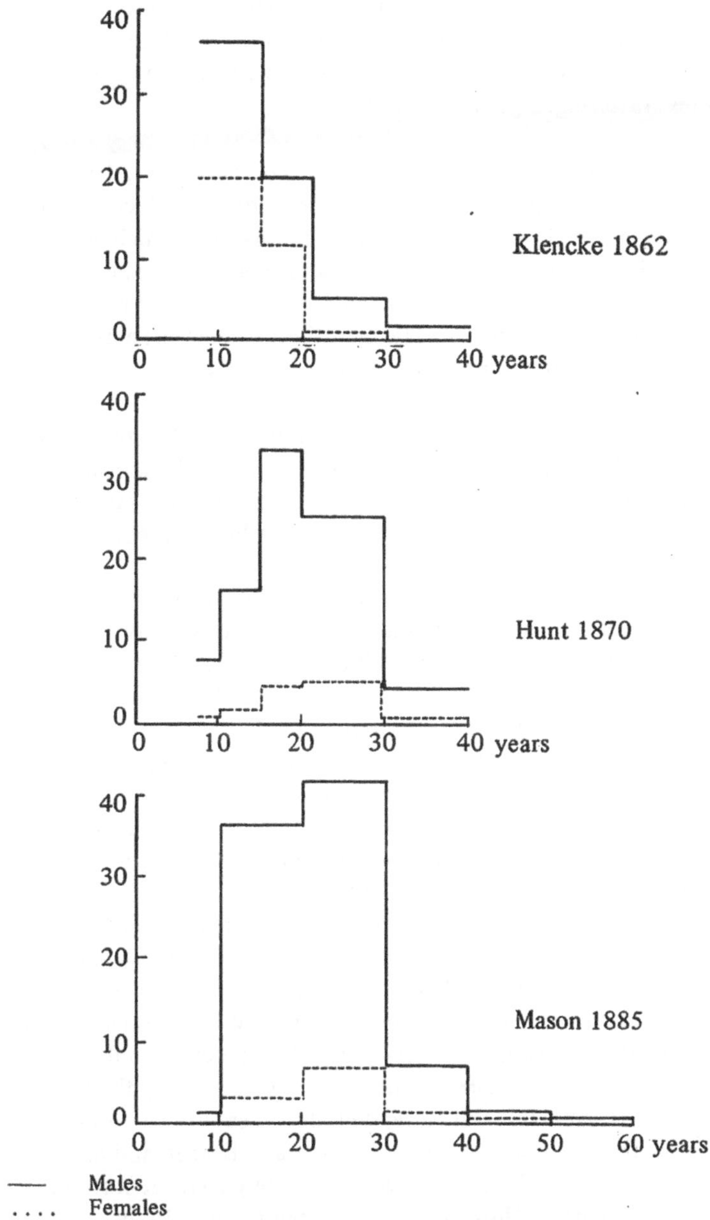

Sources: Klencke and Hunt charts from Hunt (1870), pp. 342-3, cf. Potter, p. 84; Mason chart from Mason (1885), p. 11, see Table 3.1, p. 79.

higher than contemporary ones, which set the lower limits at fifteen months to two years, the time when words are first connected.[109] Could it be that Victorians, though strict disciplinarians, were more indulgent towards hesitancies in their progeny and therefore less likely to produce problems? Alternatively, it might be a question of what constitutes stuttering, a possibility noted by Lee:

> This affection has been confounded with the hesitation, difficulty of expression, or repetition of words – *balbuties*, which commonly occurs in children in their first attempts to talk, and which generally ceases as they grow up; though, in a few instances, stammering supervenes upon it, which leads parents, and those who have the charge of them, sometimes to say, that the stammer has existed from the time they began to speak, which is not the case.[110]

With the passage of over a century, and much research, this distinction between normal dysfluencies and stuttering is still problematical, and has led one writer to state that it provides 'one of the most taxing problems with which speech clinicians have been beset in recent years'.[111]

Once language stabilises, diagnosis is easier, and for this as well as administrative reasons, school populations are the most convenient source of information on children. As Table 1.3 shows, foreign surveys preceded the British, probably partly because school medical inspections were instituted in some German regions from around 1880 and in Boston since 1894,[112] but they did not begin in England until 1908. Good agreement is found in the school estimates of sex, with Hartwell and Walter Yearsley reporting 24.84 per cent and 25 per cent of girls respectively. There is also broad agreement between the percentages in Table 1.3 and modern studies.[113]

Statistics for whole populations present more difficulties (Table 1.4). The first, and methodologically probably the best, estimate was that of Otto, in 1830, which was calculated from official returns of several Prussian regions and was widely quoted in this country throughout the century. British figures appear to have been largely conjectural, or extrapolations from clinical experience, which was possibly the basis of Hunt's map (Figure 1.1). When reading this, it should be borne in mind that his father's practice was in London and Dorset, and his own in London and Sussex. Hence, they were less likely to meet stutterers from northern counties. Hunt fully appreciated the paucity of information on the incidence of stuttering compared with deafness,

Table 1.3: Percentage and Proportion of Stutterers in Several School Populations

Foreign				
Place	Date	No. examined	%	Stutterers/ Normals
Russia	Before 1884	22,878	1.58	1/63
Germany	1886-90	252,312	1.12	1/89
US, Boston	1893-4	129,060	0.77	1/129
English				
Jews' Free School	1890	3,367	0.83	1/120
Lancashire	1909	50,000	0.578	1/173

Sources: Foreign – Gutzmann, pp. 141-3, Hartwell, pp. 101-4; English – Blake, pp. 10-11, W. Yearsley, p. 29.

which had been well quantified since the 1851 census;[114] and he hoped the Registrar-General would make good this deficiency. His wish has never been realised.

Foreign statistics, though extensively noted in English literature, are difficult to interpret due to inadequate reporting, and the computation of percentages from what material is provided is further aggravated by changes in population and national boundaries over a given period. This is particularly true of Chervin's projections for the whole population, which were based upon his well-documented military statistics for ten-year periods between 1850 and 1869.[115] At this time, the French had conscription ballots and so a large number of 20-year-old men came under review each year. It seems that amongst those given speech tests were men most at risk of stuttering, and the French figures bracketed in Table 1.5 indicate the projected number of stutterers, had all recruits' speech been evaluated.[116] Commenting on Colombat's figure of one stutterer to every 2,500 males, Chervin says that this is too low because only severe cases were exempted from military service. The actual number, he suggested, must be at least 3 to 5 per 1,000 recruits.[117]

Figure 1.1: Map Showing the Geographical Distribution of Certain Stutterers that Came to James Hunt's Notice

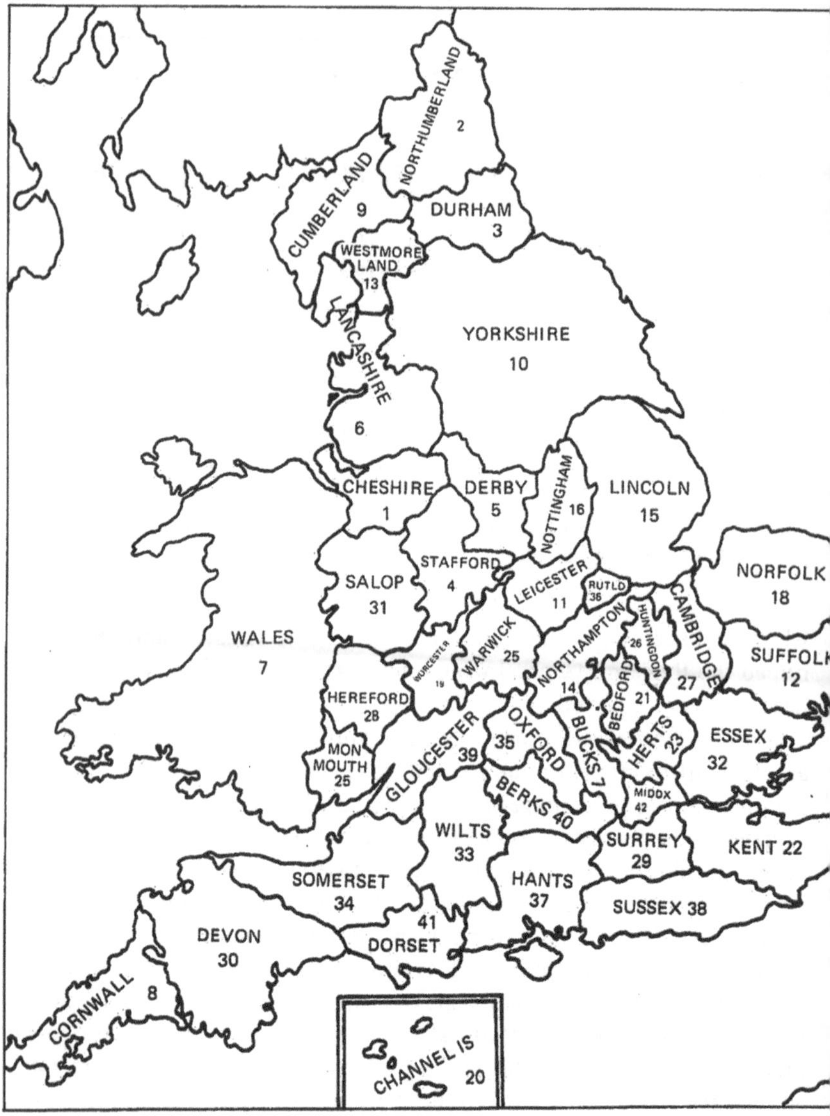

Source: Reproduced from James Hunt's *Stammering and Stuttering* (1870), opp. p. 341.

Table 1.4: Percentage and Proportion of Stutterers for Whole Populations

Foreign			
Country	Date	%	Stutterers/ Normals
Prussia			
Otto	1830	0.2	1/500
Gerdts	1883	0.13	1/766
France			
Colombat	?	0.0185	1/5,397
J. Débats	1870s	0.096	1/1,040
British			
Cull	1841	0.028	1/3,500
Hunt	1870	0.3	1/333.3
Bernard	1889	0.1	1/1,000
Abbotts	1894	0.1	1/1,000

Sources: Figures for Otto, Colombat, Hunt taken from Hunt (1870), pp. 339-40, 341; figures for Gerdts taken from Gerdts, p. 49; figures for Colombat and Cull taken from *Penny Cyclop*, p. 434; figures for *J. Débats* taken from Shuldham, p. 20; figures for Bernard taken from A. Bernard, p. v; figures for Abbotts taken from Abbotts, pp. 14-15.

What was the situation in Britain? Was Bartlett's book derived from experiences in the King's Own Light Infantry, to which he was assistant surgeon? In addition to Yearsley's patient noted above, other stuttering soldiers existed,[118] and we know that Beasley was a member of the 1st Warwick Volunteers.[119] However, during the earlier part of the century there may have been some sanctions, since a former patient of Poett, who became a Royal Artillery Medical Officer, was told that this position would not have been open to him, had he still stuttered.[120]

The British, with a strong navy, and small standing army relying on unemployment to fill its ranks, were in a rather different position from the French. They realised that French conscription provided an ideal sample for quantitative analysis lacking to them, since recruits selected themselves and were accepted or rejected according to demand.[121] Nevertheless, annual medical reports were organised in 1861 and

Table 1.5: Percentage and Proportion of Recruits Rejected From Foreign Armies Because of Stuttering

Country	Date	%	Stutterers/ Normals
France	1850-69	0.633* (0.325)	1/158 (1/307)
US (Civil War) Americans	1861-5	0.136	1/735
Frenchmen		0.308	1/324
Russia	1876-82	0.12	1/833
Austro-Hungary	1884	0.05	1/2,000
Italy	1884	≑ 0.05	≑ 1/2,000
US Second World War	–1943	0.5-0.8	1/200-125

Note: *Represents the percentage of conscripts actually examined, and the bracketed figure the projected percentage, had all been examined.

Source: Hartwell, pp. 101-2; Gutzmann, p. 142; Johnson, cited in L. Travis (ed.), *Handbook of Speech Pathology and Audiology* (New York, Appleton-Century-Crofts, 1971), p. 627.

information on returns became available from 1864. A man might be rejected on medical grounds for any of 38 disabilities. One was voice, the test being whether he could articulate loudly: 'Who comes there?'[122] This category appears to have embraced a number of impediments, but probably comprised chiefly stuttering, since those with deafness and intellectual impairment would have been rejected already, these tests preceding those of speech. In certain years, of those applying, the total number of men exempted was sometimes over 40 per cent, of which approximately 0.34 per cent had speech defects, slightly less than those with deafness.

British speech correctionists seemingly knew nothing of these reports, displayed in Table 1.6. Possibly this was because they were limited to army medical personnel, unlike in France, where Chervin was not only a well respected speech correctionist, but a member of the statistical society of Lyon.

Stutterings may have reminded Dickens' Sissy of statistics,[123] but from the foregoing discussion it is evident that no one thought of subjecting the defective utterance itself to quantitative analysis. The British were generally slower than their Continental neighbours, and

Table 1.6: Percentage and Proportion of Recruits Rejected From the British Army in Selected Years, on Account of Speech Impediment

Date	No. inspected	No. rejected	% rejected	Defectives/ Normals
1864	27,754	37	0.133	1/751
1875	25,878	16	0.062	1/1,612
1887	72,249	104	0.144	1/694
1895	55,698	102	0.183	1/546

Sources: 'Statistical Report on the Health of the Army in 1864', *Parliamentary Papers*, 43 (1866), pp. 31-2 [41-3]; 'Army Medical Department Report for the Year 1875', *Parliamentary Papers*, 44 (1876), p. 63 [533]; 'Army Medical Department Report for the Year 1885', *Parliamentary Papers*, 51 (1887), p. 28 [360]; 'Army Medical Department Report for the Year 1895', *Parliamentary Papers*, 52 (1896), pp. 28-9 [350-1].

specialists often knew more of studies in foreign countries than in their own. As regards anecdotes, however, they could hold their own. By mid-century, most of the basic questions concerning the phenomenology of stuttering had been raised and a small step taken towards delineating the problem.

Notes

1. A. Bernard, p. 16.
2. For Thelwall's adaptation of this poem, see Rockey (1977), pp. 88-9.
3. W. Abbotts, *Stammering, Stuttering, and other Speech Affections* (1894), pp. 42-3n. This book is probably a later edition of *Impediments of Speech: Stammering and Stuttering their Causes and Cure* (1869 and thereafter) by a William Abbotts Smith. In the *Medical Directories* of 1868-73 this man is listed as Abbotts Smith and in 1878 he appears to be known as William Abbotts. He was centred chiefly in London, but moved around a good deal, dying in Hastings between December 1900 and November 1901. Hereafter referred to as Abbotts and references will be to the 1898 edition unless otherwise stated.
4. 'Stammer' in *The Penny Cyclopaedia*, p. 403. Hereafter, just the *Cyclopaedia* will be noted.
5. Gerdts, p. 65. A variant of Abbotts' story appears on pp. 34-5 and turns on a dispenser who sang out a warning to the apothecary that his cellar was about to be consumed by flames. Charles Dickens and Alexander Bell also favoured the fire version.
6. Yearsley (1843-4), p. 246.
7. *As You Like It*, Act 3, Sc. 2. Cf. T.S. Clouston's description of a type of speech that resembles 'a torrent of half-articulated words, following each other like peas running out of a spout' in *The Neuroses of Development* (Edinburgh,

Oliver & Boyd, 1891), pp. 32-3. This is interpreted as a description of cluttering by Wyllie, pp. 139-40.

8. Lee, p. 4. Apart from a few additions, the first section of his book is essentially the same as his series of articles 'On stammering, and the methods proposed for its removal', *London Medical Gazette*, 2 n.s. (1840-1), 267-9, 301-6, 349-52, 385-90, 416-19.

9. Thomas Hardy, *Far from the Madding Crowd* (1874), ch. 10.

10. Wyllie, p. 30.

11. Derek Hudson, *Martin Tupper. His Rise and Fall* (London, Constable, 1949), pp. 39-41.

12. *Charles Kingsley*, ed. by wife (London, Kegan Paul, 1888), pp. 7, 168, 282.

13. M.F. Tupper, 'Of Speaking' in *Proverbial Philosophy* (London, Joseph Rickerby, 1838), pp. 133-6. The key passage has been cited recently by Van Riper, pp. 157-8.

14. *The Aldine Half-Holiday Library*, 3, no. 65 [1894].

15. Pisistratus Caxton, *What Will He Do With It?* (London, Routledge, 1875). This novel first appeared as a monthly serial in *(Blackwood's) Edinburgh Monthly Magazine*, vols 81-5 (June 1857 to January 1859).

16. According to the British Museum catalogue, the author was James Malcolm Rymer, who also used the pseudonym Errym Malcolm, a rearrangement of the last two names.

17. Minute Philosopher, p. 4.

18. 'Psellism', *Household Words*, 14 (1856), 468-9. Hereafter journal only cited.

19. Première, Prague, 30 May 1866. First performed in Drury Lane, 1895.

20. Première, Opéra Comique, Paris, 9 December 1865. Composer F.E.J. Bazin, librettists Labiche and Delacour.

21. Shuldham, pp. 40-1.

22. T.E. Pemberton, *A Memoir of Edward Askew Sothern*, 2nd edn (London, Richard Bentley & Son, 1890), pp. 24, 63, 72, 319, 321.

23. Not to be confused with Niccolò Tartaglia (c. 1501-57), the Italian mathematician, whose speech impediment resulted from a mouth wound.

24. 'Commedia dell'Arte', *Encyclopaedia Britannica*, 4 (Chicago, Macropaedia edn, 1974), p. 982.

25. *The Spectator*, no. 371 (6 May 1712) reproduced in *The Spectator*, ed. Donald Bond (Oxford, Clarendon, 1965), pp. 396–9.

26. Ernst von Feuchtersleben, *The Principles of Medical Psychology*, trans. H. Evans Lloyd (London, Sydenham Soc., 1847), p. 264. Cf. Palmer, p. 55 ff, sections of which are quoted in the review of his book, *Medico-Chirugical Review*, 12 n.s. (1830), 300-1 (289-313); cf. Hunt (1870), p. 353.

27. Shuldham, p. 44.

28. A.C.H. Jones, *The Nature of Stammering* (London, Central Pub. Co., 1908), p. 4.

29. R. Clarke, 'Remarks on the Topography and Diseases of the Gold Coast', *Transactions of the Epidemiological Society of London*, 2 (1863), pp. 104, 114 (76-123). Cf. R. Clarke, 'Short Notes on the Prevailing Diseases in the Colony of Sierra Leone', *Journal of the Statistical Society of London*, 19 (1858), p. 73 (60-81); Colman (1895), p. 1420.

30. Hunt (1870), pp. 349-55; 34-5. Cf. 'Statistics of Stammering in France', *British Medical Journal*, 1 (1880), p. 426; Kussmaul, pp. 855-6.

31. Abbotts, p. 14.

32. Cazalet, p. 6.

33. Ibid., pp. 5-7.

34. George Catlin, *Shut Your Mouth and Save Your Life*, 4th edn (London, Trübner, 1870), p. 1 and *passim*.

35. Smith, *Impediments*, p. 16.
36. Abbotts, p. 13.
37. Wendell Johnson, 'The Indians have no Word for It' in *People in Quandaries* (New York, Harper & Bros., 1946), pp. 439-66.
38. Edwin M. Lemert, 'Sociological Perspective' in Sheehan (ed.), pp. 170-87.
39. Van Riper, p. 6.
40. *DNB*, vol. 12, p. 455.
41. McCormac, pp. 93-4.
42. Physician, pp. 67-8, cited in *Mind, Breath*, p. 39 and Bacc. Med. Oxon., p. 40.
43. Potter, p. 84.
44. Abbotts, pp. 41-2. For this reason Yearsley (1843-4), p. 290 recommends that stutterers learn a wind instrument, music also assisting the sense of rhythm.
45. Colman (1895), p. 1419.
46. Physician, pp. 66-7, cited in *Mind, Breath*, p. 39 and Bacc. Med. Oxon., p. 40.
47. Hunt (1870), p. 348-9.
48. Wright (1835), p. 22.
49. Charles Darwin, 'Preliminary Notice' in E. Krause, *Erasmus Darwin*, trans. W.S. Dallas (London, John Murray, 1879), p. 81.
50. Bartlett, pp. 78-9. Cf. Colman (1895), p. 1419; A. Bernard, p. 6.
51. Abbotts, p. 44.
52. Caleb, p. 136.
53. Beasley (1905), p. 133.
54. Abbotts, pp. 15-16.
55. Hunt (1870), p. 353.
56. William R. Wilde, *Practical Observations on Aural Surgery* (London, Churchill, 1853), p. 436.
57. M'Minn, p. 13.
58. Abbotts, p. 15; Smith, *Impediments*, p. 7.
59. Hunt (1861), pp. 38-9. Cf. Beasley (1905), pp. 133-4.
60. Physician, p. 68.
61. Hunt (1870), opposite p. 340; 'Statistics . . .', *British Medical Journal*, 1 (1880), p. 426. Cf. E.J. Seltman, 'On Stammering', *Physique*, 1 (1891), p. 136 (136-40), who attributes the lesser frequency in southern latitudes to their 'gentle moods'.
62. Shuldham, pp. 20-1, 44.
63. *Household Words*, p. 465.
64. C. Darwin in *Erasmus Darwin*, pp. 38-9.
65. *Charles Kingsley* (1901), vol. 2, p. 45. I have been unable to verify the assertion in 'The Obviation of Stammering', *British Medical Journal*, 1 (1875), p. 86, that Bishop Wilberforce stuttered in his youth.
66. Hudson, *Tupper*, p. 31. Cf. *Life and Letters of J.H. Shorthouse*, ed. by wife (London, Macmillan, 1905), vol. 1, p. 402.
67. Martin Tupper, *My Life as an Author* (London, Sampson Low & Co., 1886), p. 74.
68. Beasley (1905), p. 27.
69. A.M. Bell (1900), p. 110.
70. Beasley (1905), p. 28.
71. *Unspeakable*, pp. 32-3, 40.
72. Hunt (1863), p. 209.
73. Beasley (1905), p. 28.
74. Lytton Strachey, *Eminent Victorians* (London, Collins, 1959), pp. 174-201.
75. Bartlett, p. 2. Cf. Physician, p. 37.
76. George Andrew Lewis and George B. Hynson, *The Practical Treatment of*

Stammering and Stuttering (Detroit, George Andrew Lewis, 1902), p. 71.

77. Coën, 'By what methods can propagation of affections of speech be prevented?' Report of 6th International Congress for Hygiene and Demiography, Vienna, 2.10.1887. *Journal of Laryngology and Rhinology*, 2 (1888), p. 86.

78. Charles Lamb, 'Christ's Hospital five-and-thirty years ago' in *The Essays of Elia*, new edn (London, Moxon, 1869), pp. 18-34.

79. *The Autobiography of Leigh Hunt; with Reminiscences of Friends and Contemporaries* (London, Smith Elder, 1850), vol. 1, p. 143. Cf. p. 124.

80. *Unspeakable*, p. 79.

81. Butterfield, p. 337. Eton College has no record of Butterfield, who probably negotiated directly with parents or pupils.

82. Tupper, *My Life*, pp. 14-15.

83. *The Correspondence of Thomas Carlyle and Ralph Waldo Emerson 1834-1872* (London, Chatto & Windus, 1883), vol. 2, letter 17 November 1843, pp. 47-8. The James in question is Henry Snr, father of Henry and William James. The l'Estrange reference is to *The Reign of King Charles* (London, 1655), p. 1, concerning Charles I's speech impediment.

84. Beasley (1905), p. 86.

85. Claude Abbott, *The Life and Letters of George Darley* (London, Oxford UP, 1928), p. 151. Quotation from a letter to Miss Mitford dated 22 August 1836.

86. Haward, p. 112. Cf. Colman (1895), p. 1419.

87. Thelwall (1810), p. 68.

88. Bacc. Med. Oxon., pp. 39-40.

89. McCormac, pp. 41-2. Cf. Shuldham, p. 69; Wyllie, p. 22.

90. Lee, p. 27. Cf. Physician, pp. 14-15. I have been unable to trace the source of their quotation, but similar sentiments appear in Rousseau's section on Woman in *Émile*.

91. Major Greenwood, *Medical Statistics from Graunt to Farr* (Cambridge, University Press, 1948).

92. Michael Cullen, *The Statistical Movement in Early Victorian Britain* (Sussex, Harvester Press, 1975).

93. Compare the reports of Hunt (1870), pp. 339, 342-3; Shuldham, p. 69; Potter, p. 83; Kussmaul, p. 834; Romberg, p. 363.

94. Bloodstein, pp. 72, 82-4. Cf. William Perkins, 'Physiological Studies' in Sheehan (ed.), pp. 191-2.

95. Blake, pp. 10-11.

96. Hunt (1870), p. 343; [Mason] (1885), p. 11.

97. Yearsley (1843-4), p. 246.

98. Cull (1835), p. 5. His *Stammering* was reviewed in *Medico-Chirurgical Review*, 25 n.s. (1836), 319-22.

99. *Penny Cyclop.*, pp. 430-1.

100. Review of *Du Bégaiement . . .*, p. 463.

101. McCormac, pp. 39-40.

102. Lee, p. 19.

103. Physician, p. 16.

104. Poett snr (1828), p. 5. According to the British Museum catalogue, the early books were written by Poett senior and after 1856 by the son. Both appear to have taken an interest in the subject, for each states he began lecturing on or treating stuttering, in Dublin, during December 1827. One Joseph Poett became an MRCS in 1809 and another of that name in 1827, after apprenticeship to his father. The latter also became a LSA, in 1831, aged 22. Despite priority claims in the early editions, the son makes no mention of these books and announces that he is expounding for the first time in any language the 'true theory of stammering' (1858, pp. vii, 34). Cf. *Household Words*, p. 468.

105. Catlin, *Shut Your Mouth*, p. 98.

106. Yearsley (1843-4), p. 246.

107. Romberg, p. 363; *Penny Cyclop*., p. 431 from which a short passage is quoted by Forshaw, p. 5, without acknowledgement.

108. McCormac, pp. 38-9.

109. Bloodstein, pp. 74-7. Cf. Van Riper, pp. 62-8, 260.

110. Lee, p. 17. The term *balbuties* was also used for one variety of stuttering (Physician, p. 31) and for an enunciatory disorder involving labials (Good, p. 574).

111. Bloodstein, cited in Bloodstein, p. 234.

112. *Annual Reports of the Chief Medical Officers of Education* (1911), pp. 18-20. In those instances in Table 1.3 where Gutzmann and Hartwell appear to be referring to the same studies, some of their figures tally exactly, while others are only approximately the same. Both authorities report on findings dating from 1886. However, though probably familiar with Gutzmann's article since he mentions *Physique*, the author of 'The Treatment of Stammering', *Lancet*, 2 (1891), p. 362, states that the collection of German statistics began 16 years earlier, i.e. 1875. Some of the time, at least, statistics were gathered through circulars issued to schoolmasters, see 'Medical News', *British Medical Journal*, 1 (1889), p. 1329.

113. Beech and Fransella, pp. 12-13; Van Riper, pp. 36-9.

114. 'Deaf and Dumb', *Encyclopaedia Britannica*, 9th edn (Edinburgh, Adam & Charles Black, 1877), vol. 7, p. 12.

115. Some reports state that he began in 1852. Hunt (1870), p. 340 writes that between 1852-62, 6,773 conscripts were exempted from military service, and in 'On Stammering', *British Medical Journal*, 2 (1879), p. 502 the number between 1850-69 is put at 13,215. Cf. Table 1.5, p. 40.

116. Hartwell, pp. 101-2.

117. M. Chervin, Aîné, *Bégaiement considéré comme vice de Prononciation* (Paris, Librairie, Classique de Jules Delalain et Fils, 1867), pp. 34-5. (Mémoire lu à la Sorbonne, le 5 Avril, 1866).

118. Blathwayt, p. 575; Blake, pp. 20-1; Urling, p. 38.

119. Beasley (1885), p. 62. This is a letter from a captain testifying to the severity of Beasley's own stammering in his youth.

120. Poett snr (1828), p. 15. Cf. Urling, pp. 84, 87, 89.

121. 'Copy of Report of the Committee on the Preparation of Army Medical Statistics, &c . . . ', *Parliamentary Papers*, 37 (1861), 11-12 [465-6].

122. 'Statistical Tables Relative to Recruiting for the Army and Militia', *Parliamentary Papers*, 43 (1875), 14-15 [626-7].

123. Charles Dickens, *Hard Times* (1854), ch. 9.

2 A NEW PROFESSION

In 1801, after various false starts, John Thelwall looked towards elocution for his livelihood and, in so doing, succeeded in changing his personal fortunes and in setting a new discipline in motion. Though some sporadic speech correction had been carried out previously, Thelwall was the first to see it as a discipline in its own right, distinct from the management of deafness or mental retardation. Aside from his astute clinical observations, he could claim novelty for defining it as a science as well as an art; for stressing that theory should be founded upon practical experience with patients; and for drawing attention to the relevance of physiology, a subject hitherto neglected by elocutionists. Those that followed him broadly adhered to this framework, and this still holds, though the normative aspects of elocution are now the concern of other specialists.

At the turn of the nineteenth century, rhetorical studies had an importance they no longer enjoy and the medical profession had yet to attain its present pre-eminence.[1] Consequently, it was not difficult for Thelwall, a former medical student, to conceive of his new science as spawning an autonomous profession, distinct from medicine, and branching off from the noble tradition of rhetoric. But it was not to be. The medical profession gained greater power, elocution became trivialised and much of its intellectual content lost to the growing science of phonetics. Thus, the 'abstract knowledge' so important for the acquisition of professional status was lacking and lay speech correctionists had to look to other disciplines – linguistics and physiology – for their conceptual bases and advances. Thelwall's projected discipline embraced all manner of speech problems, but in practice stuttering seems to have been the prime object of therapeutic endeavour. It was not till later in the century that diagnosis was sufficiently developed to reveal the potential scope of such activity and to necessitate the construction of a technical vocabulary. This problem was compounded by the diversity of people drawn to speech pathology, which itself created tensions that ultimately further restricted Thelwall's vision. Amidst such dissensions, the useful conditions for acquiring professional status – standardised educational curricula, licensing, establishment of ethical codes and a common state of mind[2] – were lacking. Hence, while dentists, teachers, midwives and the doctors themselves were taking steps to institutionalise their activities through professional societies, training programmes and legislation, speech correctionists remained a largely diversified and unorganised group. Nevertheless, to the extent that they agreed upon the discipline's theoretical foundations and tackled many of the impediments now within the jurisdiction of speech therapy, they were setting in train this new profession.

Origins and Evolution

The work of Holder, Wallis and Bulwer in the seventeenth century stimulated education of the deaf in this country and in due course schools were established and special teaching techniques debated. Such instruction required a particular understanding of speech and these men, together with other linguists, began describing and classifying articulatory sounds, and it was this aspect of their work that fostered Thelwall's new discipline, since it was taken up by the elocutionary movement of which he was part.[3] This movement, gathering momentum around 1750, tried to redress the imbalance that had developed within the various divisions of rhetoric, to the detriment of delivery.[4]

The elocutionists' aim was to foster eloquence and one can detect similarly high aspirations in those who branched off to specialise in speech correction. Founders of the movement gave scant attention to verbal impediments but, nevertheless, their activities were seminal. Finding difficulty in teaching the finer points of enunciation without reference to some objective yardstick, minds turned increasingly towards orthoepy. The varieties of English speech posed problems for anyone seeking to establish a norm and irregular orthography further complicated matters. Pronunciation dictionaries were therefore notable achievements, and those produced by Thomas Sheridan in 1780, and John Walker in 1791, made particular impact and embodied the prescriptive attitude to language prevalent in the eighteenth century.[5] The information they contained might help children to read, foreigners to perfect their accent, and provincials to divest themselves of obtrusive sounds. Only a small step remained: the application of orthoepic principles to impediments of speech.

The combined interest in lexicography and speech pathology continued through the nineteenth century in the persons of Benjamin Smart, who produced *Walker Remodelled*, and Richard Cull, who was responsible for pronunciation in John Ogilvie's various dictionaries. Preoccupation with phonetics was much more widely spread, however, and while pertinent to some disorders, it tended to constrict speculations on stuttering.

In the early 1800s there were perhaps only half a dozen specialists concerned with remedial speech training. Exact numbers cannot be determined for we know only those whose names appeared in print, but it is certain that with a population of 10½ million they can scarcely have scratched the surface of the problem. It was not until the late 1820s that therapeutic activity began to expand and medical men entered the scene, but by then the problem had grown also. In present day society, where treatment is available for all types of impediment and to all classes, it is gauged that six therapists are needed for every 100,000 inhabitants.[6] Since many elocutionists took normal speaking pupils, there was a limit to the time they had available for instructing the handicapped. Working on a minimum of one in a thousand of the population being afflicted, there would have been 10,500 stutterers at the turn of the nineteenth century and over 35,000 in its final decades. Hunt, however, estimates that there were 54,978 in 1860.[7] The percentage of Victorians able to afford help was obviously small and hence the demand proportionally diminished, but it must have been far in excess of the 30 patients a year that any one full-time practitioner might be expected to treat. Although by mid-century Dickens states that scores of people advertised their services,[8] hundreds would have been necessary to grapple with this one speech problem. In the absence of reputable assistance, stuttering patients were easy prey for the quack or sharp practitioner.

Who contributed to Victorian speech correction? For an answer one need only look to the many facets of speech itself. Contrary to Continental developments, educators of the deaf played a minimal role compared with those in the elocutionary tradition, who, imbued with the principles of rhetoric and often endowed with histrionic ability, saw how these skills might be adapted to those less gifted. Thus, orators, actors and orthoepists became involved, together with clergymen. Similarly, singing teachers, concerned with the voice, might be faced with its disorders and thus led to other forms of impediment. Sometimes interest was generated accidently, or passed from father to son. Former stutterers had special cause to become involved and some of their number were medical men, but doctors and dentists had other reasons for attending to speech problems.[9] Pathology could throw light on normal functioning, it was intellectually provoking, whilst patients themselves provided a practical challenge. To complicate the picture still further, some of these specialists were active in various learned societies and were therefore also known as anthropologists, phrenologists, and philologists. Richard Cull, for example, was all three.

It was difficult for so heterogeneous a group to come together. Though primarily middle-class self-made men, they differed in therapeutic experience, technical education, professional aspirations and financial expectations. One consequence of this was that they failed to acquire a common occupational title. Dickens refers to them as 'psellismologists' or 'balbutists',[10] but no one followed suit and laymen continued with the imprecise designation 'elocutionist'. This difficulty in naming the profession reflects a fundamental problem of identity which continues today, members still disputing whether the title 'speech therapist' should be changed, but unable to agree upon an alternative. Another consequence was that in England no professional society was founded and there was no formal training programme. Furthermore, there was no one journal taking special note of speech impediments, in contrast to America, where *Werner's Voice Magazine*, started in 1879, printed a wide range of articles, reported on Continental developments and carried translations, and to France, with Chervin's *La Voix Parlée et Chantée*, founded eleven years later.

Publications nevertheless abounded and their variety reflected the gamut of speech correctionists' interests. Although physicians wrote most, it would be wrong to assume that they outnumbered elocutionists. Medical men were professionally inclined to record interesting cases, write for advice over puzzling patients and report on scientific experiments or discoveries. Their audience was assured. But this did not mean that their insights were more profound or their opinions based upon greater experience. Sometimes they wrote for textbooks, and made only passing mention of stuttering, which was but one of the intriguing phenomena touching their lives. Should its solution be unforthcoming, they passed on to other things.

Provision was also made for the public, with items being carried by local or national papers and magazines. For the speech handicapped themselves there was no journal such as the deaf had, nor any equivalent of the brief running American *Phonometer* (1897-1905), directed principally at stutterers. However, some of the more academic papers were also addressed to them, as well as therapists. These writings chiefly took the form of small treatises or pamphlets which, whether written by an elocutionist or physician, were usually prefaced by an explanation of phonetics and anatomy. On this, the basis of speech pathology, they were agreed, for, as Wright put it: 'Nothing can more successfully aid the progress of any art or science, or the object of any inquiry, than a clear and distinct knowledge of its constituent parts, and the employment of concise and proper definitions.'[11] Thus, alongside the anecdotes, was a serious attempt to understand speech processes, which, it was believed, would provide a reliable structure to underwrite theory and indicate a rational plan for treatment.

Linguistic and Anatomical Foundations

In addition to deaf education, seventeenth-century linguistics had been stimulated by the search for a universal language, a method of shorthand, a phonetic alphabet and a revised spelling system.[12] Victorians witnessed a resurgence of interest in these subjects, to be augmented by the impetus to record and transmit coded or spoken speech through mechanical means, which resulted in the typewriter, telegraph, gramophone and telephone. Furthermore, breathing, voice and articulation could themselves be scrutinised by various apparatuses and techniques, not least photography.[13] Little application of these was made to the analysis of speech impediments, though in France, Féré, with a 'glosso-dynamomètre' began the sort of physiological experiment that became frequent in the twentieth century.[14]

Understandably, minimal attention was paid to phonemics, research being directed towards laying the groundwork for acoustic and articulatory phonetics. Not only were machines of value in furthering this work but articulating automata in particular had played a unique role in prompting such enquiries. Speaking machines were not peculiar to modern Europe. They had been produced in antiquity, but it is thought that they were largely based upon deception until the late eighteenth century when it was discovered that vowels could be simulated by a series of pipes and reeds, and moving parts could modify these sounds to approximate some consonants, the air flow being provided by bellows.[15] Most of the machines were Continental, but one was constructed by Erasmus Darwin,[16] and possibly one also by Professor Wheatstone, who, together with Willis, devoted considerable attention to vowel acoustics.

Though many Victorian elocutionists did little more than repeat a simple classification of sounds, some of them made more penetrating enquiries. The Bell family exemplify this broader approach, its members making outstanding contributions to science, practical elocution and, later, deaf education in America. When Alexander

Graham Bell invented the telephone in 1875, he brought to fruition studies that extended over three generations and he was only too willing to acknowledge the debt to his grandfather, who had made good the gaps in his education and influenced the future direction of his life when, as a lad of fourteen, he had stayed with the old man at his London residence in Harrington Square.[17]

Alexander senior was born to a Scottish family of shoemakers in 1790. Like his sons and grandson after him, he had striking histrionic gifts which attracted him to the stage, but he did not pursue the theatrical profession for long, his attention being turned to public readings of Shakespeare's plays, the teaching of English diction and correction of defective utterance. After a successful career in Scotland, he moved to London leaving one son, Melville, to continue the Edinburgh practice. The elder son, David, had gone to Dublin, and it was through this branch of the family that Shaw's interest in phonetics was aroused and the seeds sown for *Pygmalion*.[18]

It was lack of classical learning that Alexander senior most deplored in his grandson, who at that time wanted to be a professional pianist, having inherited musical talent from his mother. This was not encouraged and whilst in London, Alexander Graham improved his literary knowledge, observed speech teaching classes, and made good use of the library on acoustics in Harrington Square. On the death of Alexander senior, in 1865, Melville took over the London practice and Graham continued the family tradition in Scotland, where his fascination with acoustics expressed itself in experiments on resonant pitches. His results were communicated to Alexander John Ellis, who acknowledged them in his translation of the third edition of Helmholtz's *The Sensations of Tone as a Physiological Basis for the Theory of Music* (1875).[19] Significant research on this subject had already been carried out by Dondern, in Holland, but the German school was generally in the lead because investigators were principally physicists or physiologists, rather than practical linguists. Max Müller later popularised their work in Britain.[20]

The real 'grandfather of the telephone', however, was James Murray, editor of the *Oxford English Dictionary*, who taught Graham about electricity around 1857. Murray had attended Melville Bell's elocutionary course in Edinburgh with the view to learning something about the correction of pronunciation through Visible Speech.[21] He subsequently became friendly with the family and contacts were renewed once Melville moved to London. At this time, Melville also started associating with the distinguished linguist Prince Louis-Lucien

Bonaparte, nephew of Napoleon. Furthermore, he became a professor of elocution at London University and a member of the Philological Society, of which Ellis was president.[22] Among Ellis' other interests were spelling reform and shorthand, and he championed Pitman's work in these areas. He also spent much time trying to evolve a universal alphabet, but gave generous recognition to Melville Bell, who with his superior system of Visible Speech had 'done more for phonetics than all his predecessors put together',[23] and had virtually founded scientific alphabetics. Ellis found Bell's achievement of depicting how the sound is produced in the very form of the symbol 'really astonishing'. He applauded the way dialectal vowels could be recorded and said that he had never before come across 'such perfection of analysis and symbolization', at once both 'original' and 'apparently exhaustive'.[24]

Those trying to find a system for depicting speech sounds accurately had either devised organic alphabets, which were illegible to the uninitiated, of they had modified the Roman alphabet. Bell's system was of the former type, being based upon a physiological analysis of the speech organs' actions. It was widely promoted both in this country and America and though attracting much attention, it failed to achieve lasting popularity and was eventually replaced by the more comprehensible International Phonetic Alphabet, which utilised more familiar symbols from the Greek and Roman scripts.

Melville Bell did not look upon Visible Speech as merely a clever invention but, amongst other things, as a remedial tool for assisting those speech defectives and the deaf who had particular difficulty grasping the proper pronunciation of words, on account of being misled by both sound and spelling. He placed stutterers in this category and when the family left for North America in 1871, Graham established a school of vocal physiology in Boston, for 'the correction of stammering and other defects of utterance',[25] using his father's system.

It is not difficult to see how interpretations of stuttering were influenced by articulatory phonetics, but no one in England followed Béclard's lead in prefacing his account of stuttering with diagrams of articulatory postures. Attention to anatomical phonetics began in the seventeenth century and subsequently various people attempted to describe the action of the speech organs during sound formation, not least Erasmus Darwin, whose speaking machine and stenographic work caused him to make a detailed analysis of articulatory mechanics.[26] Darwin made no move to apply this to stuttering, but many specialists did depict the problem as an inability to master the requisite movements. Melville Bell, for example, gave detailed descriptions of the pathological enunciation of each letter, explaining how incorrect actions bring on extraneous movements that are not limited to the mouth.[27] The consequence of this line of thinking was a mechanical approach to treatment, directed at teaching the correct articulatory positions.[28]

Etymologically, vowels were 'calling sounds' usually defined as those capable of standing alone and of extended articulation. Since many consonants were also continuous, Thelwall criticised this definition, and suggested that vowels were those sounds modified by the mouth 'without any contact of the enunciative organs'[29] – a description with a modern ring. Speech pathologists were concerned with the characteristics of vowels and consonants because they thought that therein lay the key to why some sounds provided a greater barrier to stutterers than others. Emotion, through its intimacy with the voice, tended to be conveyed through vowels, yet stutterers, despite their reputed nervousness and emotional problems, found these sounds easier to make. This was particularly evident in song.

Whereas acoustic phonetics was primarily concerned with vowels, classificatory systems centred upon 'con-sonans', originally conceived as sounds which could be pronounced only with a vowel, but defined by Thelwall as 'an element formed by the contact, or combined action of two organs'.[30] In this particular paper he was dealing with the euphonic aspects of sound formation, over which much difference of opinion existed. Some grammarians contented themselves with a twofold division of mutes and semi-vowels. The former, now called plosives, such as *b* and *d*, had no length and their formation was analogous to the lipping of musical notes on a wind instrument or the dampers of a piano. Semi-vowels, now designating only *w* and *y*, were all other consonants capable of protraction.[31] This limited view was obviously unsatisfactory and other classificatory criteria were sought.

One contributor was Neil Arnott, who was probably the first to present his ideas in tabular form so that the 'euphonic' characteristics of consonants could be related to their anatomical locus (see Table 2.1). In other words, he was comparing their manner and place of articulation. Fifty-four years later, Wyllie prefaced his book with a similar chart of this 'Physiological Alphabet', which he also saw as having clinical application.[32] Its popularity continued into this century, through the writings of Langwill[33] in Britain, and Makuen in America, who thought it constituted 'the basis for the phonatory and articulatory treatment of stammering' and other defects.[34]

The influence of dividing sounds anatomically may be seen in some

Table 2.1: Table of Articulations

Labial	Palatal	Guttural		
P	T.L	K		Mute
B	D	G		Semimute
M	N	ng	on	Semivowel or nasal
F	th.S.sh.	ch	H	Aspirate
V	th.Z.J	gh		Vocal Aspirate
pr	R	ghr		Vibratory

Source: Neil Arnott's *Elements of Physics*, 2nd edn (1827), p. 583.

classifications of stuttering. According to Thelwall, there exist 'distinct species of impediments referable to distinct Organs'.[35] Hunt took this contention to extraordinary lengths in his classification, containing 22 subdivisions. For example, *pneumo-laryngo-glosso-cheilomania* signified 'Defective action of the respiratory apparatus, the larynx, the tongue, and the lips, as required in *lap*'. He himself questioned the utility of such a system, but he maintained that its merit lay in directing attention to those organs requiring regulation, which 'must be the object of any method of treatment that can hope for success'.[36] Though far from the minds of Thelwall and Hunt, the inherent danger of this approach was that the organs themselves might be thought defective and in need of mechanical or surgical intervention. Indeed, such an assumption underlay James Yearsley's classificatory system. He formulated eight categories: the respiratory, laryngeal, gutteral, lingual, labial, facial, choreal and mixed, which provided a basis for therapeutic flexibility and ammunition against elocutionists, whom he castigated for treating stuttering as '*one* affection, and as such requiring *one* remedy'.[37]

In addition to phonetics, it was argued that the nature of stuttering could be revealed through a knowledge of 'the audibility and mechanism of utterance'[38] and an elucidation of the natural laws of voice and speech.[39] The gross anatomy of the head and neck posed no

Figure 2.1: Diagrammatic Section Through the Head and Neck From James Hunt and Charles Plumptre

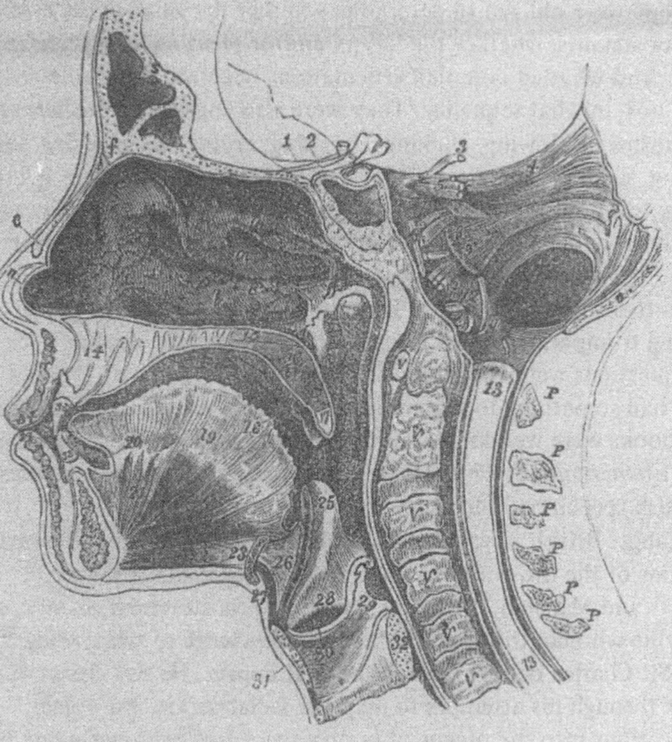

Median section of the head; *F*, frontal bone; *S*, frontal sinus; *B*, bone of the nose; *C*, cartilage of the nose; *N*, external nostril; *U*, upper spongy bone; *M*, middle spongy bone; *L*, lower spongy bone; *O*, occipital bone; *V*, vertebræ; *P*, the spinous processes; 1 to 12, the cranial nerves; 13, the spinal cord; 14, superior maxillary bone; 15, hard palate; 16, soft palate; 17, uvula; 18, tonsil; 19, tongue; 20, fraenum; 21, genio-glossus; 22, genio-hyoideus; 23, hyoid bone; 24, palato-pharyngeus, 25, epiglottis; 26, hyo-epiglottic ligament; 27, hyo-thyroid ligament; 28, superior ligament of the glottis; 29, arytenoid cartilage; 30, inferior ligament or vocal cord; 31, thyroid cartilage; 32, cricoid cartilage; 33 33, incisors 34 34, lips.

Source: Hunt (1959), p. 82; Plumptre, p. 54, fig. 9.

problems, since it had been known from antiquity. Many treatises included illustrative diagrams, one of the clearest being that in Figure 2.1 reproduced by both James Hunt[40] and Charles Plumptre.[41]

Far more difficult to assess was how the parts functioned, individually and in combination. On this point physiologists could contribute, since they were obliged to determine whether the vocal cords needed to close for sonants, whether the larynx and/or pharynx gave impulse to sounds, and whether complex articulations occurred simultaneously and, if not, in what sequence. They were also engaged in explaining the mechanisms of blowing, clicking, coughing, crying, hiccoughing, kissing, laughing, sighing, singing, sniffing, sneezing, snoring, snorting, spitting, sucking, swallowing, whispering, whistling, yawning and ventriloquism, the latter proving particularly fascinating. Constant analogies were invoked to explain the workings of individual organs, the larynx being likened to a variety of musical instruments, and the pharynx to a speaking trumpet. Amongst Continental physiologists dealing with these questions were Richerand,[42] Magendie[43] and Müller,[44] all of whom had something to say about stuttering in one place or another. Their books were well known in this country, unlike Béclard's work in *Traité Élémentaire de Physiologie Humaine*, which was not mentioned by British speech pathologists.

Amongst British physiological publications dealing with the various functions of the oro-vocal mechanism were those of Carpenter,[45] Kirkes[46] and Marshall,[47] who all touched upon stuttering as, of course, did Wyllie who contributed so much to knowledge of whispering.[48] But it was Sir Charles Bell who made the first impact. He was drawn to the subject through his attempts to map the facial nerves. Previously, investigations into the organs of human voice had been neglected by the Philosophical Society and amongst the many topics covered in his own paper was the pharynx which, by trapping sounds and controlling their emission, could act like the lungs as a force in the production of consonants.[49] He had made mention of stuttering even earlier, however, in 1827, when in lecturing to the College of Surgeons he had expressed the hope that medical men would take note of the problem and find some rational means of cure.[50] In the event, his words at that time seem to have been heeded most by the elocutionists James Wright and Richard Cull.

Many commentators drew a distinction between voice and articulate language, which resulted from modification of vocal sound by the oral structures. These Cull set out in tabular form (see Table 2.2), probably on information derived from Thelwall.[51]

Table 2.2: Classification of the Articulatory Organs

Single	Double		Active	Passive
Tongue	Lips		Tongue	Teeth
Uvula	Gums	or,	Uvula	Gums
Palate	Teeth		Lips	Palate, or roof of the mouth

Source: reproduced from Richard Cull (1833), p. 17.

Whereas Thelwall defined the vocal and enunciatory mechanism functionally,[52] the general tendency was towards an anatomical division. Voice or 'audible breath' was seen as deriving its raw material from the lungs, exhalation acting like the force that drives a windmill's sails.[53] Melville Bell also distinguished between the production of material for speech and moulding that material by articulation, but he drew upon a different analogy:

> Two entirely different sets of organs are brought into operation in the two acts: as different as the furnace, boiler, and other *steam* apparatus of a locomotive, are, from the piston, rods, and wheels, to which the steam communicates *motion*.[54]

The neurologist John Bristowe preferred to bring the distinction between vocalisation and respiration into sharper focus and, rather like Hunt's classification of stuttering, he proposed a threefold division, stressing the complexity of co-ordinated movements found in normal speech:

> For its successful performance it is necessary that three distinct and complex mechanisms – the respiratory, the phonetic, and the articulatory – shall act with precision and in exact concordance; that the lungs shall be expanded at suitable intervals, and to a suitable degree, and that the force of expiration shall be regulated with nicety; that the rima glottidis shall be opened or closed according as surd or sonant letters are to be produced, and that the tension of the cords shall be accurately adjusted to the pitch of the musical tones required . . . and the movements of the lips, jaws, tongue, and

> soft palate shall be accurately adjustable for each literal sound, and capable of passing from one set of adjustments to another with rapidity and smoothness.[55]

All this was required for one sound, which then had to be joined into syllables and words. The scope for breakdown was enormous and gave rise to speculations that stuttering represented a breakdown in the co-ordination process.

Very little comment was made upon the neurophysiology of speech. Kussmaul spoke of the 'syllabic co-ordinating apparatus' without explaining what this was.[56] Caleb distinguished between the sound generators (air-expelling and sound-producing mechanisms), the sound modifiers (resonance chambers and articulatory organs), and the 'governing nerve-influence' which acted as co-ordinator, but whose location, if an anatomical entity, was unknown.[57] Behnke and Rosenthal, however, seemed to assign the medulla the task of harmonising the activities of the lungs, larynx and articulators.[58] Even less attention was paid to the psychology of speech, so theorists had the unenviable option of explaining stuttering in terms of what they knew best – the peripheral mechanism – or venturing into uncharted regions. Many chose the former course.

Conceptual and Terminological Barriers

During the initial stages of a science, notions are indistinct and words largely inherited from the vernacular, but as a body of knowledge accumulates, concepts become refined and the discipline advances. To aid this process, the vocabulary must keep pace with new ideas. Traditional words, if they are to be useful labels for experimental groups or theoretical constructs, must be divested of many old connotations.[59] No one appreciated this better than Thelwall. As an orator, he appealed to the imagination, introducing few details, making part stand for the whole, and individual traits for complex aggregates. But in science, he asserted, language should speak to the understanding:

> there must be no pretence of synonymes; not only every aggregate idea, but every component part of such idea, must have its specific name: there must be but one term to indicate one idea; and but one idea indicated by any one term.[60]

Further, 'the signification of these must be fixed, not by arbitrary, but by strict logical definition'. The desire to put distance between everyday and technical use of language was common in scientific circles at the time. Thelwall strove for consensus by urging that terms be defined 'according to their inherent, or their analogous signification' and this must be preserved especially when a new science borrows words from another.[61] Thelwall put this into practice with his own prosodical terminology but he was in no position to delineate the majority of speech problems and those that followed him became enmeshed in terminological and conceptual confusions that continued well into this century. Indeed, it was not until after the founding of the College of Speech Therapists in 1945 that some authoritative statement on nomenclature could be made.[62]

The task facing early speech pathologists was formidable since the vocabulary was inadequate for the growing number of diagnostic categories. Particularly ambiguous was *stammer* which, together with *lisp*, had served to describe abnormal speech from at least the eighth century[63] to the fourteenth or fifteenth centuries, when the verb *stut* appeared, to be followed by the noun *stutter* around 1529.[64] Thus, although there was no suggestion that hard-of-hearing people had spasmodic utterance, we read that those 'which be halfe deafe do speak but stutteringly',[65] and three centuries later a biblical translation was still describing deaf speech in terms of stammering.[66] Widening the signification still further, Richerand wrote at the turn of the nineteenth century of stammering:

> This is a corruption of pronunciation too well known to require a definition. A tongue too large and thick; a considerable diminution of irritability, as in ebriety, in the commencement of apoplexy, or certain fevers of a bad type; an unusual length of the frenum of the tongue, by impeding the facility of its motions, become causes of stammering: it may likewise be produced by the deficiency or bad arrangement of several teeth.[67]

Indeed, Poett tells us that the word *stammer* has been 'applied to every species of Impediment'.[68] Nor was this surprising since, being popularly defined in terms of faltering, hesitant or laborious speech, it could describe almost any defect. Detailed analysis is beyond the scope of this chapter, but as the unsuspecting historian may be led astray, it is pertinent to untangle some of the confusions which underlay many false conclusions on theory and practice. In essence, Victorians were facing formidable diagnostic problems, some of which have yet to be fully resolved.

Despite some suggestions that stutterers were highly intelligent, Clouston reported 'spasmodic stammering' and 'Dundreary type speech' amongst the inmates of the Edinburgh Lunatic Asylum.[69] Wyllie also considered stammering to be a factor in 'the deranged speech of imbeciles and idiots' and some modern statistics, indicating a relatively high incidence of the disorder in mentally retarded populations, lend support to this view.[70] As with the dysfluencies of infants, however, much turns on the definition of stammering.

In 1773, Herries asserted that every speech impediment 'results from pronouncing one or more of the articulate sounds imperfectly'.[71] Granting a certain truth in this statement, it is easy to see how stuttering could be classed as an articulation disorder,[72] especially as many patients found particular sounds an impossible hurdle. Of course, there was a difference between enunciating the sounds and joining them together, but since *articulation* literally referred to the latter process, it was inherently ambiguous. The metaphor describing stutterers as 'tongue-tied' further associated their problem with some pronunciatory error of organic origin. Constant reference to Demosthenes added another complication. Though some were aware that he probably mispronounced sounds,[73] and it was suggested that he spoke nasally,[74] most preferred to think of him as a stutterer.

In Germany, some early attempts to distinguish between stuttering and articulation defects were made by Schulthess in 1827[75] and later by Merkel, who also differentiated *stottern* (alalia syllabaris) from *stammeln* (alalia literalis or anarthria literalis); so by 1878 Kussmaul could confidently assert that no one should mistake them, as diagnosis was easy.[76] However, Hunt was well aware that this distinction had not crossed the Channel:

> The terms 'stammering' and 'stuttering' are in this country synonymously used to designate all kinds of defective utterance. In no English work written upon this subject has the exact discrimination between these disorders, which differ both in kind and origin, been laid down with scientific correctness. From this confusion of terms have arisen many errors in theory and in practice, for no treatment can be efficacious unless our diagnosis be correct.[77]

He therefore defined the terms, *stammering* being:

> characterised by an inability or difficulty of properly enunciating some or many of the elementary speech-sounds, accompanied or not, as the case may be, by a slow, hesitating, more or less indistinct delivery, but *unattended with frequent repetitions* of the initial sounds, and consequent convulsive efforts to surmount the difficulty.

By contrast, *stuttering* was:

> a vicious utterance, manifested by *frequent repetitions* of initial or other elementary sounds, and always more or less *attended with muscular contortions*.[78]

This distinction would have been useful had it been widely adopted. As it was, though Hunt had a few followers, *stammering* continued to be the more popular term for spasmodic hesitancy and is still favoured by modern British speech therapists.

Hunt's definition of *stammering* was itself ambiguous, since it embraced organic disorders, the functional defects of children and imbeciles, the hesitancies of old age, and impediments consequent upon cerebral disorders, including paralysis. Indeed, Bristowe employed this wider sense of the term.[79] Sometimes verbal symptoms arising from neural lesions might be called *stammering*.[80] To the neurologically uninitiated there were good reasons for mistaking the festinance of Parkinsonism, still called 'pseudo-stammering', the scanning or staccato speech of disseminated sclerosis, and the 'syllable-stumbling' of general paresis for true stuttering. But even good diagnosticians tended to conceive of these conditions as one category, as evinced by the terms *anarthria spasmodica*[81] and *dysarthria syllabaris*,[82] which were used synonymously for stuttering. The common denominator leading to their identification was spasm, which deeply impressed Victorians and led Graves to state that it 'is evident to any one who observes the interrupted and spasmodic efforts which paralytic persons make when speaking' that 'they are in fact all stutterers'.[83] Cramps and convulsive movements also induced many to categorise stuttering with epilepsy and chorea.[84] However, it was carefully distinguished from the rare disorder *aphthongia*, a spasmodic and fluctuating condition of muscles in the distribution of the hypoglossal nerve, which rendered the sufferer inarticulate.[85]

Fleury, who first named this disorder in 1865, also called it 'reflex aphasia'. Aphasia itself had only just been named, the consequence of which was to generate interest in language disturbances and provide theorists of stuttering with new scope for speculation. Since antiquity, speech breakdown had been recognised as a precursor of apoplexy but it was not until the latter half of the nineteenth century that stuttering was tenuously linked with cerebral pathology. It – or what one writer believed physicians called aphasia – was a symptom of fevers,[86] which were also known to precipitate genuine cases of stuttering. In some instances, stuttering was associated with 'true' aphasia.[87] Several Continental writers postulated a similar underlying pathology,[88] and Trousseau even contended that some patients with right hemiplegia were actually stutterers rather than aphasiacs.[89] Victorians were disinclined to pursue these speculations and it was Bluemel, in this century, who argued the case not only that stuttering often begins with aphasia but is actually a manifestation of its subcortical or motor variety.[90] This issue is still alive, especially amongst those who favour an organic basis for the impediment,[91] and is not without serious therapeutic implications.[92]

Aside from repetitions, interpolations and strained enunciation, stutterers and aphasiacs were similar in that both might be 'lost for words'. Idiots were in an analogous state, as were those with organic or psychic confusion. Inability 'to choose or recollect a word correspondently expressive of an idea' Wright called *mental stammering*, which he defined as 'interruptions of thought, occasioned, possibly, by timidity, temporary abstraction or forgetfulness, on the one hand, and, on the other, slowness of intellect, blended with inattention, with pride and self-conceit'. It was something to which everyone is subject and is characterised by 'ums' and 'ahs'. This he distinguished from stuttering, though it might be its precursor, especially in children exposed to pressures during periods of uncertainty.[93]

Rather different is *cluttering*, a disturbance more clearly associated with language deficit and possibly of organic origin, now postulated as holding something of an intermediate position between aphasia and stuttering.[94] Differential diagnosis is still problematical, however, as the recent term 'clutterstuttering' indicates.[95] That a distinction should have been mooted at all in the nineteenth century is therefore surprising. Once again, much credit goes to Continental writers, who appear to have recognised its chief distinguishing features and mode of alleviation.[96] In England, relatively little was said about this complaint, though Thelwall had made early note of it[97] and he was followed by Hunt, who described it as 'an anomalous enunciation, which consists in pronouncing words and sentences with such rapidity, that the syllables appear only half articulated, and the speaker becomes, consequently, unintelligible'.[98] He pointed out that it was an habitual vice, not to be mistaken with the attention gaining *pattering* of actors, which is a feat. Despite these guidelines, it is likely that Victorians often mistook clutterers for stutterers and treated them accordingly, as may still happen.[99]

Finally, the larynx might lure unsuspecting practitioners into misdiagnosis, since vocal disorders of either physical or emotional origin were comparable with stuttering. A faltering or interrupted voice may signal epilepsy or apoplexy, or be a symptom of old age, intoxication, fevers and various neurological disorders.[100] Whether spastic dysphonia falls into the latter category or is of psychogenic origin remains in question, but characteristic symptoms have led to it being described as 'stuttering of the vocal cords'.[101] Possibly this is the same impediment as Dr James described in 1879. He certainly drew a close analogy between it and stuttering,[102] and though one correspondent believed them to be distinct,[103] Holmes appears to have identified the two conditions.[104] As the larynx is a most sensitive emotional indicator, stutterers and other nervous people are liable to 'lose' their voice or be 'struck dumb'. At least this is the impression severe stutterers may convey, when even their vowels become arrested. Indeed, the impediment can be a legacy of fright. Occasionally it is an hysterical reaction, which may also be operative in spastic dysphonia, but then one would expect a preponderance of females. Whatever the case, an hysterical form of stuttering was known in the last century.[105]

The crux of these diagnostic problems, yet to be resolved,[106] is whether the term stuttering denotes a symptom, common to an heterogeneous group of disorders, or whether it refers to an aetiological category. If the former, then all manner of disorders will come under its banner and are liable to be confused. If the latter, then theorists are faced with the formidable task of elucidating its pathology with precision.

Notwithstanding the pitfalls of this conceptual labyrinth, the experienced practitioner should have discriminated between simulated and genuine stuttering. He was at least forewarned:

> In the looseness of language resulting from inexact knowledge, all kinds of difficult and defective utterance are misnamed stammer, as the difficult utterance of the intoxicated, the faltering utterance of the paralytic, the imperfect utterance of deep emotion . . .

> malformed organs of speech, and the hesitation in discourse when the suitable word fails to present itself to a speaker's mind. Such affections . . . are distinct from stammer.[107]

This solution had been provided by Thelwall long before: precise definitions and commensurate nomenclature. Attempts at the former usually amounted to descriptions that failed to exclude other disorders. With the advance of neurological knowledge, terms certainly proliferated, but they were used inconsistently and with some impediments the situation approached verbal anarchy. As regards *stammering*, *stuttering*, *psellismus*, *balbuties* and *hesitation*, these were used either synonymously, as generic terms, or as labels for distinct complaints. In addition, the first two were employed in a classificatory manner, with *stammering* generally denoting the more advanced and *stuttering* the repetitive stage of the disorder.[108] Furthermore, they might have an anatomical connotation, *stammering* depicting the more posteriorly placed vocal difficulties and *stuttering* referring to repetitive action at the front of the mouth.[109] All of these meanings must be borne in mind when reading the literature.

Stuttering: A Disease?

Given these numerous uncertainties over the nature of stuttering, the way was open for disputes concerning the composition of any profession directed to its alleviation. From the outset, the discipline's twofold theoretical foundation provided an inherent source of friction, but diagnostic confusions and doubt over whether the impediment was physically based or resulted from mislearning added a further dimension to discord. If stuttering had some organic or physiological basis, then speech correction should form a new medical specialty. If the problem was primarily a bad habit or vice, then re-education was required. Representative statements illustrate the two extremes. First, a medical view: 'Stammering should invariably be treated not as a fault but as a disease';[110] the corollary being that it fell 'within the province of the healing art'.[111] Elocutionists demurred:

> the treatment of speech defects, by those who have made them their special study, no more intrudes upon the province of the medical man than do the services of a drill-sergeant in a school. The one teaches to walk well and the other to talk well.[112]

This argument placed speech correction on a didactic rather than a remedial footing.

Though some doctors forwarded their claims with an intransigence proportional to their ignorance, their position was not without substance for, in the event of misdiagnosis, cases labelled stuttering may well have been genuine medical problems. Also, aetiological misconceptions, frequently the result of too limited experience, led to hasty correlations being drawn between stuttering and anomalies which certainly did lie within the physician's jurisdiction, such as tongue-tie and epilepsy. Furthermore, if classified as a 'nervous' or spasmodic affection, it could be argued that it was 'fully as much requiring medical aid as chorea, catalepsy, or any other convulsive disease'.[113] Lastly, there was general agreement that stuttering was frequently accompanied by poor health. Thomas Hunt, however, denied that this was its cause:

> I deny that stammering is *a disease*. It is an imperfection occasioned by organic, physical, or accidental causes – the want of some proper regulation of use, and not a disease, though the fruitful source of many diseases; some of which, by reaction, may be confounded with the original cause. Such, for example, as palpitation of the heart, derangement of the nervous system, pulmonary affections, all inducing constitutional debility, both physical and mental, and frequently ending in premature death. These are the effects of stammering . . . [114]

So important did his son James consider the question that he devoted a chapter of his book to it.[115]

The strength of the doctors' position was that all medically unqualified people could be designated 'empirics' and so reputable elocutionists became bracketed with unscrupulous charlatans, whose activities they were arguably justified in curtailing, and for which they could claim the highest motives. Quackery was decried as a public 'crime' and 'inimical to public safety', even when some good ensued. Amidst these noble sentiments, however, baser instincts were at work, since any such chicanery was also condemned as a 'robbery of the profession' and elocutionists were accused of dishonesty because they came in 'like a wolf over the wall' and took guineas from men who had 'invested a large amount of time and capital in acquiring diplomas'.[116] This was the situation over a decade before the Medical Act of 1858, after which there was considerable rivalry between doctors themselves over fees.[117] It also reveals that altruistic motives were not the guiding principle of professional men, as was sometimes suggested.[118]

Since neither group could claim to have found a permanent or universal cure, it may seem strange that each was so anxious to reserve treatment to itself, for the inevitable failures would tarnish reputations and ultimately affect the pocket. To justify any monopolistic hopes, medical men should have demonstrated the superiority of their remedies and explained why patients resorted to elocutionists or quacks. Actually, they merely conceded that their profession had been insufficiently interested in the subject, and it deserved censure for failing to set standards and leaving the field open to unlicensed practitioners:

> On this account, as far as the Elocutionists are concerned, the literature of this subject, if it deserves the name, manifests, I do not hesitate to say, a greater amount of ignorance than any other allied to the medical profession. The egotism of this class is not less remarkable than their ignorance. Each has promulgated his own views as original discoveries, and all are in opposition the one to the other, a pretty sure criterion of their merits individually.[119]

The equal diversity of medical opinions and priority claims seems to have escaped this writer's notice. Any ignorance of the impediment in medical circles was put down to neglect: there was never any suggestion that the problem outwitted them. Only through neglect was stuttering an 'opprobrium on the character of the profession'[120] and a 'disgrace to the science of medicine'.[121] Conveniently overlooking the numerous medical publications which had appeared by mid-century, and wishing to rescue treatment from the 'unmerited obloquy' of 'mere' elocutionists, the younger Poett sought to enlighten medical minds through his treatise, which was purported to be 'the first practical effort to bring the disease within the legitimate domains of medicine'.[122] Why this should have been necessary when his father had brought the matter to its 'fullest perfection' in 1828 is left unexplained.[123]

In the event, Poett's contribution neither deflected the elocutionists' purpose nor provided the unequivocal answer his profession so needed. Over the following years, other medical minds were brought to bear upon the subject but, on Abbotts' own admission, they said nothing new.[124] Nevertheless, he felt justified in reasserting medical jurisdiction over the impediment and cited the words of the Continental physician, Klencke, in support of his position:

> The cure of stammering should not be undertaken merely by teachers, elocutionists, decayed actors and music-masters, who possess no physiological knowledge, who have no notion of the causes and complications and functional derangements, and who apply only a mechanical method, without reference to individual cases.[125]

In reality, reputable elocutionists were not the ignoramuses that Abbotts and others suggested. Most were familiar with the anatomy of speech and some were exceedingly well-informed. Thelwall had studied medicine under Hunter, Cline and Babington.[126] Cull had been a pupil of Thomas Pettigrew until an injured arm put paid to his surgical career.[127] Graham Bell had taken an anatomy course at University College London,[128] and James Hunt had been a medical student early in his career.[129] Indeed, Hunt's grasp of numerous matters relating to speech was hardly open to question; his *A Manual of the Philosophy of Voice and Speech*, his review of speech localisation in *The Anthropological Review*, together with his writings on stuttering, were superior to anything published by physicians treating the impediment.

Laymen hit back with some vituperous comments. For instance, Dr Bishop's *On Articulate Sounds*, the one book Abbotts found meritorious,[130] was described as 'bare-faced' plagiarism.[131] But by and large, elocutionists were on the defensive and it was unfortunate for them that three of the men intellectually and educationally best equipped to present their case – John Thelwall, James Hunt and Melville Bell – were either dead or out of the country by the time the medical profession became a more unified force. Though the role of medical auxiliaries was far from their minds, they were in the position that such groups experience when trying to raise their occupation into an autonomous profession: they had to find some area of activity over which they could claim and maintain monopoly.[132] This was not easy, in view of their theoretical reliance on oro-vocal physiology and the increasing evidence that neurological and other organic pathologies underlay several related speech problems. Even the phonetics they called upon was of the anatomical variety, commonly discussed by medical men. Thus, their task was to establish the independence of a subject that was increasingly coming within the orbit of medicine. Separating the treatment of stuttering from other speech problems was no long-term solution. Nevertheless, elocutionists put their case, arguing that speech was learned through imitation and people wishing to develop their verbal skills should apply to those who provided the best models, who understood the art of delivery, and who had developed the appropriate teaching techniques. Stutterers were in just as much need of such guidance as those aspiring to oratorical excellence.

At no time during the polemics was the basic issue debated – what constituted disease? And Bristowe, the one man who was concerned both with its definition and with speech impediments, made no effort to apply his criteria to stuttering. Anyway, Bristowe's conception of disease as a complex of symptom and cause[133] – a 'deleterious agency action upon the body' – would hardly have solved the controversy, since what constituted that agency was open to personal interpretation.

Despite much acrimony, the relations between doctors and elocutionists were not always stormy. Thelwall was on good terms with a number of physicians. And several publications were directed towards leading doctors. After Thelwall's *Letter* to Mr Cline came two treatises from Richard Cull, one addressed to Pettigrew and the other to George Birkbeck, and Alexander Bell's book dedicated to 'a surgeon', whilst Sir Charles Bell was the recipient of James Wright's *Three Letters*. Many doctors – Benjamin Brodie and Astley Cooper amongst them – either referred patients or were consulted where appropriate. Occasionally medical journals would carry articles by elocutionists and review their books favourably. Further, Dr Lennox Browne and Emil Behnke were joint authors of a book on the voice. The two men had been closely associated for twelve years and after Behnke's death Browne defended his voice training system against certain charges.[134] Both Behnke[135] and Wright[136] spoke to medical audiences, while James Hunt impressed them by print. Referring to his *Manual*, Duncan Gibb said that he had seldom 'perused one so full of useful and really valuable instruction'[137] and Gordon Holmes adjudged his treatise on stuttering to be 'the most elaborate and systematic'.[138] Testimonials also spoke eloquently, such as the note of Mrs Behnke's work[139] and the various ones received by Thomas Hunt, amongst others. The doctors in question, however, could afford to be impartial as they themselves were not directly involved in treating speech impediments. But there were others who found hobnobbing of this sort unacceptable and the *Lancet* invited its readers to provide it with the names of doctors supporting the 'quackery' of elocutionists, either by referring patients or testimonials, so that they could be placed before the profession.[140]

Since the two groups were not radically distinguished by their therapeutic activities, the debate was not really over the disease status of stuttering. This merely provided a respectable front behind which the real battle could be fought: who would get the financial pickings.

With the widening gap between the remunerative expectations of physicians and elocutionists, the dispute subtly shifted from money to one over power. This change was perhaps just discernible by late Victorian times, after which lay practitioners found themselves increasingly in the position of paramedical workers. That is, they came under the sway of the medical profession, which having control could afford to be benevolent: activities that were once derided as quackery became acceptable.

With the fluid state of the medical profession in the early part of the century there was ample scope for territorial claims. Seen in the broader context, arguments of this kind were particularly liable to erupt over those problems which had traditionally been handled by laymen and whose success with them was equal or superior to that of their medical counterparts. Indeed, the *Lancet* attack on Thomas Hunt was because of his success; had he been inept he would have posed no threat. Analogous debates were going on in fields as diverse as obstetrics and psychiatry. The office of midwife was in jeopardy as men entered her domain and doctors strove for control.[141] Meanwhile, the growing inclination to see the mind in material terms and to interpret insanity as a disease rather than a sign of sin or demoniacal possession, moved psychiatry towards medicine. Hence, the favourable responses to moral treatment obtained by laymen like Samuel Tuke were received with mixed feelings by the mad-doctors, who were still relying heavily on blood-letting and purges.[142] As Bynum notes: 'If physicians *qua* physicians could do nothing for the lunatic except treat his bodily afflictions, then the medical man had no special claim to a unique place in the treatment of mental illness. Their income, prestige and medical theories were all threatened.'[143] This statement applies equally to the medical man in relation to stutterers.

Notes

1. Freidson, p. 5.
2. Ibid., pp. xix, 76-7.
3. Rockey (1979), pp. 156, 163-4.
4. Wilbur Samuel Howell, 'Sources of the Elocutionary Movement in England: 1700-1748', *Quarterly Journal of Speech*, 45 (1959), 3-18.
5. Arthur Bronstein, 'Nineteenth-Century Attitudes Towards Pronunciation', *Quarterly Journal of Speech*, 40 (1954), 417-21.
6. Department of Education and Science, pp. 80-1.
7. H – T (1860), p. 534.
8. *Household Words*, p. 464.

9. For a more detailed discussion, see below pp. 167-9.
10. *Household Words*, p. 464.
11. Wright, *Treatise*, p. 12.
12. Vivian Salmon, *The Works of Francis Lodwick* (London, Longman, 1972), pp. 12-24 and *passim*.
13. G. Panconcelli-Calzia, 'Earlier History of Phonetics' in *Manual of Phonetics*, ed. L. Kaiser (Amsterdam, North-Holland, 1957), ch. 1, pp. 13-17 (3-17).
14. Ch. Féré, 'Note sur l'exploration des mouvements de la langue', *Comptes Rendus*, 1 n.s. (1889), 278-80; Ch. Féré, 'Note sur l'influence de l'exercice musculaire sur l'énergie, la rapidité et l'habileté des mouvements volontaires de la langue chez un bègue', *Comptes Rendus*, 2 n.s. (1890), 676-7.
15. Hunt (1859), pp. 138-47.
16. Erasmus Darwin, *The Temple of Nature* (London, printed for J. Johnson, 1803), p. 120 of 'Additional Notes'.
17. Catherine Mackenzie, *Alexander Graham Bell* (New York, Grosset & Dunlap, 1928), pp. 13, 15, 29.
18. Ibid., 13-14, 18-19, 83.
19. Ibid., 37-8.
20. Henry Sweet, *A Handbook of Phonetics* (Oxford, Clarendon Press, 1887), pp. vi-vii.
21. K.M. Elisabeth Murray, *Caught in the Web of Words* (New Haven, Yale UP, 1977), pp. 49-50, 72-4.
22. For an assessment of the contribution of these phoneticians, and earlier ones concerned with deaf education, see J.R. Firth, 'The English School of Phonetics' in *Papers in Linguistics 1934-1951* (London, Oxford UP, 1957), ch. 8, pp. 92-120.
23. Sweet, *Handbook*, p. vii.
24. A.J. Ellis's 'Estimate of Visible Speech' in A.M. Bell (1900), pp. 284-96.
25. Mackenzie, *Bell*, p. 53.
26. E. Darwin, *Temple*, pp. 107-20 of 'Additional Notes'.
27. A.M. Bell (1900), pp. 158 ff.
28. See below p. 228.
29. 'Mr. THELWALL'S LECTURE. – On the Harmonic Qualities of the Literal Elements, and their classification according to their musical and other inherent properties', *Panoramic Miscellany*, 1 (1826), 41-2 (41-6); 'Mr. THELWAL'S [*sic*] LECTURE on the Elements of Euphony', ibid., 194-5 (193-8).
30. Ibid., pp. 41, 195.
31. Borthwick, pp. 6, 9-11.
32. Wyllie, pp. ii-iii, 6, 24, 31. Cf. Colman (1895), p. 1419; (1899), p. 449.
33. See, for example, H.G. Langwill, 'Stammering and its Treatment', *Practitioner*, 85 (1910), 568-82.
34. G. Hudson-Makuen, 'The Physiology of Language in its Relation to the Treatment of Stammering', *New York Medical Journal*, 84 (1906), p. 1262 (1261-3).
35. Thelwall (1812), p. lxiii.
36. Hunt (1870), pp. 241-3.
37. Yearsley (1843-4), pp. 289-93.
38. *Penny Cyclop.*, p. 429.
39. Cull (1835), pp. 27-9.
40. Hunt (1859), p. 82.
41. Plumptre, p. 54, fig. 9.
42. Richerand, pp. 366-77.
43. F. Magendie, *An Elementary Compendium of Physiology*, 3rd edn, trans. E. Milligan (Edinburgh, printed for John Carfrae & Son, and London, Longman, 1829), pp. 128-53.

44. Müller, pp. 972-1058.
45. Carpenter, pp. 334-53; William Carpenter, *A Manual of Physiology*, 4th edn (London, Churchill, 1865), pp. 725-34.
46. *Kirkes' Hand-Book of Physiology*, 11th edn, W. Morrant Baker & Vincent Harris (London, John Murray, 1884), pp. 246-9, 518-33.
47. John Marshall, *Outlines of Physiology* (London, Longman, Green, 1867), vol. 1, pp. 268-9.
48. Wyllie, pp. 33-8, 463-84.
49. C. Bell, pp. 306-14, 319.
50. Cull (1835), p. 27.
51. Thelwall (1812), p. xxxiii.
52. Ibid., pp. xxviii-xxxiii
53. Abbotts, pp. 19, 41.
54. A.M. Bell (1900), p. 255.
55. Bristowe (1882), p. 1513.
56. Kussmaul, p. 835.
57. Caleb, p. 148.
58. E. Behnke (1893), pp. 15-16; Rosenthal, p. 133. Cf. below p. 137.
59. Denyse Rockey, 'Some Fundamental Principles for the Solution of Terminological Problems in Speech Pathology and Therapy', *British Journal of Disorders of Communication*, 4 (1969), 166-7 (166-75).
60. 'THELWAL'S LECTURE . . .', *Panoramic Miscellany*, p. 193.
61. Ibid., p. 194.
62. 'Terminology . . .', pp. 35-9.
63. Thomas Wright, *Anglo-Saxon and Old English Vocabularies*, 2nd edn (London, Trübner, 1884), pp. 8, 9, 37, 39, 161, 314.
64. Thomas Finkenstaedt, Ernst Leisi, Dieter Wolff, *Chronological English Dictionary* (Heidelberg, Carl Winter, Universitätsverlag, 1970), pp. 297, 420.
65. Helkiah Crooke, *A Description of the Body of Man* (London, 1618), p. 701.
66. William Tyndal, *The New Testament* (London, Samuel Bagster, 1970), pp. 297, 420.
67. Richerand, p. 373. (The term used in the French is *bégaiement*, see *Nouveaux Eléméns de Physiologie*, 2nd edn (Paris, 1802), p. 338.)
68. Poett snr (1833), p. 81.
69. Clouston, *Neuroses of Development*, pp. 12, 30, 31, 32, 33.
70. Bloodstein, pp. 132, 134-5.
71. John Herries, *The Elements of Speech* (London, Edward & Charles Dilly, 1773), p. 53.
72. Bishop (1851), p. 46. Cf. Good (1829), pp. xxx, 565; John Mason Good, *A Physiological System of Nosology* (London, printed for Bensley & Son, 1817), pp. 98-9.
73. Hunt (1861), pp. 26-7; Kussmaul, p. 849; A.M. Bell (1900), p. 250.
74. Caxton, *What Will He Do With It?*, vol. I, p. 318.
75. Kussmaul, pp. 826-7; Colman (1895), p. 1419, (1899), p. 448; Coote, p. 611.
76. Kussmaul, p. 837.
77. Hunt (1861), p. 12.
78. Ibid., pp. 12-13; cf. M.D., 'Periodic Stammering', *British Medical Journal*, 2 (1893), p. 1311 [1311-12].
79. Bristowe (1892), pp. 1191-3.
80. Pershing, pp. 779-81; cf. Bastian, pp. 57-9; Kussmaul, pp. xv, 661, 664-6, 805-9; Romberg, p. 363; Rosenthal, p. 134; Julius Mickle, *General Paralysis of the Insane* (London, H.K. Lewis, 1880), pp. 13-14, 29, 143-4; Report of a paper by Auguste Voisin on 'The Pathology of Lesions of Speech in the General Paralysis

of the Insane', *British Medical Journal*, 2 (1874), p. 288.

81. Pershing, p. 777.

82. Kussmaul, p. 826. Cf. p. 633.

83. Graves, p. 658.

84. See below pp. 130-3.

85. Bastian, pp. 59-60; Bristowe (1882), p. 1513; Kussmaul, pp. 825-6, 843. Cf. Wyllie, pp. 19-20; Romberg, vol. 2, 304-5 on 'glossoplegia'.

86. M'Minn, p. 15.

87. Wyllie, p. 23.

88. R. Arend, L. Handzel and B. Weiss, 'Dysphatic Stuttering', *Folia Phoniatrica*, 14 (1962), 55-6 (55-66).

89. James Hunt, 'On the Localisation of the Functions of the Brain, with Special Reference to the Faculty of Language', *Anthropological Review*, 7 (1869), p. 213. This article appeared in instalments; 6 (1868), 329-45; 7 (1869), 100-16, 201-14.

90. Bluemel, vol. 1, pp. 206-31.

91. Van Riper, pp. 344-5. Cf. Arend *et al.*, *Folia Phoniatrica*, 14, pp. 59-64.

92. See below p. 217.

93. Wright (1835), pp. 20, 23, 24-5, 35-6.

94. Deso Weiss, *Cluttering* (Englewood Cliffs, N.J., Prentice-Hall, 1964), pp. 19-63.

95. R. Luchsinger, 'Inheritance of Speech Defects', *Folia Phoniatrica*, 22 (1970), 223-9 (216-30).

96. Kussmaul, pp. 816-18.

97. Rockey (1977), p. 89.

98. Hunt (1861), pp. 33-4.

99. Luchsinger, *Folia Phoniat.*, 22, p. 224.

100. Physician, p. 16.

101. Margaret Greene, *The Voice and its Disorders*, 3rd edn (London, Pitman Medical, 1972), pp. 208-18; Herbert H. Dedo, 'Recurrent Laryngeal Nerve Section for Spastic Dysphonia', *Annals of Otology*, 85 (1976), 451-9.

102. Prosser James, 'Stammering of the Vocal Cords', *Lancet*, 2 (1879), 726-7.

103. R. Locke Johnson, 'Stammering of the Vocal Cords', *Lancet*, 2 (1879), p. 899.

104. Gordon Holmes, 'Stammering of the Vocal Cords', *Lancet*, 2 (1879), p. 820.

105. Pershing, pp. 801-2.

106. Robert West and Merle Ansberry, *The Rehabilitation of Speech*, 4th edn (New York, Harper Row, 1968), pp. 115-23.

107. *Penny Cyclop.*, p. 429.

108. Beasley (1885), pp. 23-4; A.M. Bell (1900), p. 234; M'Minn, p. 12.

109. Abbotts, p. 22. Cf. Thelwall (1812), p. lxiii; 'Emil Behnke on . . .', p. 257.

110. Physician, p. 37. Original in italics.

111. Editorial (1846a), p. 557. Cf. Blake, p. 3. For a more recent revival of this argument, see correspondence in *British Medical Journal*, 1 (1922), pp. 546, 666.

112. Mason, (1884), p. 11n.

113. Poett jnr, p. 35.

114. Thomas Hunt, letter to the editor of the *Lancet* which he declined to publish and which appeared in *The Literary Gazette*, no. 1532 (1846), p. 503.

115. Hunt (1861), pp. 120-8.

116. Editorial (1846a), 557-8.

117. Noel Parry and Jose Parry, *The Rise of the Medical Profession* (London, Croom Helm, 1976), pp. 134-5.

118. Ibid., pp. 29-30.

119. Physician, p. v.
120. Poett snr (1828), p. 9.
121. McCormac, p. 31. Cf. Blake, p. 4.
122. Poett jnr, pp. 5, 7, 34.
123. Poett snr (1828), p. 58.
124. Abbotts, p. 9.
125. Ibid., p. 11.
126. Rockey (1979), p. 165.
127. Towards the end of his life, Richard Cull was unable to work because of ill-health, was rendered indigent through investment failures, and was obliged to seek financial aid from the Royal Literary Fund in London, by whom permission to inspect the material was kindly given. His application sketches events relevant to his literary career, see Registered Case File no. 2139, 1882.
128. MacKenzie, *Bell*, p. 43.
129. Presidential Address, *Journal of the Anthropological Society of London*, 8 (1870-1) (*Anthropological Review*, 1870), p. lxxix (lxxviii-lxxxiii).
130. Abbotts, p. 9. The book was also well received by the *British and Foreign Medico-Chirurgical Review*, 8 (1851), 527-9 and the *London Medical Gazette*, 12 n.s. (1852), 1118-19.
131. *Unspeakable*, pp. 137-9. Material reputedly taken from Dr Latham.
132. Freidson, p. 66.
133. J.S. Bristowe, *A Treatise on the Theory and Practice of Medicine*, 4th edn (London, Smith, Elder, 1882), pp. 3-17.
134. Lennox Browne, letter to *Professional World*, 2 (1893), p. 138; Behnke [1893], Appendix, p. vii.
135. Behnke's article in the *Journal of Laryngology and Rhinology* was based on a talk given at the Central London Throat and Ear Hospital. Cf. E. Behnke [1893], Extract, pp. 1-31 (following p. 48).
136. Wright's article in the *Lancet* was based on a talk given at St George's Hospital School of Medicine.
137. G. Duncan Gibb, *On Diseases of the Throat and Windpipe*, 2nd edn (London, John Churchill, 1864), p. 190. Cf. Review of Hunt's *Manual* in *British and Foreign Medico-Chirurgical Review*, 25 (1860), 140-4.
138. Holmes, p. 96.
139. F.L. Nicholls, letter to *British Medical Journal*, 1 (1893), p. 1043.
140. Editorial (1846), p. 664.
141. Donnison, ch. 3 and *passim*.
142. Bynum, pp. 317-34.
143. Ibid., p. 325.

3 NOTIONS OF CAUSALITY

Causality has been central to discussions on speech impediments because it is generally assumed that once their origin is known a rational and effective course of treatment will be ensured. Such an assumption implies the convertibility of agent and effect. Imbued with this notion, Thelwall stated that to remove the active cause was to conquer the disease,[1] a sentiment echoed through subsequent decades and 80 years later reiterated by Ball. Joining the swelling ranks of those who claimed to have solved the riddle of stuttering, he asserted that past therapeutic failures were due to erroneous views on causality, not one writer having come 'within measurable distance of the truth'.[2]

If the treatment record was poor, it would be untrue to say that no stutterers had been cured. Modest, or even startling successes, were on record, some originating from most unlikely quarters and through quite unexpected means. But though this might occasion the patient to rejoice, it was not necessarily applauded by professionals. The respectable, scientifically-oriented practitioner was always anxious to disassociate himself from any taint of quackery and the best way to do this was to base treatment upon theory, which served to vindicate his actions even where these produced indifferent results. Victorians hardly realised the tenuous connection between aetiological hypotheses and efficacious cures, and it is only recently that the value of the former has been questioned:

> present theories . . . do not deserve that label in a serious sense of the term; for they are little more than favored speculative notions supported by partial observations, preferred facts, and contrived explanations. Many widely accepted viewpoints embody concepts and principles which are internally inconsistent, contrary to many facts, lacking in support from either research findings or therapeutic results, and most regrettable of all, seemingly impervious to reasoned analysis.[3]

This critique is even more apt of views in the last century, when hypotheses were often based upon scanty or erroneous facts, cemented by faulty logic and promulgated with a zeal fired by wish-fulfilment.

Speech pathology rarely initiated its own aetiological concepts, but applied those already existing in medicine, psychology and linguistics. Until the seventeenth century, medical influence predominated in the form of the humoral theory, which had shaped thinking on speech impediments from the Hellenistic era, through the medieval Arabs to Renaissance Europe.[4] Hence writers like Francis Bacon were still attributing stuttering to excessive coldness and moisture of the tongue. This traditionally organic interpretation of speech impediments was inherited by later generations and in Thelwall's time was still commonly accepted, though the organic conception of aetiology had shifted from the humidity or calorific state of the tissues to their structure. Thelwall called such defects 'natural', but he argued that they were much rarer than generally supposed, for where the organisation of the parts was adequate for life it was also adequate for speech.[5] His contention was that most defects were 'habitual', that is, they arose from 'moral' causes, which roughly equated the category later designated 'functional'.

The concept of moral causation did not signal a radical departure from Greek thought since it stemmed from the Aristotelian doctrine of harmonising the emotions, and it was to these that Pinel and his successors directed their attention. Moral problems were imputed to aberrant emotional forces and insanity consequently was ascribed to disturbances of the 'passions' or 'affections' rather than to the intellectual functions of memory, imagination and other faculties.[6] The former might arise from exhaustion and disturbing experiences, whilst the latter had an ideational base.[7] Both might underlie speech problems, as Thelwall promptly realised, and where faulty habits of learning were involved he used the terms 'mental', 'intellectual' and 'educational' cause.[8] In the case of stutterers, it was not only their emotions, but also their judgment, imagination and attention that provoked comment.

The category of 'functional' causes, into which speech defects are now commonly placed, had broader implications. Gall and his followers focused attention upon mental faculties and their supposed organs by laying particular stress upon their activity or 'function', a term having either a psychological or physiological sense. In so doing, phrenologists not only impressed this concept upon later psychologists,[9] but steered psychology away from metaphysics and towards biology.[10] Since cerebral activities were often clearly disturbed, it was not long before the notion of a 'functional' cause was introduced. This has been attributed to Andrew Combe, who attempted to overcome the phrenologists' inability to demonstrate that mental disturbances invariably arose from pathology, whether of physical or psychological origin, in those organs of the brain upon which all thought and feeling depended.[11] However, the term was certainly in use before this. Following closely Itard's paper of 1817, McCormac depicted stuttering as a 'functional disease'[12] and the next year Palmer asserted that 'impeded elocution' was a functional defect wholly independent of 'mal-formation, or any morbid change in the structure, of the organs of speech' but resulting 'simply from derangement of their functions'.[13] Combe rejected the term 'moral' because this had reference to the mind and associations of immateriality. His concern was with the brain, which, he asserted like Jones,[14] and others after him, could well harbour abnormalities undetectable by contemporary techniques. These ideas were outlined in his *Observations on Mental Derangement* written in 1831.[15] Two years later, Cull, a fellow phrenologist, was describing stuttering as a functional disturbance,[16] and within the decade others were following suit.[17] For Cull, like Palmer, 'functional' in this context seemed to imply absence of any organic defect in the peripheral speech organs. Later, when used with the ambiguous word 'nervous', no clear picture emerges as to whether writers were envisaging the presence of undetected neural pathology or a psychogenic disturbance.

While subscribing to the natural-habitual or organic-functional dichotomy, most investigators concentrated on elaborating a classificatory system which depicted several causes operating in an hierarchical fashion. Thelwall set the pattern when he adopted an aetiological system based on an unnamed school of philosophy introduced to him by his former anatomy tutor, Henry Cline.[18] It was widely used in medicine but there was little agreement amongst speech pathologists over specific details; indeed, consensus was lacking over such basic issues as which factors associated with stuttering were causes and which effects. The theoretical questions entailed were formidable and their magnitude and implications were barely grasped, as investigators had little awareness of the assumptions under which they were operating or the method, if any, that they were employing.

Theoretical and Methodological Considerations

The empirical observations, or spontaneous and intuitive impressions, which Bernard saw as the precursors of scientific medicine, and to some extent its constant companions,[19] were amply provided by the numerous anecdotes on stuttering behaviour. The task was to find an explanatory model which could accommodate the variations in hesitancy with sex, age, language and class; its erratic manifestation in differing phonetic, verbal, physiological, environmental and social situations; and its absence in singing and unusual modes of speaking. Furthermore, any theory had to account for the disorder's course, something which featured little in Victorian thinking. For Bernard, a theory was a 'scientific idea controlled by experiment', formulated without appeal to authority and confirmed by counterproof after having been subjected to uncompromising doubt.[20] By these criteria, speculations on stuttering hardly ranked as theories. Factual impressions were not empirically tested, the need for verification apparently not having occurred to investigators. While sceptical of rival postulates, they were uncritical of their own. And their dogmatic pronouncements, based largely on *a priori* opinions, were not conducive to fostering impartial and objective enquiry; nor were they in tune with that scientific spirit which should have served to differentiate the legitimate practitioner from the quack.

In lieu of any attempt to isolate and examine those factors which might play a special part in the onset or maintenance of stuttering, the enquiring Victorian chose to catalogue the numerous phenomena that chanced to co-exist with the complaint. Obviously, as experience with patients grew, the list was liable to increase and show a growing diversity of content. There is no evidence that the passage of time was attended by greater perspicacity, for as late as 1894 we find Abbotts listing the 'non-surgical' causes of stammering as:

> delibility, paralysis or spasm of the muscles of the larynx and tongue, wrong position of the tongue during speaking, excessive secretion of saliva, imitation of other stammerers, speaking too rapidly or in too low a tone, not filling the chest sufficiently with air, keeping the mouth open, various affections of the throat and lungs, and nervousness, etc.[21]

This was not the casual speculation of someone untutored in stuttering pathology, but the serious reflection of a man with 30 years' experience, who had been physician to the Hospital for Affections of Speech and Ear.

As untold phenomena could be associated with the disorder, lists such as Abbotts' rendered the term 'cause' almost meaningless. Little effort was made to determine whether a significant connection between stuttering and other factors actually existed and, if so, whether positive correlations implied a causal relationship. Plainly, speech pathologists defaulted on Bernard's criteria for scientific inference:

> proof that a given condition always precedes or accompanies a phenomenon does not warrant concluding with certainty that a given condition is the immediate cause of that phenomenon. It must still be established that, when this condition is removed, the phenomenon will no longer appear. If we limit ourselves to the proof of presence alone, we might fall into error at any moment and believe in relations of cause and effect when there was nothing but simple coincidences . . . coincidences form one of the most dangerous stumbling blocks encountered by experimental scientists in complex sciences like biology. It is the *post hoc, ergo propter hoc* of the doctors, into which we may very easily . . . be led, especially if the results of an experiment or an observation supports a preconceived idea.[22]

Apart from falling into this trap, therapists also succumbed to the temptation of arguing from therapeutic success to aetiology. If surgical alteration of the speech musculature was followed by an amelioration of stuttering, it was gratuitously assumed that oral anomalies underpinned the problem and due consideration was not given to the multiplicity of factors that might have effected the cure, should this, in fact, have had any permanency.

Although useful statistical techniques were not devised until Galton and after, there was no reason why raw data on variables associated with stuttering could not have been collected. Aside from information on sex, age and frequency given in Chapter 1, and some figures on the various causes operating in different cases (Tables 5.1 and 5.2, p. 144) Mason's chart alone provided readers with some quantitative data (Table 3.1). Compared with the information currently available in psychiatry,[23] for instance, this was a meagre contribution, but nevertheless it represented an advance upon pure conjecture.

Another yardstick by which the standards employed in stuttering investigations may be gauged is provided by phrenology, which itself contributed to speech pathology in several ways. Each employed the anecdotal method, was impressed by unusual rather than average cases, and was concerned with behavioural characteristics, for which no standardised quantitative tests were available. Moreover, one suspects that speech pathologists, like phrenologists,[24] selected examples that supported their preconceived positions, and explained away awkward cases. But while phrenologists systematically collected an array of

Table 3.1: Coincidence of Various Factors With Stuttering According to Sufferers' Age and Sex, 1882-5

Age	Cases	Bad Health	Not from Childhood	Total Abstainers	Moderate	Excess	Non-Smokers	Moderate	Excess	Not Nervous
Males										
Under 10	7			7			7			
10 to 20	235	8	19	164	71		160	72	3	28
20 to 30	272	6	18	120	151	1	113	150	9	21
30 to 40	46	1	6	18	28		19	24	3	3
40 to 50	10			4	6		5	4	1	1
50 to 60	3			1	2			3		
Total Males	573	15	43	314	258	1	304	253	16	53
Females										
10 to 20	22		3	15	7					2
20 to 30	44	5	3	27	17					
30 to 40	9	2		4	5					
40 to 50	1			1						
Total Females	76	7	6	47	29					2
Total Males	573	15	43	314	258	1	304	253	16	53
TOTAL	649	22	49	361	287	1	304	253	16	55

Source: Reproduced from *The Elocutionist*, 3 (1885), p. 11, in N.H. Mason's *The Natural System for the Cure of Stammering and all Defects of Speech* (n.p., n.d.), unpaginated.

skulls and measured prominences, speech correctionists were merely apt to blame the patient's lack of diligence for failing to respond to a particular remedial system. The validity of the system remained unquestioned, at least by its proponents. It was not unknown for hypotheses about stuttering to be derived from observations on a handful of patients; indeed, Neil Arnott's original conjecture was based upon experience with one case.[25] Excellence in other areas of science was no safeguard against naivety or blatant theoretical errors when it came to stuttering.

It must be admitted that the correlations concerning phrenologists were easier to establish than those relating to stuttering. For a start, much of their data was normative, if unusual, and one variable – cranial topography – could be specified precisely, conserved for future reference, and measured with some degree of accuracy. Stuttering, conversely, was ill-defined and evanescent. True, recording equipment was available towards the end of the century and might have been used in speech analysis, but even so, there was no certainty that a diagnosis of stuttering was accurate. A few rudimentary criteria and unstandardised tests were used to differentiate the so called 'continued'[26] or 'physical'[27] stammer from its functional counterpart. The former was a permanent condition, indifferent to the weather and the presence of listeners and manifesting itself only on certain letters, apparently as a consequence of diminished lingual flexibility. If, according to Bishop, the stutterer 'could articulate any sentence whatever' then his complaint was not of this type.[28] Specific test items were of the pattern adopted in *Le Voyage en Chine*: tongue-twisters and alliterative phrases. More specifically, as surgery on the tongue could be justified only if lingual sounds were affected, Bennett Lucas screened patients with sentences containing *t, d, n* and *l*, for example: 'two teetotalers [[29]] taking tea together'.[30] Once again, this demonstrates the influence of phonetics upon the analysis of stuttering throughout the century. By its close, Wyllie had systematised the tests. He employed sentences graded from the easiest, those containing vowels, e.g. 'Eels ail amid ocean ooze', to those containing difficult voiceless plosives, e.g. 'Two poor comrades'. In addition, the clinician could make use of phrases supplied in *Peter Piper's Practical Principles of Plain and Perfect Pronunciation*.[31] In assessing the malady, little thought was given to its severity, as indicated by the form and length of hesitancies, the degree and distribution of extraneous movements, or the extent to which sufferers began modifying their behaviour by avoiding painful situations.

In certain quarters, there was a dim awareness that the aetiological conclusions, so glibly bandied about, had a shaky basis. For calling nerves, ill-health and the like 'causes' of stuttering, theorists were charged with failing to demonstrate a 'constant coincidence', which implied an invariable, if not necessary, connection between the two.[32] As Thelwall pointed out, regarding speech defects in general:

> many persons who have equal irritability of fibre and delicacy of constitution, have no impediment; and many persons, also, have impediments, of the same, or very similar descriptions, who have, otherwise, no mark or semblance of such constitutional defect . . . nervousness, then, and . . . debility, are not the sole, the necessary, or the immediate causes.[33]

Even Bennett Lucas, an advocate of oral surgery, had to admit that if everyone with morbid tonsils stuttered, then the number of hesitant speakers would be very great indeed,[34] and would leave unexplained why boys were more frequently affected than girls, both being equally liable to tonsillar infection. Similar objections could be levelled at other factors linked with stuttering. It may seem to be precipitated by the dryness of air in summer and winter,[35] but whole populations do not fall victim to these climatic changes: hesitancy is no meterorological barometer. Philosophers may argue whether the bond between cause and effect is one of ontological necessity or statistical probability, but writers on stuttering had not even succeeded in establishing a significant connection between the impediment and any phenomena, excepting sex, and no one attempted to formulate a theory on that basis.

The contemporary European debate on scientific methodology by such men as Comte, Herschel, Whewell, J.S. Mill and Claude Bernard[36] passed by elocutionists and physicians, who were more concerned with consolidating their professional practice than in philosophical disquisition. Nevertheless, Bernard did not allow the confusing situation in medicine – as exemplified in the quotation from Abbotts (p. 77), to escape comment. In treatises on pathology:

> By no means all the circumstances enumerated are causes; at most they are means or processes by which a disease can be produced. But the real and effective cause of a disease must be *constant* and *determined*, that is unique; anything else would be a denial of science in medicine.[37]

In actuality, the scientific status claimed for speech pathology was more verbal than real, it being one tactic by which professionals endeavoured to distinguish themselves from mountebanks. Granted, the discipline's foundation upon oral physiology was widely recognised, thus fulfilling one of Bernard's criteria for science.[38] But the necessity for fact gathering, and the controlled manipulation of variables, leading to predictability, was almost unknown, partly because that desirable constituent of any experiment[39] – the happy combination of head and hand, of theorist and practitioner – was hard to find. Some elocutionists were frankly unimpressed by academic enquiries, which they regarded as having little therapeutic value. Blathwayt, for example, obviously considered he was being complimentary when reporting that in Beasley he could detect 'nothing scholastic' and 'nothing of the pedant'.[40]

Theorists may not have got far with their speculations, but practical men were apt to err in another direction, for they failed to substantiate their much publicised successes, to relate these to contemporary scientific advances, or to record their methods, which, when shrouded in secrecy, died with them. Consequently, some of the best placed to assist in building a body of knowledge contributed less than the clinically inexperienced theorist, whose erroneous hypothesis at least indicated unfruitful lines of enquiry.

Pathologists of stuttering may have been unaware that a philosophy of science was emerging in their midst, but they were not impervious to current aetiological language. Between them, they employed approximately 40 adjectives to qualify 'cause', the majority of which clearly had a scholastic source.[41] This is not strange when one considers that many of the Aristotelian–Scholastic causal concepts and nomenclature lingered on in vestigial or altered form until late Victorian times.[42] Though heirs to this philosophic lexicon, they had little idea of the original meaning and context of the terms, which they employed in cavalier fashion. This compounded existing terminological confusions in their discipline. Some qualified causality in more detail than others. Thelwall, for example, used nearly a score of adjectives, whereas Shuldham limited himself to exciting and immediate causes. By and large, the vocabulary was more prolific at the beginning of the century than in its final decades, but no clear pattern emerges. If a specific theory was being proposed, the writer might restrict his discussion to one type of cause; but those taking a broader view, and wishing to explain the manifold factors associated with stuttering, found the concept of a casual hierarchy more useful. However, little effort was made to determine how one cause interacted with another, nor was there consistency in the number invoked. For a simple overview, three aetiological categories have been chosen for discussion – the proximate, predisposing and exciting – as these seem most representative. They were in common medical use and were incorporated in the title of the younger Poett's *Treatise*, the only book explicitly directed to their elucidation.

Proximate Cause

To the extend that those in the vanguard of contemporary philosophy and science searched for causes over and above laws, they gave most credence to the 'proximate' category, these being 'true' causes in that they alone were responsible for the production of a given effect. The combination of two volumes of hydrogen to one of oxygen, for example, provides the sole essential prerequisite for water: such necessary and immediate antecedents fell within the ambit of science.[43] In pathological bodily states, where deprivation of due function is being investigated rather than the production of some new entity, similar certainty was the aim. Bernard admitted that in medicine it was very much more difficult to obtain but for that reason all the more desirable;[44] and because physico-chemical processes offered the surest opportunity for certitude, he virtually equated scientific medicine with physiology.

There is no indication that writers analysed the causal concepts they employed or that these corresponded with contemporary usage in the philosophy of science. Proximate or immediate causality remained ill-defined, though one physician did describe it as the 'actual state of the parts originating the symptoms'[45] and another as the manner in which the ultimate cause 'manifests itself in producing stammering'.[46] It was most usually ascribed to the oro-vocal structures, these being the final and best understood point of the speech chain. By virtue of their function, these structures were inevitably implicated in all speech action and so came closest to Bernard's stipulation that 'true' causes be singular and necessary, that is, uniquely responsible for the symptom and essential to it.[47] In this way, theorists arrived at some form of universal explanation for the morbid hesitancies, as well as partially accounting for their severity, which could be seen as a direct reflection of the length and intensity of muscular energy used in articulating.[48] Finally, proximate causality found favour because it provided a point of certitude where this was hard to find, for, as Wright said, it could not be denied that stuttering is brought about by vocal and respiratory stoppage.[49]

During stuttering the lips may hold fast, the tongue cleave to the roof of the mouth or the voice become caught in the throat, all the result of 'trying to speak in an impossible manner',[50] that is, 'without the proper use of the natural and efficient causes of fluent speech' which occasions effort and struggle 'to accomplish what, under particular circumstances, is decidedly impossible'.[51] Everyone agreed that these symptoms reflected abnormal muscular activity, but there was disagreement over whether this was a consequence of malformation or misaction of the speech organs. Certain surgeons made play of the former, commonly designated 'mechanical' or 'structural' causes; the term 'physical' was likewise used,[52] though this could refer to a patient's constitutional disposition. A more dynamic interpretation of stuttering was taken by those attributing proximate causality to functional muscular derangement, described by Wright as a 'physiological' cause,[53] which, being central to the impediment, might also be called an 'essential' cause.

A further point at issue was which of the various structures was principally responsible for the defect. Palmer, for example, attributed it to the chest, larynx and mouth,[54] but others concentrated on individual organs. Rather than debating which muscles were implicated, another approach was to examine the nature and reason for the irregularities themselves. This led to consideration of innervation with Poett junior ascribing proximate causality to excitability of the motor nerves[55] and Carpenter ascribing it to the 'nervous centres'.[56] Thelwall was even less specific in looking upon 'mental embarrassment', whether of organic or psychological origin, as the immediate and necessary precursor of stuttering.[57]

So closely were peripheral irregularities associated with the impediment in some minds, that the two became identified,[58] and it is therefore pertinent to note Hooper's definition of proximate cause, which 'may be said to be in reality the disease itself. All proximate causes are either diseased actions of simple fibres or an altered state of the fluids.'[59] But if 'stuttering' was merely shorthand for 'spasmodic action of the phonetic organs sufficient to arrest speech', then any distinction between the two statements is more verbal than real. Consequently, such spasms hardly rank as antecedent phenomena or 'true' causes. Rather, they are symptoms or effects and hence it was tautological to maintain that the key to successful therapy lay in removing these proximate causes.

Remote Causes

Philosophers of science remained agnostic about 'ultimate' or 'primary' causes, which they considered beyond the reach of experiment and therefore unknowable through induction.[60] Science could only elucidate *how* phenomena occurred, that is, their immediate and determining cause, but was forever ignorant of *why* they happened,[61] which was a question for theologians.

These aetiological terms were ambiguous in writings on stuttering: 'ultimate' usually referred to 'remote' causality, but 'primary' might be used in this sense or for proximate causality. Whatever the case, their connotation was rather different in medical and philosophical circles. It is true that Bernard considered sex, age, race, the state of the digestion and so forth, as influencing the constitution of the inner environment and hence coming within the domain of proximate causality,[62] but more often these factors were interpreted as a 'predisposing' cause, which, together with the 'exciting' cause, comprised the two divisions of Hooper's category of remote causality. Hooper does concede, however, that:

> The distinction between the predisposing and the proximate cause is not always obvious, since what is called the predisposing cause is often hardly to be discriminated from an obscure degree of the disease itself.[63]

This was less true of aetiological discussions on stuttering, as peripheral irregularities were commonly distinguished from constitutional dispositions, the latter being either congenital or the consequence of unfavourable environmental circumstances.

Predisposing causes

Many people have similarly shaped mouths, and share a common social and educational background, yet not all stutter. It was therefore reasonable to postulate that certain individuals have some intrinsic susceptibility or diathesis, making them more liable to speech breakdown. Such an in-built predisposition was defined medically as 'that which renders the body susceptible to disease . . . The most frequent predisposing causes are, the temperament and habit of the body, idiosyncracy, age, sex, and structure of the parts'.[64] Among the constitutional factors purportedly disposing towards stuttering, only sex was backed by quantitative evidence. A modicum of facts was gathered on the role of heredity (Tables 5.1, 5.2, 5.3, pp. 144-5) but alongside these objective stirrings pure speculation persisted. Paralleling myths relating to mothers' marks, such as a cleft palate or lip having been produced when a pregnant woman's path was crossed by a hare, Ball, as late as 1890, suggested that if a mother was exposed to a stutterer before birth, the speech problem could be transmitted to her infant.[65]

More serious conjectures turned upon the nature of sufferers' unfortunate proclivities. Cull thought they may have an unchecked imitative faculty or be subject to uncontrollable passion,[66] whereas Palmer believed their problems stemmed from an 'uncommon ardour of mind' or an 'exquisite susceptibility of moral impressions'.[67] This was akin to the belief that stutterers were more 'sensitive', implying that they had either greater intelligence or a particularly impressionable personality, principally on account of an inherently excitable nervous system.

Delicacy of constitution might be acquired though external forces acting physically or psychologically. Poor food, uncleanliness, moist climate and so on, might weaken the frame and render it less able to withstand pressures.[68] However, rather than demonstrating the prevalence of stuttering in depressed districts, the existing evidence pointed to the contrary. While general bad health might make someone liable to speech breakdown,[69] it was more dramatic events like fevers and terrors that could directly increase nervous susceptibility,[70] and there were many accounts of stuttering beginning after shocks to the system. Once established, similar factors acted as 'aggravating' causes, though these were often interpreted as exciting causes.

Predisposing causality was one of the few subjects provoking a minimum of dispute. Only Thelwall made any serious comment upon it:

> these physical causes have . . . an influence . . . upon those mental and moral causes, which I conceive to be the principle sources of Impediments of Speech; as, also, of many other species of derangement and non-development of the organic faculties. But every predisposition does not necessarily produce a specific disease; – nay it is never the *producer*! – nor, is the disease incurable, because the original constitutional predisposition cannot be entirely eradicated.[71]

In sum, if the disorder could be rectified while the constitution remained unaltered, the latter was hardly a cause, taken strictly. It helped explain certain features of stuttering, but since none of the predisposing agents were its consistent precursors, they could be looked upon as merely conditions. The same might also be said of the many phenomena described as 'exciting' causes.

Exciting Causes

Given the propensity to stutter, it was still necessary to postulate the existence of some activating agent which precipitated it at any given moment. Generally called the 'exciting' cause, this arose either from internal or external sources,[72] and was defined by Hooper as 'that which actually produces the disease, thus, exposure to cold or damp air is the exciting cause of catarrh'.[73] Catarrh, of course, persists well after the patient has removed himself from chilling draughts. Likewise stuttering might be the legacy of some distant, perhaps forgotten, trauma, which led Mason to distinguish between the event or 'originating' cause, initially responsible for the complaint, and the factor that later acted as trigger, for which he reserved the term 'exciting' cause.[74] For many, this category embraced the moral and educational causes.

To Hunt, the mind was the exciting cause of speech and so lack of mastery over the articulatory organs could be ascribed to mental agitation or lack of self-control.[75] In this passage, Hunt appears to identify exciting and original causes, which, he says, are of little consequence, since they have ceased to exist, an apparently absurd contention also proposed by Beasley.[76] Elsewhere,[77] Hunt specifies the exciting causes of stuttering more precisely – affections of the brain and spinal cord, abdominal conditions, irritation of the nervous system, solitary vices, spermatorrhoea, mental emotions, mimicry and involuntary imitation – these presumably acting through their undesirable effect upon the mind. In addition, fright, accidents, fevers, passions, worms, carious teeth and uncleanliness were also seen as originating or exciting causes by some writers.

These phenomena, often being only transitory, were sometimes described as 'occasional' causes, which obliged theorists to explain why stuttering persisted in their absence and sometimes failed to appear in their presence. For a start, some account of how the various aetiological categories interacted would have been helpful, but the problem was not faced squarely, nor perhaps recognised. It was much easier to list causes and hypothetical correlations, than to produce a theory of the processes by which they actually operated. A few embryonic theories did emerge, however, and these will be covered in the following two chapters.

Cause and Effect

The trouble with most theories, according to one physician, was that they were 'grounded on consequences rather than causes', and these consequences he appeared to identify with proximate causes.[78] The question of cause and effect was well known to philosophers, the problem being, as Herschel saw it, that:

> in a great number of natural phenomena, the effect is produced gradually, while the cause goes on increasing in intensity; so that the antecedent of the one and consequence of the other becomes difficult to trace, though it really exists. On the other hand, the effect often follows the cause so instantaneously, that the interval cannot be perceived.[79]

Here he limits causes to temporal rather than ontological priority. In any event, medical and psychological sciences were faced with peculiar difficulties, because a symptom, usually equated with an effect, was not necessarily the unique product of one agent and therefore not convertible with it. Certainly unique physico-chemical processes may be necessary precursors to an itch or specific form of tremor, as an appropriate combination of hydrogen and oxygen is for water, but these processes are rarely what physicians mean by cause, because they are not always diagnostically helpful, even if known. The responsible lesion may lie at some distance from the source of cutaneous irritation or muscular weakness.

Arguments over cause and effect embraced both the physical and psychological aspects of stuttering. Where an hypothesis hinged upon a particular interpretation of causality, its proponent was bound to take a definite stand, but a few other commentators chose to remain agnostic. For example, regarding the tendency of stutterers to reverse the normal breathing process, Borthwick wrote:

> whether this mode of effecting the respiration necessary for the production of speech be the primary cause of the impediment, or merely an effect induced by ill-directed efforts to continue the expiration . . . cannot be positively determined. Neither can it be determined, from this fact, whether the error lies in deficiency of effort, or in rigidity of muscle. In all probability, it will be sometimes attributable to one, sometimes to another, or perhaps to all of these causes combined.[80]

Furthermore, he took the unusual course of suggesting that, therapeutically, this doubt was of no great moment. He was content to devote his efforts to improving respiration, one of the oldest focuses of treatment. The implication that correct theory was not an essential prerequisite for therapeutic success was not, however, an idea prompted, or even contemplated, by those most anxious to divest themselves of associations with empiricism.

Thelwall agreed that in practice it was often difficult to distinguish cause from effect,[81] because 'circumstances in which physical and moral phenomena run a circle . . . become alternately cause and effect'.[82] Thus:

> In cases where there is an evident mixture of physical or constitutional derangement, it seems to be equally necessary to remove the disease, in order that you may cure the impediment, and the impediment, that you may cure the disease . . . The consolation . . . is . . . causes that have acted in a circle, will re-act in a circle, also.[83]

Doctors, then, had a part to play. There was relatively little discussion on circular causation, but half a century later, Potter was informing his American colleagues that: 'Cause and effect are constantly found changing places, or passing, the one into the other.' He made special mention of nervousness which 'is often a cause, but more frequently an effect, the consequence of the affection'.[84]

Nervousness was a subject upon which many words were spent, because it was so commonly held to be at the root of stuttering. Amongst those who did not agree was Wright:

> Stuttering, doubtless, causes and afterwards increases nervousness; on the other hand, nervousness, so caused, increases stuttering; and in proportion to the quality and quantity of hesitation, so, at all times, seems to be the nervousness of the stutterer.[85]

But Yearsley, anxious to exclude psychological factors and thereby lend justification to his surgical treatment, was more dogmatic:

> The supposed nervous character of stammering I believe to be most erroneous . . . How much more rational and allied to truth would it be, to consider the *nervousness* as *an effect* of the infirmity, whether deafness, stammering, or any other human malady, rather than *the cause*! I fear the vague theory of *nervousness, nervous irritability,*

> or by whatever name it may be denominated, has proved a sad drawback to the advancement of medical science.[86]

He laid blame squarely upon stricture of the throat, but those opposing a physical causation argued that if such abnormalities existed, they were a legacy of the chronic muscular irregularities characterising stuttering. Mason's figures (Table 3.1 p. 79) certainly lent support to the view that stutterers were nervous, and though this could be symptomatic of their whole personality and border on despair, it was also taken as a reaction limited to speaking situations only and one which would disappear once the problem was resolved. Indeed, some patients were the 'bravest of brave'.[87] Another objection to a nervous aetiology was that children, at an age when the complaint most usually appeared, were seldom nervous,[88] and that notwithstanding the greater prevalence of this trait amongst women, they stuttered less.[89] No one offered a definition of nervousness and Mason's figures were probably based on subjective reports from patients. Furthermore, lacking the requisite technology, scant attention could be paid to the physiological accompaniments of nervousness. Observations were limited to gross changes, chiefly of the respiratory and cardiac systems; it is only in recent decades that extensive physiological data have become available, though whether investigators have been measuring a constitutional disposition towards stuttering, or its inner effects, is by no means certain.[90]

To sum up: the Victorian period witnessed a turning away from the humoral interpretation of speech problems. For the first time, the behavioural complex associated with stuttering was being recognised but lack of agreement over the classification of causes, particularly the predisposing and exciting, and what factors these contained, together with the question of which phenomena were causes and which effects, compounded existing confusion over terminology and diagnosis. Had some thought been given to scientific method, to the quantification of facts, the manipulation of variables, to prediction and verification, as applied in the natural sciences and certain areas of medicine, some way out of this tangle may have been found. As it was, Victorians made do with the postulate of a casual hierarchy, which proved to be a poorly thought-out device for answering certain questions posed by the impediment. Their notion of multiple aetiology bore little resemblance to Aristotelian multi-causality, to which it was terminologically allied, nor to the various modern concepts.[91] Today, instead of calling related phenomena 'causes' they may be referred to more cautiously as 'factors'[92] or 'conditions'[93] that predispose, precipitate and perpetuate the problem, and under these heads are gathered all manner of things from twinning and diabetes to biochemical reactions and anxiety. Unlike the crude efforts of Victorians, current hypotheses are formulated within a more sophisticated experimental and philosophical framework; hence they are more coherent and intellectually satisfying. But despite these speculative advances, progress is still limited, if we are to judge from one contemporary authority, who concedes that 'we as yet have essentially no conclusive evidence to show that *any* of the current theories of stuttering is wholly or partially valid'.[94]

Notes

1. Thelwall (1810), p. 57. Cf. Bishop (1851), p. 76; *Mind, Breath*, p. 15; Sandlands, p. 8.
2. Ball, p. 23.
3. Wingate, pp. 3, 4.
4. Denyse Rockey and Penelope Johnstone, 'Medieval Arabic Views on Speech Disorders: Al-Razi (c. 865–925)', *Journal of Communication Disorders*, 12 (1979), 229-43.
5. Thelwall (1810), p. 62.
6. Kathleen Grange, 'Pinel and Eighteenth-century Psychiatry', *Bulletin of the History of Medicine*, 35 (1961), 442-53.
7. D. Hack Tuke, *A Dictionary of Psychological Medicine* (London, J. & A. Churchill, 1892), vol. 2, pp. 696, 1205.
8. Thelwall (1810), frontispiece, pp. vi, 44, 57, 60-1, 64-5, 71, 84-5, 128, 142-3, 146, 152, 251.
9. K.M. Dallenbach, 'The History and Derivation of the Word "Function" as a Systematic Term in Psychology', *American Journal of Psychology*, 26 (1915), 474-84.
10. Young, pp. 12-13, 17-37, 50-3, 159-60, 250-2.
11. Hunter and Macalpine, pp. 812-20.
12. McCormac, p. 26.
13. Palmer, pp. 63, 64, 66. Palmer was an admirer of Gall and Spurzheim, but not committed to their doctrine (ibid., pp. x, 11-14). His planned 'philosophical inquiry into the causes, the phenomena, and treatment, moral and physical, of impeded utterance' (ibid., p. 67n) appears not to have been published. Possibly he took the advice of his book reviewer 'not to publish his intended Treatise', *Medico-Chirurgical Review*, 12 n.s. (1830), p. 304 (289-313).
14. C. Handfield Jones, *Studies on Functional Nervous Disorders*, 2nd edn (London, Churchill, 1870), p. 3.
15. Andrew Combe, *Observations* . . . (Edinburgh, Anderson, 1831), pp. 62-86, 130-2, 142, 149, 157, 285-7.
16. Cull (1833), p. 23. Cf. *Penny Cyclop.*, p. 433.
17. See, for example, the discussion by the Medical Society of London (1840-1a, b) on the appropriateness of surgical treatment.
18. Thelwall (1810), p. 56.
19. C. Bernard, pp. 6-7, 12-13, 27, 32-5, 191, 198 and *passim*. (Original French edition published in 1865.)
20. Ibid., pp. 26, 35-43, 48-52, 203.

21. Abbotts, p. 28.
22. C. Bernard, p. 55. Cf. ibid., pp. 56, 194.
23. See, for example, Tuke's *Dictionary*, vol. 2, 1194-207.
24. Young, pp. 30, 35, 36, 37, 39, 40-1, 43, 53, 62, 73.
25. Arnott (1827), pp. 585-6.
26. Bacc. Med. Oxon., pp. 31-3.
27. Lee, pp. 24-5, 48-9.
28. Medical Society of London (1840-1a), p. 25.
29. A stutterer, Richard Turner, a Methodist plasterer, is said to have originated this term at a Temperance Society meeting in Preston during Septembei 1833, when he declared he would 'be reet down out-and-out t-t-total for ever and ever'. Brian Harrison, *Drink and the Victorians* (London, Faber & Faber, 1971), pp. 125-6, 429. For references relating to disputes over the word's origin see also the *New English Dictionary*.
30. Lucas (1840-1), pp. 389-90. Cf. Mr Lucas, 'Operation for the Cure of Stuttering', *Provincial Medical and Surgical Journal*, 1 (1840-1), 366-7.
31. Wyllie, p. 17.
32. Thomas Williams in Westminster Medical Society (1840-1b), p. 79.
33. Thelwall (1810), pp. 56-7.
34. Lucas (1841a), p. 14. Cf. Lee, p. 28.
35. Romberg, p. 364. Cf. Abbotts, p. 25, who says it is worse in cold, wet weather, Lee in Westminster Medical Society (1840-1b), p. 78, who believes wet and hot weather to have the more deleterious effect.
36. Wallace, pp. 76-160.
37. Cited by Wallace, ibid., p. 149 from C. Bernard, p. 83.
38. C. Bernard, pp. 1-2, 66, 76, 92, 99 and *passim*.
39. Ibid., pp. 1-3, 6, 7-10, 12, 16, 26-7, 57, 205-18.
40. Blathwayt, p. 574.
41. Compare the causes listed by Bernard Wuellner in *A Dictionary of Scholastic Philosophy*, 2nd edn (Milwaukee, Bruce, 1966), pp. 41-4.
42. Wallace, pp. 77, 85, 134, 154-5.
43. Ibid., pp. 99, 104, 111, 131, 136-7, 143, 148-9, 156-7. Cf. C. Bernard, p. 83.
44. C. Bernard, pp. 2-3, 59 and *passim*.
45. Poett jnr, p. 41.
46. Bacc. Med. Oxon., p. 33.
47. C. Bernard, pp. 56, 83.
48. Cazalet, p. 19. Cf. Poett jnr, p. xxix.
49. Wright (1839), p. 25.
50. Beasley (1885), p. 23. Cf. Bishop (1851), p. 60; Poett jnr, p. 15.
51. Wright (1850), p. 287.
52. Lee, pp. 28, 66.
53. Wright (1839), p. 31.
54. Palmer, p. 65.
55. Poett jnr, p. 20.
56. Carpenter, p. 352.
57. Thelwall (1810), p. 58.
58. Foster [1885], p. 22.
59. Robert Hooper, *Lexicon-Medicum*; or *Medical Dictionary*, 4th edn (London, Longman, Hurst & Co., 1820), p. 721.
60. Wallace, pp. 104, 142, 150, 156-7.
61. C. Bernard, p. 82-3.
62. Ibid., p. 99.
63. Robert Hooper, 'Aetiologia' in *Lexicum Medicum*; or, *Medical Dictionary*, 8th edn, rev. Klein Grant (London, Longman, 1848), unpaginated.

64. Hooper, *Medical Dictionary* (1820), p. 717.
65. Ball, p. 9. Cf. Gerdts, p. 53.
66. Cull (1833), pp. 19-20.
67. Palmer, p. 65.
68. Poett jnr, pp. 20-1.
69. Abbotts, p. 24.
70. Cull (1833), p. 19.
71. Thelwall (1810), p. 57.
72. Hooper, *Medical Dictionary* (1820), p. 341.
73. Hooper, *Medical Dictionary* (1848), 'Aetiologia'.
74. Mason (1884), pp. 10-11.
75. Hunt (1863), p. 178.
76. Beasley (1905), p. 135.
77. Hunt (1861), p. 24.
78. Bacc. Med. Oxon., pp. 21-2.
79. J.F.W. Herschel, *A Preliminary Discourse on the Study of Natural Philosophy*, new edn (London, Longman, 1830), p. 151. Also cited by Wallace, p. 108. Cf. ibid., pp. 133, 344.
80. Borthwick, p. 22.
81. J. Thelwall, 'On Difficulty of Speech', *Medical and Physical Journal*, 15 (1806), p. 175 (172-5).
82. Thelwall (1810), p. 66.
83. Ibid., pp. 66-7.
84. Potter, p. 79.
85. Wright (1835), p. 21.
86. Yearsley (1841), pp. 21-2. Cf. A.M. Bell (1900), p. 236.
87. Poett snr (1833), pp. 24-5.
88. Beasley (1885), p. 24. Cf. Wright (1839), p. 46.
89. Borthwick, p. 25.
90. Bloodstein, p. 14.
91. For a summary, see ibid., pp. 66-9.
92. Muriel Morley, *The Development and Disorders of Speech in Childhood*, 2nd edn (London, E. & S. Livingstone, 1965), p. 394.
93. Perkins in Sheehan (ed.), pp. 191-219.
94. Bloodstein, p. 67.

4 IRREGULARITIES OF THE PERIPHERAL SPEECH ORGANS

By its nature, stuttering entails abnormal activity of the phonatory and articulatory organs, and so it was appropriate that these be amongst the first objects of investigation, especially as they are reasonably accessible. Though the demise of humoral pathology had shifted emphasis away from the tissues, increased understanding of the oro-vocal mechanism justified an examination of stuttering in light of peripheral physiology, if not structure. However, lacking both scientific methodology and the clinical acumen derived from experience, certain writers ranged well beyond the legitimate bounds of evidence and logic to form unwarranted conclusions, in which they placed remarkable confidence. Rigid preconceptions further inhibited penetrating or wide-ranging enquiry, with the result that several hypotheses were proposed which interpreted stuttering primarily or solely as a peripheral anomaly. Various ideas were formulated. It was explained in structural terms, occasionally with ambiguous references to 'deranged function'; as physiological malaction; and as the end result of reflexes. Some writers conceded, at least implicitly, that moral factors might be operative, but as a rule these played less part in their thinking than did the proximate causes.

To describe some of the conjectures recorded in this chapter as theories or hypotheses of stuttering is justifiable in an historical rather than scientific context, as many of the patients adduced in evidence laboured under some other malady. Lee's 'physical' or 'permanent' stammerers appear to have had an articulation defect, possibly of structural origin, but despite contrasting them with 'nervous' stammerers, he failed to make a clear, specific distinction between the two groups. Indeed, because of the ambiguity in the word 'stammer', surgeons saved face over their misplaced operative treatment by asserting that this was justified in certain instances. In reality, even the number of 'physical' stammerers to benefit must have been small, as this group probably embraced various dysarthric conditions, the neurological basis for which was most obscure during the early decades of the century. Ignorant of central speech processes and confronted by spastic, flaccid or fibrillating tongues that not only functioned poorly but, like other paralytic muscles, appeared structurally defective, it is not difficult to see how inexperienced practitioners might be led into supposing that the responsible lesion lay in the periphery.

Over-emphasising the role of peripheral structures in genuine cases of stuttering incurred the risk of reducing a complex psychological problem to a simple organic one. Therapeutic measures might accordingly be limited either to didactic treatment of a purely symptomatic kind, or to mechanical intervention in the form of surgery or gadgets. With advances in neurophysiology, psychology and psychiatry, the underlying pathology of an increasing number of speech disorders could be identified. Correspondingly, the number of defects assignable to structural deviations diminished and has gradually been reduced to such gross conditions as cleft palate. Over the long term, this trend has been in one direction, masking the periodic backsliding. Lacking a traditional body of knowledge and an organised profession, investigators often started from scratch and previous warnings went unheeded, with the result that erroneous notions reappeared, often to be presented as new discoveries or great insights. This was particularly true of those suggesting a physical reason for the impediment. In 1762, Sheridan declared that amongst stutterers and malpronouncers 'there is not one in a thousand, which proceeds from any natural defect or impediment'.[1] Fifty years later, Thelwall was reiterating that structural defects could have no direct causal connection with stuttering, and hence surgery could never be an appropriate remedy.[2] And again, in 1817, Itard was called to comment: 'Some modern anatomical writers instead of throwing new light upon the subject, have rather withdrawn our attention from the real seat of the affection, as they considered stuttering as a consequence of organic defects.'[3] Yet a quarter of a century later, leading medical men were not only seriously debating the issue, but were subjecting patients to a variety of operations.

If psychologically naive, not all discussions on the physiological aspects of stuttering were misguided. In the first instance, it was quite legitimate to examine certain associated phenomena within the peripheral context: respiration, vowel fluency, singing, whispering, the anatomical locus of spasms and their linguistic selectivity. Contemporary oro-vocal physiology and motor phonetics might well have provided reasons for some of the behavioural characteristics of stuttering.

Lungs and Breathing

One of the most compelling, universal and ultimately distressing accompaniments of stuttering is some form of breathing disorder. So it is understandable that this should have been a focus for speculation as well as scientific enquiry. Victorians had good reason to concern themselves with respiration: recording equipment facilitated lung measurements, the new chemistry threw light on metabolism, and distressing social conditions focused attention on ventilation. These factors each had some bearing on stuttering, though they played little part in the genesis of McCormac's widely discussed theory.

The mechanics of external respiration, or breathing, had been elucidated by Borelli and others during the seventeenth century and presented no particular obscurities to the student, but more accurate assessment of lung capacity was made possible by the spirometer, built by Hutchinson in 1844. This was valuable in establishing norms,[4] which provided ammunition for those fighting against habits contrary to health, such as the widespread use of stays, found to reduce breathing by one third.[5] This was of concern to Lennox Browne and Behnke, who reproduced a chart on the distribution of breath capacity and chest girth from data collected by the Anthropometric Committee of the British Association for the Advancement of Science,[6] the medical investigator being their colleague Charles Roberts. Spirometric readings on stutterers showed that they were unable to attain more than a half to two thirds of mean capacity and X-ray photographs revealed diaphragmatic abnormalities.[7] The duration of at least one patient's inspirations was timed by Blake, who also measured chest girth before and after treatment,[8] as did Gerdts,[9] whose more detailed findings are recorded in Table 4.1. In 1855, respiratory movements were recorded on the pneumograph, which was probably first used on stutterers in Britain by the Behnkes,[10] whose failure to publicise their work has meant that they were overshadowed by researchers like Scripture, then in the United States.[11]

Elucidation of internal respiratory processes rested upon an understanding of combustion, which Lavoisier realised depended upon a new gas he called oxygen, discovered independently by Joseph Priestley and Carl Scheele in the last quarter of the eighteenth century. Priestley, himself a stutterer, was one of many radicals and dissenters with a social conscience also interested in science. Appalled by conditions in slave ships, prisons and hospitals, reformers sensed a connection between health and atmospheric conditions, realised that physiological chemistry was the key to elucidating this relationship, and gave an urgency to questions of lighting and ventilation, the latter becoming fashionable largely because of the miasmic theory of disease. Edinburgh University, in the person of Cullen, was in the forefront of chemical experimentation,

Table 4.1: Changes in Chest Circumference and Lung Capacity in Stutterers as a Result of Treatment

Circumference of the chest of patients in drawing a deep breath:					
Before the cure:	77,	82,	91,	94	
After the cure:	82,	86,	95¼,	99½	Centimeter
Then more:	5,	4,	4¼,	5½	
Inhaled air from deep drawing of breath:					
Before the cure:	1672,	1946,	2154,	2240	Cubic-
After the cure:	2248,	2820,	2854,	3376	Centimeter
Then more:	576,	874,	700,	1136	

Source: A. Gerdts, *The Impediments of Speech* (1883), p. 48.

which was furthered by his pupils, amongst whom was John Bostock, who linked respiration to 'animal chemistry' or metabolism.[12] Paradoxically, Bostock's celebrated article on stuttering (p. 193) had nothing to do with respiration, but he did provide a detailed review of one of its 'remote effects', namely, the formation of voice. And he made the interesting point that until mid-eighteenth century, so little was known about respiration that Haller believed its chief function was voice production.[13]

Stuttering must affect internal respiration, for if breathing is shallow and erratic, gaseous exchange diminishes, as does the renewal of energy to nervous and muscular tissues, making relaxation more difficult and continued spasm more likely. In recent times, biochemical studies have probed not only the respiratory effects of stuttering but its influence on mineral levels, sugar and so forth in the blood.[14] The Victorians got no further than commenting upon the inadequate oxygenation of the lungs, which, like poor digestion, Kingsley saw as a consequence of bodily fatigue following upon depression.[15]

Apart from these physiological concomitants, faulty breathing could participate in a circularity of causes entering the psychological domain, and this was a feature of Gerdts' analysis:

> Chronic cramp of the diaphragm, which engenders fear, and the thought 'You stutter', this operates on the nerves of the diaphragm,

> so that the same is convulsively drawn up, pressing against the lungs and heart, checking the small blood-vessels and thereby engendering a feeling of anxiety and accelerated heart-beatings, which makes it impossible for the stutterer to apply the breath to speaking.[16]

He believed this vicious circle originated with the diaphragmatic cramps, which were the 'one sole reason for stuttering'. These cramps first began after illnesses like whooping cough and 'nerve fever', fits, 'unreasonable blows on the back' and rarely psychic traumas, all of which concussed the diaphragm and strained the respiratory organs.[17] A disturbed pattern of breathing ensued even during rest,[18] and as breath is the first element in speech production,[19] its irregularities have grave consequences.

Borthwick also saw the lungs as the chief or active agent in speech production,[20] but was less certain about where in the psycho-physical sequence the spasms actually began. Sometimes they were purely physical, especially in young children, and the presence of muscular deficiency could be inferred if symptoms improved under stimulants or anger.[21] He did not minimise the mental element, however, as fear specific to speech was common and heightened with repeated stuttering:

> This feeling, by reacting on the respiration, causes an increase of the evil. The emotion of fear rises in proportion, producing a further accumulation of the impediment; and thus, *though the original defect may be actually decreasing*, the impediment is gradually heightened by a system of action and reaction between the mind and the respiration, until it becomes such an object of dread as to produce the most inveterate symptoms even on the most ordinary occasions.[22]

What Borthwick did controvert was that the problem arose from generalised nervousness and here he differed from another writer, who otherwise proposed similar ideas on the interdependence of thought and respiration a decade later, unaware that anyone before had 'publicly or privately taught' or 'shewn the connexion between the mind, the breath, and speech'.[23] Bryan believed the immediate and physical cause of stuttering to be irregularity of breath, but he placed greater emphasis upon the disruptive powers of the agitated mind, the antecedent cause, which acts upon the breath 'in the same manner that the air or atmosphere is violently, suddenly, and irregularly acted upon by a gust of wind'.[24]

Breathing inadequacies were ascribed to functional disorders or physical weaknesses of the lungs. No one actually suggested that these irregularities in stuttering flowed from organic disease, though phthisis pulmonalis, or pulmonary consumption, was said to be a frequent attendant.[25] In an age when tuberculosis was prevalent, sometimes in epidemic proportions, many sensitive people and those in poor health succumbed, and it appears that stutterers were often amongst their number. According to Melville Bell, pulmonary disease was a consequence of the speech impediment with its associated shallow breathing, which resulted in the lungs adhering to the chest wall. Lack of mechanical inflation led to a closing up of the small air pockets, which then became a site for tubercular infection.[26] For Poett senior, these potentially serious if not fatal consequences of stuttering extended beyond the lungs to the liver and heart on account of circulatory deficiencies. Muscular spasms so constricted the carotid arteries and jugular veins that venous blood was retained in the brain and arterial blood correspondingly diminished to the facial region. Engorgement of the veins was one of the similarities between stuttering and epilepsy, and if interruptions to the blood flow became chronic they would predispose the patient towards apoplexy and aneurysm.[27] McCormac, likewise, commented upon circulatory problems, believing the blood to be 'less organised' in stutterers, who, because of their contracted chests, were also more liable to lung disease.[28]

It was Henry McCormac who focused greatest attention upon the lungs and, along with Neil Arnott, provoked the first widescale debate on stuttering aetiology in this country. McCormac passed his professional life in Belfast, but had previously studied in Dublin and Paris before graduating from Edinburgh University in 1824. His book on stuttering, written four years later, was the first of many publications and the numerous manuscripts he left attest to his interest in philology and insanity. McCormac, father of Sir William MacCormac who distinguished himself as a surgeon in both the civil and military spheres, became physician to the Belfast District Lunatic Asylum and it is perhaps surprising that he did not expand his early views on stuttering to say more of its mental pathology. The Asylum lost no patients during the 1832 cholera epidemic, an achievement attributed to McCormac's prophylactic dietary and sanitary regime. He subsequently applied preventive medicine to consumption, stressing the importance of pure air.[29] The seeds of this concern with respiration were sown early in his career, as his interpretation of stuttering indicates.

After graduation, McCormac travelled to Africa and also visited New

York in 1826, where he learned of the celebrated Mrs Leigh's work with stuttering; it was she who gave him food for thought. In the absence of any British treatise on the subject, he later read some Continental publications, but his own theory was established independently of others and resulted from a discovery that came to him quite suddenly while trying to imitate the disorder. It was simply that stuttering arose from speaking with the lungs in a state of 'collapse' or, less frequently, from speaking on inhalation with the lungs fully expanded. In arriving at this conclusion, McCormac had reached the acmé of his desires, acquired the first insight for thousands of years, and through his *Treatise*, placed this invaluable information 'within the compass of even the most abject poverty'. Such florid descriptions of the system's value were to characterise Victorian writings on stuttering, and McCormac was more modest than most, merely asserting that though he may not have been the first to make this discovery, he was the first to communicate it.[30] The theory certainly became linked with his name and stimulated considerable debate.

The substance of McCormac's idea, sketched in brief before his book appeared,[31] was reiterated by certain commentators.[32] Others, usually with theories of their own, were doubtful. Some queried his facts. In over 300 patients, Poett had not seen a single case of depleted lungs;[33] Borthwick observed that, far from speaking with collapsed lungs, stutterers 'oppress themselves with too great a quantity of breath', which they were unable to release in a continuous fashion;[34] and Wright argued that if the lungs were collapsed, then all the letters would be equally affected.[35] In Good's experience, stutterers often spoke with so strong a voice it was untenable to postulate a paucity of breath.[36] While he assigned the difficulty to improperly controlled articulators, another colleague blamed thoracic mismanagement, the latter noting that very little air was required to sustain voice and that singers' lungs came near collapse during the feat of *sostinuto* [*sic*] without a diminution of vocal quality. Furthermore, stutterers could sing easily, an activity said to require greater control of the lungs than speaking.[37]

Though not always discussed in the context of McCormac's theory, its second aspect, speaking on inspiration, was also a matter of dispute, the underlying question being whether good speech rested primarily on proper inspiration, or expiration as Gerdts believed.[38] Von Meyer was amongst those arguing that both acts were defective in stuttering, the 'root' of which lay in spasmodic inhalation, like hiccoughing, but in the former a long contractile condition of the diaphragm also prevented exhalation.[39] Arnott doubted that stutterers ever actually spoke while drawing air in,[40] but this was not the experience of Cull,[41] Abbotts[42] or Poett who thought inspirational speech was one ruse by which they endeavoured to side-step past failures.[43] The sudden bursts of speaking were supposed by Borthwick to be a desperate attempt to utilise any air available,[44] Cazalet adding that speech was initially made possible by a release of tension following upon spasmodic exhaustion. Injudicious expenditure of air resulted in lung collapse and, if the patient wished to continue speaking, he was liable to do so on the following inhalation.[45] Unvocalised inspirational gasps at inappropriate moments during utterance, designed to keep the lungs fully stocked, were another common feature of the complaint.[46] In addition to their effects upon speech, opinion was united that all these symptoms could contribute towards the subjective feelings of suffocation, discomfort or even pain, and towards stutterers' digestive troubles.

Speech was believed to be held in abeyance during stuttering by a conflict between the breath and those organs modifying it somewhere along the respiratory tract. The first point at which it could be arrested was the larynx, a structure of interest to a wide range of specialists.

Vocal and Related Structures

If, as Aristotle says, the meaning of a word is evident from its etymology,[47] we can infer from *ischnophonos* that stuttering signified, to the Greek mind, some defect of voice. This aspect of the disorder generated relatively little interest over the following centuries and it was only after Neil Arnott's publication that serious thought was given to the larynx. His theory proved erroneous and the larynx itself was consequently assigned a diminishing role in the aetiology of stuttering. Recent technology, however, has enabled its mechanism to be viewed afresh, and the experimental work of Wyke[48] demonstrates that the laryngeal contribution to stuttering is still a live issue.

It is not difficult to see why speculations on the larynx should have found such a ready audience amongst Victorians. They pointed to stutterers' fluency with vocalic sounds, singing and speaking melodic languages. This appeared to be linked with phonation and it was therefore reasonable to enquire whether abnormal hesitation was not a sign of laryngeal pathology. The extraordinary potential of the human voice was of more than theoretical interest to elocutionists, theatrical teachers, performers and public speakers, all of whom were engaged in developing its range, flexibility, quality and carrying power. The physiological mechanisms underlying these abilities had long been a mystery but animal experiments[49] and new instrumentation promised to alter the horizons of laryngology. Here was a meeting point for the medical and theatrical professions and the common ground they shared is exemplified in the partnership between Lennox Browne and Emil Behnke, which flourished until the latter's death in 1892. One fruit of this union was the joint publication of *Voice, Song and Speech* (1883), which ran into a score of editions.

Browne was descended from James Boyer, who had dealt so harshly with the stuttering young Leigh Hunt. He studied medicine at Edinburgh, St George's and the Middlesex hospitals, and, after serving an assistantship to Sir Morell Mackenzie, he went on to become co-founder of the Central London Ear, Nose and Throat Hospital and the British Larynogological and Rhinological Association, of which he was an early president. His *The Throat and Nose, and their Diseases* was a standard text and was greatly enhanced by its illustrations, which he executed himself. Browne had exhibited at the Royal Academy, and it may have been his artistic inclinations that attracted him to theatrical circles. Stage personalities made up a large part of his practice and he would also have met them in his capacity as surgeon to the Royal Society of Musicians, the Royal Choral Society and the Dramatic Sick Fund.[50] Emil Behnke also worked in this theatrical milieu. He was a singing teacher and his wife, Kate, an actress. Apart from developing his own system of training,[51] he was one of the first to succeed in photographing the larynx in action, around 1870, and his own vocal abilities made him a good subject for demonstrating various vocal phenomena.[52] As stutterers sought his help in increasing numbers and he did not wish to abandon his work as a voice trainer, his wife gradually took over their management and when she died, in 1918, the practice passed to their daughter, who had been prepared for the task from a very early age.[53] By Behnke's time, the fundamental behaviour of the vocal cords during speech was well known, and he attributed stuttering more to breathing irregularities and inco-ordination of the thoracic and oro-vocal systems than to the larynx as such.

Victorians were fond of drawing analogies between musical instruments and the larynx, whose delicate mechanism far outstripped its mechanical counterparts. From antiquity, it was known to be the organ of voice production, but it was not until the eighteenth century that significant strides were made in understanding its action. In 1700, Dodart stated that variable tension of the glottis was responsible for tonal changes and 42 years later Ferrein applied the term *vocal cords* to the lips of this aperture. Even earlier, Claude Perault had shown that the windpipe played no part in voice production,[54] but the erroneous view that pitch changes were brought about by variations in its length and width persisted into the nineteenth century.[55] Of more concern, however, was how the cords behaved during phonation. As there was no way of studying them in action, arguments were based on analogy, with opinion being divided as to whether the larynx acted as a wind or stringed instrument as Dodart and Ferrein, respectively, had suggested. In addition, Kratzenstein likened it to a drum and Blumenbach to a type of Aeolian harp.[56] These opinions were discussed in many physiological texts and mentioned in Arnott's *Elements of Physics*, the enormous success of which must have been partly responsible for the publicity his stuttering theory received.

Neil Arnott, doctor, inventor and natural philosopher, came from humble Scottish origins and rose to be physician to diplomats and royalty, as well as an original member of the senate at the founding of London University. Voyages to the Far East in his youth had stimulated an interest in meteorology and sanitation, and in later life he was in the forefront of the sanitary movement.[57] Although his section on the aetiology of stuttering in the *Physics* was short, it provoked probably more discussion than any other over the century. In the first editions, his remarks were limited to generalisations about it being a problem of association. Two years later, in 1829, his ideas had crystallised into a theory relating to the status of the glottis during spasm. This was the same year Robert Willis, of Cambridge, was making some classic experiments on the muscular control of the vocal cords and Benjamin Babington described his instrument, a 'glottiscope', designed to examine the larynx but apparently not achieving this end.[58]

Notwithstanding a lack of demonstrable evidence, the general view was that the glottis (Figure 2.1, p. 55, nn28-32) remained open during phonation. Since stuttering, as he knew it, was characterised by voicelessness, Arnott assumed that a spasmodic glottis must be hindering the emission of breath and therefore preventing the edges of the vocal cords from vibrating. A hiccough arrests the ingress of air, the glottis likewise closing during weight lifting to prevent air escaping. Arnott saw a similar phenomenon occurring in speech:

> it is that also, by the repeated shutting of which a person divides the sound in pronouncing several times, in distinct and rapid succession, any vowel, as o, o, o, o. Now the glottis during common speech need never be closed, and a stutterer is instantly cured, if . . . he can keep

it open.[59]

The fact that stutterers could sing was because a tune was continuous and so there was no occasion for the glottis to shut. Shakespeare's analogy of the emptying bottle was also well taken, for once the glottis opened the stutterer was in a hurry to say as much as he could while the opportunity remained. So convinced was Arnott that stuttering was impossible so long as the cords were apart, that he went so far as to suggest that if it were feasible to sever the nerves closing the glottis without destroying its voice producing action, then the problem would be of no consequence,[60] a strange comment in view of his earlier description of the expulsive action of the glottis during coughing.[61]

That stuttering was caused by spasmodic closure of the glottis was well received by Cull,[62] although within the decade he was indicating that the idea was outmoded,[63] as did Hunt even later.[64] Nevertheless, the view persisted[65] with writers placing the primary spasm in the glottis;[66] even at the close of the century it was said that in most stutterers the laryngeal muscles were at fault.[67] By this time, the emphasis had shifted from glottal spasm to inco-ordination of the oro-vocal mechanism. Wyllie, for example, saw the problem in most cases as 'delayed action' of the larynx *vis-à-vis* the articulatory mechanism.[68] On the Continent, Arnott received firm support from Müller,[69] and the glottis was also held suspect by Schmalz, Merkel[70] and Schulthess,[71] whose use of the term *phonophobia* indicates how he associated stuttering with both voice and emotion. If Arnott had succeeded in renewing interest in the voice, he failed to prove his own particular theory, which soon came under fire. His critics' main weapon was once again phonetics, but as glottal action during the articulation of voiced and mute sounds was not known, objectors could have been right for the wrong reasons.

James Wright, a follower of Walker's school of vocal inflection, was one that believed the accentual glides of the voice during conversational pitch changes were much more difficult than those of song. When voices break, command over the larynx is precarious, particularly for stutterers. Thus, Wright concluded that their impediment was in 'danger of being firmly rooted in what might be termed *organic defect*'.[72] Prompted by an extract from Arnott's book in *The Times*, he expressed views on this also, voicing his disagreement in a letter to the editor.[73] Taking as an example a sentence beginning 'many men . . . ', of which the stuttering version might be 'm-m-m-e-e-n-n-y m-e-e-e-en . . . ', he argued against McCormac as well as Arnott, that as a continuous sound was present even in the defective version both the breath supply must be adequate and the glottis open. If this were not so, then all sounds would be similarly affected. This point was actually conceded by Arnott[74] who, strangely, dismissed spasms of the mouth as rare and therefore not requiring accommodation within his theory. Wright also took Cull to task because, in words beginning with aspirates, like *such*, the stutterer is liable to continue with a hissing sound *ssss* indicating that the glottis must be open. Further, it was fallacious to assert that in singing the vocal stream was continuous. To the contrary, it was interrupted by all aspirated consonants as well as mutes (i.e., plosives). At some point, Wright evidently had believed the glottis to be continuously open during speech, but he revised this view and came to think that even in fluent speech it was repeatedly closed:

> not only at every pause, when a fresh supply of breath is not required, but also at the articulation of every vowel which has not a consonantal prefix; so that, according to this doctrine, the glottis is also an organ of articulation, similar in effect to the tongue which articulates notes on the flute, and renders them staccato.[75]

What Arnott had supposed was happening during the rapid repetition of vowels, as *o*, *o*, *o*, Wright applied to all initial vowels. Probably both men were unwittingly referring to glottal stops. In continuous speech, however, only the vowel beginning a sentence is strictly without a prefix.

Marshall Hall's objections were founded upon his own classification of consonants, which were grouped according to their influence upon respiration.[76] He drew attention to the laryngeal murmur frequently accompanying spasms on Class I sounds, like *b* and *t*. These are formed by a complete interruption of the breath stream, but during stuttering their silent period may be prolonged and a concomitant vocalisation heard, indicating that the cords have not approximated. The co-existence of noises during blocks on other classes of sounds led him to the same conclusion, namely, 'the larynx is not closed in stammering, and . . . that its closure and stammering are totally incompatible with each other'.[77] Ten years later he was still adhering to this position.[78] In short, paralysis of the laryngeal muscles – which Arnott had intimated might cure the malady – would have no such effect.

A third objection contained features of the last two. It was argued that on the words *a bird*, the stutterer may be unable to pass from the vowel *a* to the following *b*, or to pass from the *b* to the following *i*, and so the sound was deflected through the nostrils. Either way, the lips were at fault, in the first case because they could not be closed and in the second because they could not be opened. But the simultaneous presence of sound, whether on the protracted *a* or in the nose, indicated that the glottis was open. The ability of stutterers to sing was explained by the measured pace and lighter pronounciation entailed and it was added that, if Arnott were correct, then stuttering should be more common in women because their smaller larynx predisposes them to glottal spasm.[79]

Arnott was unable to verify his theory scientifically but he maintained that had it been possible to observe the glottis in action, stuttering would not have remained a mystery for so long.[80] Paradoxically, it was the invention of the laryngoscope that proved him wrong. A direct view of the larynx was first obtained in 1854, but although over a decade earlier he was reported to have abandoned his theory,[81] it was still featured in the sixth edition of his book, written ten years before his death and after the discovery of the laryngoscope.

From the seventeenth century, various attempts had been made to devise a system of mirrors that would enable specialists to look directly into the larynx.[82] Success came finally, not to a physician, but to the most famous singing teacher of the day, Manuel Garcia, a Spaniard resident in London, who was in a unique position to make such experiments for not only did his training enable him to hold a mirror against his palate without gagging but also to control the pitch of his voice as required whilst making these observations. His report, published in 1855, was expressed mainly in musical terms and took the form of a communication to Dr Sharpley, then secretary to the Royal Society.[83] The developed version of his instrument, the laryngoscope, was to revolutionise laryngology, but its medical significance was not appreciated at the time and a few years elapsed before the Continental physicians Türck and Czermak began publishing their findings.[84]

News of these developments soon reached James Hunt and were incorporated into the next edition of his book. There he forecast that the technique would be of little value in elucidating the activity of the glottis during 'speech',[85] by which he probably meant 'stuttering', for he later pointed out that though laryngoscopy failed to reveal any structural abnormalities amongst sufferers, the membraneous lining of their cords may be congested on account of stress.[86] Hunt's source of information, at least in part, was a fellow member of the Anthropological Society, George Duncan Gibb, a student of Czermak and one of the leading English laryngologists. The two referred to each others' work and probably had patients in common. Gibb made extensive studies of the vocal cords in their normal and pathological states, which rendered Arnott's hypothesis that fluency depended upon an open glottis untenable. However, Gibb did observe certain deviations amongst stutterers:

> Constant and irregular contraction and rapid approximation of the cords, with a tendency for the glottis to remain shut, are the phenomena noticed in cases of stuttering before undergoing treatment . . . When the person inspires and utters a continuous humming noise, the vocal cords resemble in their action a couple of strings being alternately and rapidly pulled towards one another, and striking their free borders with such apparently spastic rigidity as to produce a distinct flapping noise. All the laryngeal muscles are no doubt in a condition that might almost be compared with St. Vitus' dance, involuntarily contracting and relaxing . . . If a long or full breath is taken, to see the expansion of the glottis, the view is only momentary, for the tendency is so strong to irregular contraction of the muscles, that it is almost instantly closed.[87]

Normally, the cords would be closely approximated and vibrating steadily during phonation and remain wide open during deep breathing. As these deviant phenomena were observed during humming and deep inspiration, it indicates that the irregular laryngeal behaviour patterns of these patients extended beyond speech to disrupt non-verbal functions. Stuttering itself was difficult to investigate as the mouth needs to be open during laryngoscopy. This being so, it is probable that the 'humming' and 'isolated' sounds studied by Gibb and James, respectively, were similar, in contrast to their results, for the latter found little or no deviations amongst stutterers.[88] James was principally concerned with 'stammering' of the vocal cords, a disorder he claimed to have discovered. Browne and Behnke, however, stated that the condition was 'long understood', had been described by Kingsley, and occurred when the patient attempted to speak after having wasted his air and the lungs were empty,[89] which is presumably their reason for the symptom of words 'dropping soundlessly' from the speaker's lips. Holmes, likewise, identified the condition with genuine stuttering, the choreic movements being the cause for loss of breath and he went on to relate this fact to earlier theories of stuttering proposed by d'Alais, Bequerel, Arnott and McCormac.[90]

As well as failing to check the profligate expenditure of air, the glottis could malfunction in the opposite direction. Braid, arguing against Yearsley's view that no thoracic air escaped during spasm, asserted that stuttering was 'caused by the glottis being prevented from rising sufficiently to admit the quantity of air required, and acting with that promptitude necessary to secure free and correct enunciation'. Some air reached the mouth but the spasmodic actions, chiefly of the lips increases intraoral air pressure which affects the base of the tongue and epiglottis in such a way as to close the glottis more securely and thus reduce the airflow.[91] A somewhat similar idea had been expressed a decade earlier by Wright, who thought that during articulation of 'mute' sounds the glottis and epiglottis closed to facilitate silence by preventing the egress of air. He tentatively suggested that in uttering these consonants the epiglottis is 'taught' to close over the laryngeal cavity and that in stutterers it grew to anticipate these articulatory movements and so covered the larynx prematurely. However, he was not fully convinced by his own argument and expressed doubts that laryngeal spasms, not caused by deranged action of the speech organs, ever resulted in stuttering.[92] Wright made little of these remarks but they were possibly more widely discussed verbally: Hartley, writing in 1833, stated that it was then fashionable to ascribe stuttering to the epiglottis or collapsed lungs.[93]

The mechanism and function of the epiglottis is still being investigated. In the nineteenth century, Magendie conjectured that it was essentially an apparatus of voice, serving to prevent pitch rises as phonation swelled in loudness,[94] but later it was thought to be necessary for stopping food entering the larynx during swallowing.[95] This was clearly the belief of Ball, who was probably under the impression that its sphincteral action was strong.

Apparently unaware of previous speculations upon this structure, Ball announced that he had made a 'great discovery', the gist of which was that the stutterer was caught in a struggle between two simultaneously incompatible actions: swallowing and speaking. Swallowing was initiated by willed tongue and lip movements, the consequent muscular actions following involuntarily. As the posture for certain articulate sounds was very similar to those for swallowing, Ball conjectured that the act which followed became a matter of contest, swallowing often gaining ascendency because of its automatic character. The fluctuations of stuttering emerged as articulation endeavoured to reassert itself. Once swallowing was under way, the epiglottis closed down firmly, at least in spasmodic episodes, preventing air from leaving the lungs.[96] By this means, Ball endeavoured to explain, first, patients' 'violent expiratory efforts', and secondly, the fluency they may unexpectedly achieve:

> relief [from suffocation] comes presently from sheer necessity of preserving life . . . because, the swallowing muscles yield, with the action of the epiglottis, to the muscles of speech, and both cannot be in action at the same time.[97]

Ball's theory may be classed as a version of the anticipatory struggle hypothesis,[98] translated onto the physical sphere.

The upper portions of the larynx and epiglottis are attached to the hyoid, or tongue, bone (Figure 2.1, p. 55, n23), which had also been held responsible for stuttering by Hahn and Morgagni during the eighteenth century.[99] Their ideas did not attract support amongst Victorians and Kingsley is not to be taken seriously when attributing his 'stuttering dumbness' to 'this paralytic os hyoides of mine'.[100] But if the hyoid bone was not the object of much speculation, the same cannot be said for the organ it served to anchor – the tongue.

Tongue and Tongue-Tie

So closely has the tongue been associated with man's faculty of speech that the word signifies not only the organ itself, but articulate language. Although the etymology of *ischnophonos* suggests that stuttering was first conceived as a vocal disorder, it was soon attributed to the tongue, which, according to writers in the humoral tradition, might be too moist, swollen, cold, hot or tied down and so be unable to make the requisite movements for speech.

These notions went into decline as concepts from neurology and psychology offered more penetrating tools for analysis. Nevertheless, the articulatory patterns of stutterers' tongue movements remained suspect, either on account of habit or nervous influence. In 1841, however, the physical aspect of the tongue, along with other oral structures, again came into prominence as surgeons, anxious to find reasons for operating, looked for deviations that would justify recourse to the scalpel. Since this form of treatment began on the Continent, it was there that many of the ideas were first aired. Within a week or two reports appeared in British journals, indicating considerable interest here. The investigatory method underlying these hypotheses was clinico-pathological, the subjects were any patients that the doctors fortuitously met, and the lingual anomalies encountered ranged from deviations in length and size to asymmetry and tongue-tie. If an irregularity were found, it was causally linked with stuttering.

Apart from English summaries of foreign articles, British physicians were kept abreast of a wide range of Continental developments through the prolific publications of Edwin Lee, who might be described as a medical journalist. During his training at St George's he had visited the Parisian medical schools and he continued to travel after becoming a member of the Royal College of Surgeons in 1833. In 1846, he obtained an MD from Göttingen, which led to his election as a member of various European medical associations.[101] Five years previously he was also in Europe, this time reporting on the excitement engendered by the operative treatment of stuttering, and as he also visited surgeons' practices in London, he was in a better position than most to give an impression of the frequency and type of physical anomalies found amongst hesitant speakers.

To discuss every mention of lingual defects associated with stuttering would be both tedious and entail a good deal of repetition, partly because some writers believed that several anomalies contributed towards the impediments. For example, Baudens, surgeon-in-chief at the military hospital in Gros-Caillou, thought it was chiefly related to four phenomena: slight tongue deviation; inability to raise the tip to the upper lip except by simultaneous movement of the jaw; spasmodic lingual agitation where the tongue moved around without striking the palate; and a notable development of the genio-glossi muscles (Figure 2.1, p. 55, n21), especially where they attached to the jaw bone.[102] For clarity and brevity, lingual size and symmetry will be discussed separately, with only one or two authors cited for illustration. However, it should be noted that probably everyone who wrote on surgical treatment had something to say about the appearance of the organs upon which he was operating.

Hervez de Chégoin is said to have been the first to record a correlation between stammering and defective tongue length,[103] or its 'disproportionate' size,[104] by which was probably meant enlargement. According to Lee, this was the most common abnormality and though he did not set out the limits for normal lingual volume, he did describe an overly long tongue as one that could reach the nose. In a few individuals, namely the 'physical' stammerers, he considered such defects to be the chief causal agent, but in the majority of cases a large tongue was an 'accidental coincident' or consequence of stuttering, resulting from vigorous exercise of the muscles with their 'disordered nervous action'.[105]

Although it was most pertinent to the rationale for surgery, Lee was not alone in unwittingly equivocating over whether the argument rested upon establishing a defect in an organ's structure or in its innervation. Velpeau, for example, asserted in one place that stuttering was related to an overlong tongue[106] and, in another, that it arose from 'a deranged function of one or more of the muscles of the tongue'.[107]

Stuttering could apparently be brought about by opposite reasons, for diminished tongue length was also said to be a contributory factor. And here we have an example of the uncertain distinction between proximate causality and the disorder itself: 'I consider', said Baudens, 'the essential causes of stuttering to consist in a spasm of the tongue, and a shortening of the organ produced by that spasm, which shortening prevents its apex being carried to the palate.'[108] Frequent reference was made to the tongue's inability to reach the palate, a fact that explained why, for Bennett Lucas, stuttering tended to occur more frequently on tongue tip sounds.[109] Restricted elevation could, of course, be related to a number of factors, either directly or in combination: muscular weakness; abnormal reduction in lingual size, for whatever reason; an unusually high palate; or an unduly tight fraenum.

The fraenum, or bridle, serves a useful purpose not only in restricting tongue movements, especially in a backward direction – thus forestalling blockage of the throat and suffocation – but it also restrains unruly movements that might require a person to pay undue attention to his speech. The fraenum has, nevertheless, been traditionally blamed for speech impediments. In most instances, the patient was probably not tongue-tied but it was formerly believed that every child was born in this condition,[110] a belief that no doubt led to the frequent practice on the part of midwives of cutting the band whether or not this was imperative.

A good deal of folklore had grown up around the fraenum, but by the beginning of the nineteenth century several writers were aware that its effects were rarely as handicapping as had sometimes been supposed. Denman even maintained that severing the fraenum was unnecessary and that he had only done so under pressure from parents.[111] For this extreme position he was taken to task by Thelwall, who certainly favoured caution because he found that with appropriate training a tight ligament could be stretched, but who thought operative intervention desirable, should this not occur by the early teens. While denying that most impediments were attributable to structural abnormalities, he did admit that extreme rigidity of the fraenum might occasionally give rise to 'thick' speech or a 'sort of lisp', but not once did he mention stuttering in this connection.[112]

By the mid-nineteenth century, the fraenum was again under discussion. It was suggested that, at the least, a tight ligament would augment a pre-existing stammer.[113] But despite several accounts of patients with anchored tongues, Yearsley, wishing to restrict responsibility for stuttering to the tonsils, denied that it was ever caused by tongue-tie. Of 200 stutterers under his notice, not one had exhibited this deformity. And he rightly pointed out, like Thelwall, that when it did occur it was more likely to give rise to an enunciatory defect that could well respond to surgery.[114] Such speech seems to have been the characteristic of Lee's 'physical' stammerers and with Amussat's eleven-year-old patient, whose:

> pronunciation was thick, and articulation imperfect, but the amount of stammering slight. The fraenum was strong and hard, and seemed ready to give way when an attempt was made to elongate the tongue; there was also a deviation of the tongue to the right side, and the tongue could not be brought into contact with the upper teeth.[115]

It was the French surgeon, Amussat, who was chiefly responsible for associating lingual asymmetry with stuttering. Four of Amussat's cases were recorded in British journals and it seems likely that his hypothesis was formulated on experience with less than a dozen cases,[116] of which the 25-year-old Morton was typical. The man stuttered severely, as did his father and two brothers. His tongue deviated to the left and was unable to reach the palate, elevation tensing the fraenum. On the basis of such instances, both Amussat and Boyer concluded that stuttering depended upon the obliquity and contraction of certain lingual muscles, which impeded their free contact with the palate.[117] Amussat also provided evidence from a stuttering soldier, whom he explained at post-mortem:

> The two sides of the tongue were of unequal volume; the left side being flattened, while the right one was thick and arched. This . . . showed that one of the chief obstacles to distinct pronunciation consisted in an abnormal state of the tongue; it was too short, and deviated through irregular contraction of the genio-glossi muscles . . .[118]

One promise of surgery was that it might bring the tongue back into symmetry.

Even before the calamitous consequences of these precedures became evident, surgeons were roundly censured. The most spirited denunciation came from their French colleague, Gerdy, who disputed both their facts and their implied belief that the tongue was essential to speech:

> M. Gerdy did not hesitate to predict, that this proposed operation would prove utterly valueless; stuttering was a congenital fault, depending on very complex conditions, but not at all on shortness of the tongue, every one knew that a considerable portion of the tongue might be removed, without impairing pronunciation, which is a complex function, depending simultaneously on the lips, teeth, tongue, and fauces. Stutterers pronounce each letter of the alphabet singly, with facility, and are only embarrassed at the pronunciation of syllables, or rather certain syllables. Besides it was not the fact, that the tongue of stutterers was shorter than natural . . . the conception of this operation could only have arisen from gross ignorance of the functions of the organs of voice.[119]

Ironically, it was with such ignorance that some surgeons charged elocutionists, who also had the temerity to criticise them. Of course, Gerdy's point was well taken, but before passing judgement with the benefit of hindsight, it is pertinent to determine the extent to which 'everyone knew', or should have known, of the tongue's role in speech.

It is interesting to speculate upon whether these clinico-pathological correlations would have been modified had Edward Twisleton's *The Tongue Not Essential to Speech* been available. Twisleton, a Protestant, was anxious to disprove nine post-Apostolic miracles supported by Cardinal Newman, and so he chose to undermine the credibility of the most convincing, namely, the African Confessors, whose tongues had been severed at their roots by Huneric in 484 A.D. Their subsequent eloquence was considered miraculous, but Twisleton amassed numerous examples to show that it was unnecessary to invoke divine intervention to explain the phenomenon.[120] Of note, was a French lad from Saumur who had lost his tongue from gangrene and a Portuguese girl born without one. Both these cases had been recorded in English by Dr Conyer Middleton in 1748. Then there was the celebrated Margaret Cutting, whose diseased organ fell onto a plate when she was four. The account of her case in the *Philosophical Transactions* for 1742 barely seemed credible to some members of the Royal Society and so a Dr Parsons was dispatched to investigate further. His confirmatory findings were recorded in their journal four years later.

Other sources of information were travel stories from Persia, where excision of the tongue was a common punishment, and veterans from Waterloo. Certain of these reports may not have been readily accessible but summaries were to be found in the medical texts of Cooper[121] and Good.[122] Of more significance, however, was Bartlett's publication, written in 1839 and uncannily anticipating the controversy, which specifically set out by means of these notable case histories to show that stuttering could not be related to organic deficiencies, and he began by castigating medical colleagues for their 'vulgar error' in suggesting the contrary.[123] In short, as a contemporary book reviewer was also informed on the subject,[124] surgeons operating upon stuttering must be judged culpably ignorant:

> After proposing this [mechanical] hypothesis, the next rational step would have been to inquire whether such hypothesis strictly corresponded with the functions of the several parts in question, in reference to the production of voice and speech. Had this been previously done, we should never have heard of the many surgical mutilations of these organs, which have taken place both at home and abroad; since, even without the attainment of anything approaching to an accurate knowledge of the normal functions of these parts, it might easily have been ascertained by a little inductive reasoning, that some of the parts which have been subjected to operations could not possibly be concerned in the production of the malady.[125]

If surgeons did possess knowledge commensurate with their professional status, then their actions were to be deplored on ethical grounds.

Elocutionists also had reasons for commenting upon the tongue. Melville Bell, with his linguistic orientation, was particularly disposed to analyse the stuttering event in anatomico-phonetic terms. He described it as a fault of 'organic action', a sign of 'mechanical derangement' or mismanagement of the vocal organs, which resulted in them being incorrectly placed for articulation. With *t*, for example, the tendency of stutterers to lower the tongue tip caused an elevation of its middle, thus creating the '*very worst position for speech*'.[126] It was natural for Melville to follow his father in having ideas about optimal tongue positioning. Alexander senior had been of the opinion that stuttering was caused by breath being impeded somewhere along its path, often through erratic tongue movements. Believing an open glottis necessary for a smooth air flow, he advised stutterers to hold their tongues low in the mouth.[127] Others also had views on the subject. Describing the various undersirable lingual postures, Abbotts apparently interpreted this as one reason for stuttering.[128] More publicity, however, was given to Mrs Leigh's opinion that it resulted from the tongue being insufficiently elevated to touch the palate on speaking.[129] In England, a raised tongue tip was implicated by Bartlett,[130] but Mason demurred saying the chief problem was an inability to shift the tongue rather than its wrong positioning – hence the impression that it was 'sticking' to the roof of the mouth. The most natural position for the tip was behind the lower teeth and this was the ideal starting point for speech.[131]

From a contemporary standpoint, such debates seem trifling, while structural interpretations of stuttering appear unwarrantably misguided; so the modern commentator finds himself in accord with Thelwall:

> My experience of cases of impediment has not much increased my faith in the vast differences and caprice of Nature in the conformation of tongues. That some tongues want more regulation and government than others; that some are larger, and others smaller, cannot be denied; but, that the mere fashion and quantity of the tongue, independently of awkward tricks and habits, is a frequent cause of impediment, I do not believe.[132]

For those that did believe, certain surgical, prosthetic and elocutionary remedies were logically indicated.

Teeth

James I's queen, Anne, had just died when Cherbury went to Paris as British ambassador. Shortly thereafter, he was received by the French monarch, whose character he presents in an unsympathetic light. In addition to several unfortunate physical and psychological traits, Louis XIII stuttered severely and had a double row of teeth.[133] In view of the Victorians' partiality for anecdotes and clinico-pathological correlations, it is perhaps surprising that this information was not used to illustrate some theoretical position. In fact, there was nothing to suggest that defective teeth were directly responsible for any speech problems, though they may aggravate an existing condition or tendency. The Saumur boy spoke intelligibly despite having a double row of teeth and no tongue, amongst other oral deviations, some of which were attributed to the absence of pressure from lingual movements. Margaret Cutting also had dental problems, but her teeth were few having been infected by the same disease that destroyed her tongue. None the less, some stutterers felt their teeth some way at fault: 'Now you stammer merely because your upper teeth, like mine, shut over the lower ones', wrote Kingsley to a female correspondent, adding that she should get rid of any bad teeth.[134]

Dentists began acquiring a professional identity in the second half of the nineteenth century[135] and were undoubtedly faced with the severe problems of cleft palate, but, aside from a few individuals, they paid little attention to stuttering and those who spoke of it in relation to teeth were chiefly medical men. They saw decayed or erupting teeth as predisposing or exciting causes and it was noted that stuttering might appear temporarily at period of dentition or become worse then, as it may during puberty, exhaustion and so forth.[136] The deleterious effects of carious teeth upon a stutterer came either through a lowering of his vitality, or because they triggered certain reflex paths.[137]

The most detailed account of the ramifications of abnormal dentition in children came from John Ashburner, whose great interest was hypnotism, spirit rapping and Zoism, possibly generated in India, where he was born.[138] Stuttering, speechlessness and miscellaneous infantile complaints resulted from 'derangement of organisation' or 'entanglement of developmental trains'. His thesis was founded upon two premisses: first, that perfect development depended upon harmony – 'the norm of nature' – between bodily structures whose due proportion rests on mental and physical well-being, and, second, that the skin and nervous system are closely related.[139] Ashburner believed that many troubles arose from abnormal 'configurations' or what the French called 'vitiations', namely, diminished or excessive growth of one part at the expense of another, often consequent upon desirable social habits such as those engendered by urban life.[140] The teeth commonly suffered and being a dermoid structure, irritated the nervous tracts which in turn triggered various spasmodic disturbances, one being stammering. Both skin disorders and spasms were manifestations of nervous irritation, the latter being a sign of irritation without relief.[141] Ashburner produced case histories in support of his thesis, which Wright quotes with apparent approval.[142]

While the major thrust of his argument involved the teeth, Ashburner conceded that spasms might arise from dental malformations, as well as such irritating conditions as costiveness; stammering, indeed, could even come from a nervous diathesis.[143] He spoke of certain states of the skin and nervous system as being 'coincident', the causal priority depending upon circumstances and individual constitution, but since he believed both were largely occasioned by unhealthy environments, it is safe to infer that he saw the teeth as one of the principal exciting causes of spasmodic behaviour, including stuttering.

Against those who argued that stuttering often occurred from causes unrelated to the teeth and that the condition would be permanent, were these responsible, Ashburner states:

> Controversialists, without being aware of it, often talk great nonsense. Stammering is sometimes better and sometimes worse; sometimes linked with anormal development, sometimes not. Occasionally, like a permanent squint . . . blindness . . . deafness, it has commenced in alliance with an anormal condition of some development, and habit has fixed it incurably, or the '*temporary derangement of organization*' has become permanent. One or another particular train of events is not necessarily continuous; it may suddenly appear, and as suddenly cease. A person subject to epilepsy is not always in fits. In most cases where the process preparatory to cutting the wise teeth goes on for years, and effort at development is repeatedly made, and subsides again . . . Gradually an increase of growth takes place.[144]

The physical basis of stuttering which he outlines goes some way towards throwing light on symptomatic changes over a period of time, but it hardly explains fluctuations from minute to minute. Possibly this is accounted for by habit. Because of their neural affiliations, Ashburner assigns a special causal role to the teeth in the production of spasms. In part, however, his argument could apply to morbid conditions of other structures, like the tonsils.

Throat and Palate

Principles from physiology and phonetics, which had served to implicate the glottis or tongue in stuttering, could also be found to support hypotheses locating its primary spasm at the palate or fauces. To some specialists, stutterers' difficulties with specific sounds, and their interrupted breath and voice, was more explicable in terms of the shape of the hard palate; the activity of the soft palate (velum); the size of the uvula; the condition of the tonsils; the position of the palatine arches straddling them; or the width of the faucal orifice which they bounded (Figure 2.1, p. 55).

The French surgeon, Velpeau, claimed to be one of the first to associate a peculiarity of the palatine vault with stuttering,[145] and in England Bennett Lucas found patients in whom both these conditions co-existed.[146] As with the tight fraenum, where the palate was particularly deep and narrow, it was difficult for the tongue to make contact, which explained the frequency of stuttering on apex sounds. Years later, a similar view was advanced by Williams, a dentist, who offered the patient in question prosthetic rather than surgical treatment.[147]

To the Italians, a golden voice – *un'ugola d'oro* – refers, literally, not to the larynx but to the uvula, the idiom expressing the intimate relationship this structure was thought to have with singing. According to James Yearsley, the uvula had little function other than to separate the nose and throat during swallowing and vomiting but he did agree that singers could reach higher notes if the uvula were excised, adding that the same was true, to a lesser extent, after removal of the tonsils.[148] Physiologists, especially on the Continent, were reporting that the palate heightened and the uvula diminished in size during singing in the upper register and this caused an elevation of the larynx and lengthening of the trachea, which was the real reason why the shape of the latter varied with pitch changes. No one endeavoured to correlate this observation with stutterers' agility in song. However, since removal of the uvula had not only enabled professional singers to increase their pitch range, but made their voices smoother and more sonorous, Cull thought the procedure worth trying with stutterers,[149] despite the fact that its amputation was already proving a disappointment[150] and that the stuttering of a syphilitic woman, whose uvula had ulcerated away, continued unabated.[151]

Without mentioning anyone by name, Wright indicated that some medical colleagues believed fissures of the uvula or palate could be a cause of stuttering. His own opinion, contrarily, was that these were more likely to relieve it,[152] the reason being that by providing a permanently patent airway vocalisation would be unimpeded. The question of melodic languages is not featured in his argument but he does suggest that stuttering would not exist if all speech sounds were continuous. The logic behind Wright's reasoning is difficult to follow, probably because it is based on the dubious premiss that a stutterer's difficulty stems from his substitution of mutes for nasals. The former, by their nature interrupt the breath stream, and so he envisages the air as becoming pathologically trapped between the various points of articulation in the mouth and velum. Both sets of organs are therefore suspect. Rejecting Yearsley's limited view of the uvula's function, he asserts that apart from its biological use, it must assist the velum in sealing off the nose during speech.[153] If the velum is important in singing, its timely action is also necessary for speech. Indeed, Wright stresses its special role in the genesis of the various respiratory and vocal irregularities associated with stuttering, 'the principal mechanical and physiological cause' of which:

> arises from a sluggish, tardy, and *contrary action of the organ which closes the nasal passage*, and from the *contrary action* of those organs which are *employed* for the *proper utterance* of the *mute consonants*, and that such inefficient and contrary actions induce a sudden and untimely closing of the pharynx on all sides, and sometimes, perhaps, of the glottis itself, till the chords of the glottis be deranged, the breathing checked, and frequently, for a second or so, stopped; – when the lungs lose their orderly alternate action.[154]

The theory of Arnott and McCormac would not hold water because thoracic or laryngeal blocks would not selectively affect the mutes. In support of his argument, he postulates that patients with defective palates never stutter,[155] which accords with the experience of both Astley Cooper and Charles Bell. Through this line of reasoning, Wright comes close to conceding that snipping the uvula or palate might be useful, and he rather lamely explains his vigorous opposition to surgery by saying that such treatment is as bad as the impediment.[156]

A rather different interpretation was given by Marshall Hall, who postulated that the uvula might instigate oro-vocal spasms by irritating the tongue's surface and setting a reflex in train similar to vomiting. This basically neurological theory will be examined in the next chapter along with Charles Bell's inco-ordination hypothesis. The latter influenced with the second version of Wright's book, as did his analysis of the pharynx in speaking, which, Wright stressed, must act in concert with the velum.

As we have seen, Wright did not attribute stuttering to any organic defect in the soft palate and he made no comment upon odd reports that its arches were lower or more backwardly placed in stutterers. He did, however, controvert Yearsley's attempt to site the primary spasm at the oro-pharyngeal orifice, on account of the surrounding structures being diseased. Yearsley asserted that in the 'great majority of stammerers' the faucal opening was reduced through swollen tonsils, uvula or rear of the tongue.[157] His generalisations were based upon several hundred cases,[158] but Poett, after experience with over a thousand, found no correlation between speaking difficulty and morbidity of tonsils or uvula.[159] Nor did Lee,[160] while a Dr Chowne doubted that an elongated uvula could ever obstruct the breath mechanically. Dr Pilcher, also at the London Medical Society meeting, had reason to query Yearsley's diagnoses, noting, like Bishop,[161] that even if such defects existed they would not produce stuttering,[162] a point Yearsley himself had made in relation to tongue-tie. Many years later, however, a case was reported of stuttering being initiated by tonsillitis, at which time its cause was conjectured to be inco-ordination or reflexes.[163] It is unlikely that any significant number of Yearsley's patients had a similar problem and so, assuming that he was reporting in good faith, the divergencies in his findings may possibly be accounted for by the nature of his practice, it being more likely that patients with throat conditions would find their way to an oto-laryngologist.

Although Yearsley's hypothesis rested upon a physical disability, like Hall, he called upon the concept of a reflex arc to explain the sequence of events. As irritation or obstruction of the mucous tract resulted in coughing, sneezing and so forth, so blockage at the fauces might occasion spasmodic behaviour in the respiratory and allied muscles. In straining to surmount the obstruction, the lips could become involved, either through sympathy or an overflow of excessive nervous energy.[164] On this point, at least, his position was close to Wright's.[165]

The principles shaping Yearsley's thinking were representative of many of those wedded to a peripheral interpretation of stuttering. He aimed to highlight the point at which respiration became impeded, and attributed the fluency in singing to a patency of the airway; the specificity of stuttering for certain sounds was determined by the locus of the primary block; and other muscles became implicated by an overflow of the spasm. Finally, together with others proposing an organic aetiology, he was not always clear over whether this acted mechanically or through its effect upon adjacent nerves.

Notes

1. Thomas Sheridan, *A Course of Lectures on Elocution* (New York, Benjamin Blom, 1968), p. 23. A facsimile reproduction of the 1762 edition published in London.
2. Thelwall (1810), p. 54.

3. Cited by Hunt (1861), p. 71. For original see Itard, 'Mémoire sur Bégaiement', *Journal Universel des Sciences Médicales*, 7 (1817), p. 130 (129-44). See also Michael Clark, 'Jean Itard on Communication Disorders: A New Translation and Historical Commentary on his "A Memoir on Stuttering" . . . (1817)', in *Psychology of Language and Thought*, ed. R.W. Rieber [a volume in the series: Studies in Applied Psycholinguistics, gen. ed. R.W. Rieber] (New York, Plenum Publishing Corp., 1979).

4. John Hutchinson, 'On the capacity of the lungs, and on the respiratory functions, with a view of establishing a precise and easy method of detecting disease by the spirometer', *Medico-Chirurgical Transactions*, 29 (n.s. 11) (1846), 137-252.

5. Browne and Behnke, pp. 108-22, 179-94.

6. Ibid., p. 123.

7. Mrs Emil Behnke, *The Speaking Voice*, 12th edn (London, J. Curwen & Sons, n.d., copyright USA 1897), p. 249; Kate Emil Behnke, 'Stammering – What Is It?', *Lancet*, 1 (1922), p. 1130.

8. Blake, pp. 13, 20. Cf. Yearsley (1843-4) p. 247.

9. Gerdts, pp. 40, 54, 62.

10. K. Behnke, *Lancet*, 1 (1922), p. 1130.

11. E. Scripture, *Stuttering and Lisping* (New York, Macmillan, 1917), pp. 21, 23-36.

12. S. Smith, 'The Contributions to Science of John Bostock. M.D., F.R.S. 1773-1846' (London Univ. MSc thesis, 1954-5), pp. 15, 29.

13. John Bostock, *An Elementary System of Physiology* (London, printed for Baldwin, Cradock and Jay, 1826), pp. 213-17.

14. For a summary of this work see Perkins in Sheehan (ed.), pp. 188-238.

15. Minute Philosopher, pp. 6, 11. Cf. Gerdts, pp. 14, 48, 56-7.

16. Gerdts, p. 42. Cf. ibid., pp. 39, 40, 61, 64, 65.

17. Ibid., pp. 15, 36, 51, 52-3, 62, 64.

18. Ibid., pp. 7, 29, 30, 33, 39, 44.

19. Ibid., pp. 15, 25.

20. Borthwick, p. 2.

21. Ibid., pp. 25-7, 29, 30, 32-5, 37, 38.

22. Ibid., pp. 23-4.

23. *Mind, Breath*, p. vi. The author, a clergyman of Essex, was probably the Rev. P.W. Bryan, who wrote *Stammering considered with relation to the Management of Breath with a plan for its Remedy, and practical Observations* (London, James Maddon, 1847). A book by this title was the earlier edition of *Mind, Breath*, see frontispiece and p. v.

24. Ibid., pp. 11, 16, 18, 19.

25. Poett snr (1833), p. 23.

26. A.M. Bell (1900), p. 254.

27. Poett snr (1828), pp. 5-6, 21, 35, 48; (1833), pp. 21-3. Cf. quotation from Hunt, cited above p. 65.

28. McCormac, pp. 12-13.

29. *DNB*, vol. 12, 455-6.

30. McCormac, pp. v-x, 15, 24-5, 29-34, 71-2, 83.

31. Henry M'Cormack [*sic*], 'Outline of the Nature and Cure of Stammering, or Hesitation of Speech', *Medico-Chirurgical Review*, 9 n.s. (1828), 193-4.

32. Abercrombie, p. 258; Gray, p. 23; *Charles Kingsley* (1910), vol. 3, pp. 18, 267; Haward, p. 112; Review of McCormac's *Treatise, London Medical Gazette*, 2 (1828), 80-2.

33. Poett snr (1833), pp. 77-9.

34. Borthwick, pp. 44-5. Cf. ibid., pp. 40-2; Helmore, p. 60.

35. Wright (1835), p. 4.

36. Good (1829), p. 568.
37. Physician, pp. 19-20.
38. Gerdts, pp. 32-3, 34.
39. Georg Hermann von Meyer, *The Organs of Speech and their Application in the Formation of Articulate Sounds* (London, Kegan Paul, Trench & Co., 1883), p. 176.
40. *Supplement* to the first edition of Dr Arnott's *Elements of Physics or Natural Philosophy* (London, Longman, 1828), p. xxx. Cf. Arnott's *Elements of Physics*, 5th edn (London, Longman, 1833), pp. 648-9.
41. *Penny Cyclop.*, p. 430.
42. Abbotts, p. 55.
43. Poett jnr, pp. 17-18.
44. Borthwick, p. 39.
45. Cazalet, p. 16.
46. Borthwick, pp. 20-1, 39.
47. *Problems*, 895a 19.
48. See, for example, Barry Wyke, 'Deus Ex Machina Vocis An Analysis of the Laryngeal Reflex Mechanisms of Speech', *British Journal of Disorders of Communication*, 4 (1969), 3-25.
49. See, for example, Magendie's *Compendium of Physiology*, pp. 137-8.
50. Obituaries: *British Medical Journal*, 2 (1902), 1565-6; *Journal of Laryngology, Rhinology and Otology*, 17 (1902), 629-31.
51. This took some 20 years to perfect and led to Behnke being judged 'the most competent living authority'. After his death, there was dispute over the right to his system, see *Professional World*, 2 (1893), pp. 72, 120, 138, 150, 154.
52. Browne and Behnke, pp. 173-8, 304.
53. Kate Emil-Behnke, *Stammering, its Nature, Causes, and Treatment* (London, Williams & Norgate, 1947), pp. 5-7.
54. Stevenson and Guthrie, p. 81.
55. See, for example, Joseph Watson, *Instruction of the Deaf and Dumb* (London, Darton & Harvey Printers, 1809), pp. 6-7.
56. Bartlett, pp. 23-5.
57. William Munk, *The Roll of the Royal College of Physicians of London 1801-1825*, 2nd edn (London, The College, 1878), vol. 3, 161-6; *DNB*, vol. 12, p. 455.
58. Stevenson and Guthrie, pp. 80, 94-5.
59. Arnott (1829), p. 608.
60. Ibid., pp. 610-11. Arnott's views on stuttering were quoted *in extenso* in a review of his *Elements*, *London Medical Gazette*, 5 (1829-30), 309-11.
61. Ibid., p. 585.
62. Cull (1833), pp. 26-7.
63. *Penny Cyclop.*, p. 431.
64. H – T (1860), p. 533.
65. *Mind, Breath*, p. 16.
66. Graves, pp. 658, 659; Marshall, *Physiology*, vol. 1, p. 268.
67. Colman (1899), p. 451. Cf. ibid., p. 448.
68. Wyllie, pp. 2-3, 31-2.
69. Müller, pp. 1056-7. Cf. Hunt (1861), pp. 83-9.
70. Kussmaul, pp. 836, 837.
71. Potter, pp. 49, 71. Cf. ibid., pp. 47-8, 55.
72. Wright (1835), pp. 47-8.
73. James Wright, letter to *The Times*, 6 January 1830, n.p., reproduced in his *Treatise*, pp. 1-4.
74. Arnott (1829), p. 608.
75. Wright (1839), p. 3.

76. Hall (1825), pp. 8-16.
77. Hall (1831), pp. 253-61.
78. Westminster Medical Society (1840-1a), pp. 24-5.
79. Physician, pp. 17-19. For a criticism of this argument, see Wright (1843), pp. 12-15.
80. Arnott (1829), pp. 608-9.
81. Physician, p. 19; Yearsley (1841), p. 16.
82. For a contemporary historical survey see Browne and Behnke, pp. 140-55.
83. Manuel Garcia, 'Physiological Observations on the Human Voice', *Proceedings of the Royal Society of London*, 7 (1855), 399-410.
84. Frederick Brodnitz, 'One Hundred Years of Laryngoscopy: to the Memory of Garcia, Tuerck and Czermak', *Transactions of the American Academy of Ophthalmology and Otolaryngology*, 58 (1954), 663-9.
85. Hunt (1863), pp. 176-7.
86. James Hunt, *Stammering and Stuttering*, 6th edn (London, Longman, 1865), p. 183. Cf. Hunt (1870), pp. 308-9n.
87. Gibb, *Diseases of the Throat*, pp. 189-90.
88. James, *Lancet*, 2 (1879), p. 726.
89. Browne and Behnke, pp. 298-9. Cf. Morell Mackenzie, *A Manual of Diseases of the Throat and Nose* (London, J. & A. Churchill, 1880), vol. 1, 492-5; Bishop, p. 64.
90. Holmes, *Lancet*, 2 (1879), p. 820.
91. Braid (1840-1), pp. 116-17; James Braid, 'Stammering', *London Medical Gazette*, 1 (1840-1), p. 950 (949-51). Cf. Rosenthal, pp. 133-4.
92. Wright (1835), pp. 5-6, where he seems to be anticipating conditioned reflexes.
93. A.M. Hartley, p. 30. Cf. ibid., pp. 51-2.
94. Magendie, *Compendium of Physiology*, pp. 140-1.
95. Lennox Browne, *The Throat and its Diseases*, 2nd edn (London, Baillière, Tindall & Cox, 1887), p. 63.
96. Ball, pp. 15-21.
97. Ibid., p. 18.
98. See below p. 155.
99. Potter, p. 43.
100. Letter to Rev. F.D. Maurice, 6 August, 1855 in *Charles Kingsley* (1888), p. 168.
101. *DNB*, vol. 11, 790-1.
102. Baudens, p. 164.
103. Academy of Medicine, Paris (1841), p. 135.
104. Potter, p. 48. Cf. ibid., p. 71.
105. Lee, pp. 22, 23, 26, 38, 46. Cf. Physician, p. 13; A. Bell, p. 26.
106. 'M. Velpeau . . .', p. 197.
107. Academy of Medicine, Paris (1841), p. 135.
108. Baudens, p. 165.
109. Lucas (1840-1), pp. 389-90.
110. Thomas Denman, letter *Medical and Physical Journal*, 14 (1805), 97-8.
111. Ibid., p. 97.
112. John Thelwall, 'On Cutting the Bridle of the Tongue', *Medical and Physical Journal*, 14 (1805), p. 258 (256-9).
113. Lee, p. 21. Cf. ibid., pp. 24, 25, 44.
114. Yearsley (1841), pp. 19-20.
115. Academy of Medicine, Paris (1841), p. 135. Cf. Academy of Sciences, Paris, p. 366, where a slightly different rendering is given.
116. Academy of Medicine, Paris (1840-1), p. 381.
117. Academy of Sciences, Paris, p. 366.

118. Academy of Medicine, Paris (1840-1), p. 381.
119. Academy of Medicine, Paris (1841), p. 136.
120. Edward Twisleton, *The Tongue Not Essential To Speech* (London, John Murray, 1873), pp. 4-5, 9-10, 12, 40, 43, 165-7.
121. Samuel Cooper, *A Dictionary of Practical Surgery*, 4th edn (London, Longman, 1822), pp. 1037-9.
122. Good, pp. 543-4.
123. Bartlett, pp. 3, 35-8, 47. Cf. Abbotts, p. 36, where the writer tells of a butcher who fell on a knife and severed a large part of his tongue without undue hindrance to speech; Lee, pp. 5-6n.
124. Review of four recent publications . . . , p. 209.
125. Bishop (1851), p. 47.
126. A.M. Bell (1900), pp. 206, 239, 242.
127. A. Bell (1849), pp. 26-7. Cf. Foster, [1900], p. 21.
128. Abbotts, pp. 23, 35, 55.
129. Lee, pp. 29, 37.
130. Bartlett, pp. 54-5.
131. Mason (1884), p. 7n.
132. Thelwall, *Medical and Physical Journal*, 15, p. 174.
133. *The Life of Edward, First Lord Herbert of Cherbury* written by himself, ed. J.M. Shuttleworth (London, Oxford UP, 1976), p. 93.
134. *Charles Kingsley* (1901), vol. 3, 267-8.
135. Lillian Lindsay, *A Short History of Dentistry* (London, Bale, Sons & Danielsson, 1933), pp. 66-8, 71, 84.
136. Kussmaul, p. 835. Cf. E. Behnke [1893], p. 27; Physician, p. 13; Yearsley (1843-4), p. 288.
137. See below pp. 134-5, 137.
138. Munk's *Roll*, vol. 3, 181-2.
139. John Ashburner, *On Dentition, and Some Coincident Disorders* (London, Longman, 1834), pp. xi-xii, 5-6, 14-15, 83-4, 86, 116. See also eleven papers in the *London Medical Gazette* from 26 October 1833 to 1 February 1834, which contain substantially the same text; John Ashburner, 'On the Teeth – as a Source of Health or Disease', *London Medical Gazette*, 12 (1832-3), 425-6.
140. Ibid., pp. 3, 4-5, 12-13, 88-9.
141. Ibid., pp. 83-4, 101-2, 104-5, 111, 113, 154-5, 174-5.
142. Wright (1839), p. 6; (1850), p. 290.
143. Ashburner, pp. 104-5.
144. Ibid., pp. 160-1.
145. 'M. Velpeau . . . ', p. 196.
146. Lucas, *Provincial Medical and Surgical Journal*, 1, p. 366; Lucas (1840-1), p. 389.
147. Williams, p. 396.
148. Yearsley (1841), p. 14.
149. Westminster Medical Society (1840-1b), p. 80.
150. Ibid., p. 81.
151. Medical Society of London (1840-1b), p. 76.
152. Wright (1843), p. 11.
153. Ibid., pp. 18-26.
154. Wright (1839), p. 31.
155. Ibid., pp. 6, 30.
156. Wright (1843), pp. 26-8.
157. Yearsley (1841), pp. 15-16.
158. Ibid., p. 9.
159. Poett snr (1840-1), pp. 414-16.
160. Lee, p. 21.

161. Bishop (1851), pp. 48-9.
162. Medical Society of London (1840-1a), p. 27.
163. H. Rainsford, 'Temporary Stammering coming on with Tonsillitis', *British Medical Journal*, 1 (1890), p. 1009; Report of Dr Farquhar Matheson's paper 'Stammering or Stuttering and Naso-pharyngeal Disease', *British Medical Journal*, 2 (1888), p. 487.
164. Yearsley (1841), pp. 16-19.
165. Wright (1839), pp. 5-6.

5 NEUROLOGICAL AND PSYCHOLOGICAL INFLUENCES

Concerned primarily with the more dramatic and bizarre aspects of human behaviour, neurology and psychiatry had traditionally formed one branch of internal medicine: only gradually were these disciplines distinguished from it and each other. Alongside psychologists, who were moving nearer biology as they probed the physiological basis of behaviour, psychiatrists, many of whom had a neurological training and a commitment to the materialistic principles of phrenology, were taking a close look at brain function. Not least amongst the justifications for this trend was the discovery of an organic basis both for the psychotic symptoms of general paresis[1] and of language. Thus, though neurology and psychiatry acquired separate identities, their subject matter remained interrelated and gave a new perspective to the debate on the underlying mind-body question.

Neuropsychiatric conditions were not readily disentangled from medical and social problems, with some unfortunate consequences. As odd behaviour was not only the mark of 'lunatics' – madmen and idiots – but of vagrants, paupers, petty criminals and other social misfits, such people might find themselves under one administrative umbrella, and there was to be much legislation before things improved. Much also rested upon a new interpretation of mental problems. Hypochondriasis, almost endemic in Victorian society, was frequently treated as a somatic complaint, not every physician being as perceptive as Benjamin Brodie in detecting the emotional basis for many physical symptoms.[2] More serious nervous disorders also needed reclassifying, as is evident from Prichard's *A Treatise on the Diseases of the Nervous System* (1822), where epilepsy, chorea, vertigo and apoplexy are discussed alongside somnambulism, maniacal delirium and ecstasy. The question was how stutterers, subject to paroxysms, physical ills and appearing stupid, strange and unsociable, fitted into this medley of complaints. Having vividly portrayed the mental anguish of stuttering, theorists were faced with determining whether its numerous nervous features were best explained in terms of neurological or psychological pathology.

The peculiar difficulty in categorising stuttering arose because its root seems to lie 'in that mysterious region which we may call the neutral ground of mind and matter'; it was a nervous disorder of a most distressing type, intimately bound up with the neurological system, that intermediary between thought and action.[3] Some classed it as a 'neurosis', with other spasms, though not William Cullen, who introduced the term at the close of the eighteenth century and for whom it depicted something other than the minor psychological illnesses it now signifies.[4] It was argued that calling stuttering a 'nervous affection' was merely substituting 'one kind of ignorance for another': with all spasmodic complaints it was necessary to determine which way the nerves were affected.[5] This was a laudable if ambitious aim by mid-nineteenth century, but Cullen and his contemporaries were poorly placed to differentiate neurological from psychological disorders, as neuroanatomy and neurophysiology were then in their infancy.

One landmark in the development of neurology was Romberg's *Lehrbuch der Nervenkrankheiten des Menschen* (1840-6), translated into English in 1853 and considered the first neurological textbook. Here, stuttering is classed amongst the 'neuroses of motility', whereas it is labelled a 'spasmodic neurosis of co-ordination' in Kussmaul's *Disturbances of Speech*, the first text on verbal impediments, which appeared in English in 1878, when Ziemmsen's *Handbuch* (1877) was translated. In Britain, an important practical milestone was the opening of a national hospital for nervous diseases in Queen's Square, during 1860. In 1871, William Gowers compiled the first nosological table of its residents. The 168 patients were afflicted almost equally with paralysis or epilepsy and there was one stammerer amongst them.[6]

It was during the nineteenth century that a start was made in unravelling the neuropathology of certain articulatory and language disturbances, and the state of knowledge on dysarthria may be gauged from Bristowe's *Treatise on the Theory and Practice of Medicine*, a standard text. This touched upon several types of paralysis, including that fatal glosso-labio-laryngeal form, which had been identified by Trousseau in 1840, and later elaborated as a syndrome by Duchenne. Bristowe also recognised the speech difficulties of loco-motor-ataxy, chorea and disseminated sclerosis. Language defects are likewise described, but his classification is muddled and he fails to distinguish properly between dysarthria and aphasia.[7] There is no mention of apraxia; he does not examine the neurology of vocal defects, nor does he mention stuttering at his time.

The language disturbance now known as aphasia came into prominence following Paul Broca's celebrated paper to the Anthropological Society of Paris, in which he described the post-mortem findings on an aphasic patient. For speech pathology, the discovery had far-reaching consequences. For a start, it put the investigation of verbal handicaps firmly on the intellectual map; it also deflected the most enquiring medical minds away from stuttering. Nevertheless, this was not unfruitful as the realisation of a dominant hemisphere led to the hypothesis that stuttering might be more frequent amongst left handers, due to a conflict between the hemispheres, neither one having gained complete ascendency. None of this was cogitated, however, in British circles during the nineteenth century.

In 1890, Blake was regretting that neither general practitioners nor neurologists were giving stuttering the attention it deserved.[8] One contemporary neurologist who did not ignore the subject, however, was John Bristowe of St Thomas', a hospital where he had excelled as a student and at which he subsequently became a leading, if somewhat unsatisfactory, lecturer.[9] More popular was his medical *Treatise* and three years after its first edition appeared, Bristowe was invited to deliver the Lumleian lectures at the Royal College of Physicians. He chose speech and voice as his topic and it was at this point that stuttering briefly entered his considerations.[10] He later published several competent summaries of the problem, but they contained nothing original, probably because his practical experience was limited, and as a teacher he was more concerned with imparting current views than evolving new theories. His reviews, however, were no more sketchy than those found today in medical dictionaries or neurological texts.

In 1798, Cullen's pupil at Edinburgh, Alexander Crichton, did make a few comments on speech handicaps, but thereafter the only notable contribution on stuttering from a psychiatrist was Henry Monro's. Monro was himself a sufferer but unlike many others he kept personal experiences hidden though he did later acknowledge authorship of the book published under the pseudonym Bacc. Med. Oxon.[11] There is no indication that stuttering was a familial trait, but Henry did inherit his family's artistic ability – as is evident from his self portrait reproduced in *The Royal College of Physicians of London. Portraits* (1964) – and its concern with insanity. His departure from Bethlem for St Luke's in 1852 ended a continuous Monro association with the asylum that had begun four generations previously when James entered its precincts in 1728. A philanthropist, devoting much of his life to alleviating distress, Henry Monro also found time to participate in the institutional developments taking place within his profession. In 1864, he became president of the asylum medical officers' association.[12]

Asylums had become the focus for ever more stringent government regulations and for the new medical specialty. Spearheaded by Lord Shaftesbury, practical reforms were instituted which, primarily designed as a safeguard against unjust certification, weighted psychiatric progress towards legalism.[13] Training was almost non-existent and the formidable classificatory and administrative problems facing the profession meant that its members had little time for the subtleties of stuttering. The general indifference of psychiatrists towards stuttering is exemplified by the fact that it was the neurologist, Bristowe, who dealt with the subject in Tuke's *Dictionary*.

Psychiatrists were aware that derangements of speech and mind often accompanied one another and their materialistic orientation made aphasia of special interest. This interest was not misplaced, as sufferers risked being classed insane, even though Crichton had perceptively distinguished between patients with this 'memory' disorder and those whose dumbness or gibberish stemmed from insanity,[14] thereby diminishing their chances of being placed in a madhouse rather than a hospital. By the end of the century the situation was reversed: insane patients were liable to be diagnosed aphasic.[15] From Van Der Kolk we learn that dysarthrics were confined in Dutch asylums and no doubt this happened in Britain.[16] Stutterers were probably more fortunate, unless they had mental lapses, as did one patient who needed restraint for maniacal fits, during which she spoke fluently.[17]

What, then, was the position regarding the psychopathology of stutterers? They had been described as having a 'temporary insanity',[18] a melancholy bordering on insanity,[19] and Thelwall had compared their lack of self-mastery to derangement and idiocy, yet their verbal output could hardly be likened to the incoherencies of lunatics. Nor could they rank as hysterics, more commonly women, though Bristowe recognised an hysterical form of stuttering, characterised by the bizarre repetition of words.[20] Gerdts described it as a 'physical-psychical' complaint, the latter predominating once the child became self-conscious and fearful.[21] Aside from Cull and Monro, little was said about this developmental aspect and until the concept of a psycho-neurosis had taken root and the dynamics of irrational behaviour sketched, a psychiatric interpretation of stuttering was not on the cards. German publications indicate a move in this direction by the end of the century, but it was not until Appelt wrote his *The Real Cause of Stammering*, in 1911, that English readers were presented with a detailed psycho-analytic exposition of the disorder. To judge from a brief note in the *British Medical Journal*, a decade later, its readership was still unaware that stuttering, by then, was being classed as a neurotic condition along with hysteria, anxiety neuroses, phobias, etc., the corollary being that treatment should 'be carried out only under medical care'.[22] Both before and after this time, others also favoured a psycho-analytic interpretations,[23] it variously being argued that stuttering is a result of oral and/or anal fixation. Unfortunately, these speculations have been therapeutically unrewarding.

There was, in fact, no theoretical framework or classificatory system into which stuttering neatly fitted and which would provide a convenient substitute for the humoral theory. So imagination was given free rein and the result was a rash of opinions rather than well reasoned hypotheses. These fall broadly into five groups that are not mutually exclusive and reflect the vantage point from which the complaint was analysed. More precisely, it was viewed as a symptom, along with other spasmodic conditions; as a reflex phenomenon; as stemming from suggestion or an inbuilt disposition; and as the culmination of undesirable associations and habits.

Spasms, Cramps and Tremors

'Stammering may be defined as a spasmodic interruption in articulation.'[24] It is due neither to structural defect, faulty learning, habit, paralysis, nor mental defects, but to 'a spasm or hitch in the course of utterance'.[25] These statements, from Bernard and Bristowe, are as representative of Victorian thinking as they are ambiguous. In the major nosological systems of medicine, spasm was commonly depicted as a distinct disease category embracing cramp, convulsion, paralysis and tremor, as well as affections like tetanus, lockjaw, hydrophobia, epilepsy, hysteria, syncope, asthma, squinting, wry neck, chorea and 'psellism'.[26] In 1844, Alison was classifying convulsions, i.e. generalised spasms plus insensibility, both as symptom and as a disease, when it was idiopathic and called epilepsy.[27] It was even later that Charcot demoted tremor to the status of a symptom.[28] Clinical tests can now reveal many types of tremor and paralysis, but the situation was far from clear a century ago, when the muscular oscillations of clonic spasm, the rigidity of tonic blocks and the extraneous jerks of head and body were likened to or identified with other nervous disorders. The contortions of stuttering even bore a superficial resemblance to those of Bell's palsy, which was to have a tangential relevance to stuttering surgery.

A closer parallel could be drawn between the stutterer's mouth, fixed open or shut, and the trismus or antitrismus of lockjaw, and the influence of such analogies is evident in Colombat's classification, which was well known in Britain. He used the term 'guttero-tetanic' for tonic spasms trapping breath within the throat and 'labio-choreique' for clonic movements, primarily of the lips.[29] Epilepsy was also mentioned, either because its affect on the muscular system was similar to stuttering,[30] or because the two conditions co-existed, in one case at least, both problems arising after teasing.[31] Even today, a connection between the two complaints is mooted.[32] Whereas a common aetiology was usually envisaged for all spasmodic complaints, McCormac believed that apoplexy, paralysis, angina pectoris, hydrophobia (plus aneurysms of the heart and great vessels) themselves 'more or less' produced stammering, at least temporarily.[33]

Stuttering was also classed with cramps. Amongst Romberg's 'neuroses of motility' were gathered all manner of spasms, tremors and convulsions. Some, like writer's cramp, were located in the range of motor nerves supplying the arms, while others, like stuttering, were situated in the vocal area.[34] Later authorities adopted many different classifications. Bristowe compared stuttering and scrivener's palsy, both of which resembled the cramps of pianists and swordsmen.[35] Rosenthal, apparently impressed by Fritz' collection of patients with writer's cramp who also stuttered, classified these two, along with chorea, as 'neuroses of co-ordination', their similarity being that the individual muscles could perform normally in isolation.[36] Later, however, Poore maintained that strictly speaking stuttering could not be viewed as an 'occupational neurosis', like writer's cramp and miner's nystagmus, since there was no evidence of it arising as a consequence of loquacity.[37] Nevertheless, so close was the comparison between manual and vocal spasms that writer's cramp was also called 'stammering of the fingers'.[38] And Paget extended the connotation of *stammering* still further to 'similar affections of other organs', such as those involved in urination and swallowing.[39]

Of all spasmodic complaints, by far the commonest comparison drawn was between chorea and stuttering. Carlyle, for example, disillusioned after a meeting with Charles Lamb and his literary confrères, described the essayist's speech as wriggling 'hither and thither with an incessant painful fluctuation', mirroring the whole group's conversation, which he likened to a St Vitus' Dance.[40] Carlyle was referring to the superficiality and lack of purpose in their exchanges, and perhaps only indirectly to the physical aspect of Lamb's speech, but the analogy served, as it did for medical men and elocutionists. This line of thinking spanned the century and also embraced other speech impediments.

Around 1809, Thelwall had spoken of cluttering and chorea together,[41] and later 'choreic paraphasia' was the label used for that medley of words 'no key could unlock', characteristic of certain language disorders.[42] The serious association of chorea and stuttering began in the first half of the century and by 1890 it so impressed Blake that he entitled his treatise on stuttering *Lip Chorea*.

Chorea Sancti Viti, manifested by convulsive limb movements and mental aberrations, was prevalent in northern Europe during the middle ages. Superstition sheathed its origins, dated 1027 A.D., when some peasants were purportedly found cavorting in a churchyard during a service, for which they were cursed by the priest and doomed to continuous dancing and screaming for the following twelve months. The mania erupted periodically thereafter and the names of Saints John, Anthony and Guy were also associated with it. By the time Sydenham wrote his classic paper on 'chorea minor', in 1686, 'chorea major' was on the wane, but his choice of name served to perpetuate their association. Dancing mania was an hysterical state, Sydenham's chorea a neurological one, but medicine made no such distinctions then, and even today hysteria may be difficult to distinguish from its organic counterpart.

Resemblances with stuttering were not hard to find. Bouillaud's 'follie musculaire' of chorea became, for therapists of stuttering, an 'insanity' of the voluntary muscles. In either case, inco-ordination was paramount, although wilder movements were sometimes responsive to the will. Both were nervous affections, showing typical fluctuations, developing at an age when children were particularly susceptible, and having a peculiar affinity for sensitive people. Imitation often initiated the complaints, which were liable to run in families. Poett, following Dr Copland, maintained that not only were their predisposing conditions identical, such as nervous temperament and constitutional debility, but also their proximate cause.[43] For Marshall Hall these lay in the excito-motor system, but Poett was content to ascribe them simply to excessive irritability of the ganglionic nerves, whose impulses spilled over into the voluntary muscles. Their exciting agents were also similar, with intestinal pathology being frequently noted, and worms in particular.[44] Even as late as 1894, Wyllie believed these to be instrumental, not only in chorea but also childhood aphasia.[45] Yet there were inescapable differences. The movements of chorea were constant and, some thought, independent of the will. The stutterer was relieved of his symptom once the desire to speak ceased, the choreic patient only became still during sleep. Furthermore, boys were more prone to stutter, girls to suffer from chorea, as well as hysteria and epilepsy.[46]

The exact relationship between stuttering and St Vitus' Dance was not spelled out, but reading between the lines it would seem that some conceived of the two conditions as co-existing, others looked upon stuttering as a partial chorea, while the remainder were either speaking metaphorically or were unable to differentiate between the various types of hesitancies. What, for example, was the position with Bennett Lucas' young patient, who was being considered for lingual surgery? He had been afflicted with St Vitus' Dance for six years, had a diverging right eye and a somewhat stupid expression, though was mentally quite sound. On trying to stand, he was overcome with fits of shivering, his arms moving frequently and involuntarily. Lucas describes his articulatory problems as follows:

> This patient's stammering is very intense. It is painful to witness his attempts to describe his sufferings. The pronunciation of any word is alike difficult to him, and when he perseveres in his attempt to speak for some minutes, the movements of his body become more severe and uncontrollable and his face congested.[47]

Clearly, medical men were uncertain of the nature of the speech impediments confronting them. Even Marshall Hall appears to have been led astray, in his deduction that stuttering was caused by excessive spinal action. Since such action underlay the muscular irregularities of choreic patients, he reasoned that it must also be responsible for their speech difficulty, which he called stammering.[48] Fifty years on, Blake was still of the opinion that the majority of choreas were reflex responses to peripheral irritation.[49]

With diagnosis problematical, treatment was liable to fall into the wrong hands. If the ganglionic nerves were involved, doctors felt that patients should be under their control, and sensing a threat to their pocket they were quick to speak out. Echoing Copland's words, Poett stated that sending a stuttering child to an elocutionist was 'as absurd as sending a case of chorea to a drill-sergeant'.[50] The *Lancet* sounded a more general warning, for if the profession should weaken over this complaint, there was no telling where it would end: 'If stammering is to be given up, why not chorea? if chorea, why not epilepsy? and so on, until the quacks have had the pick (as they really have had) of the whole nosology?'[51] The prospect was clearly alarming.

Reflexes

This is not the place to examine the history of reflexes, which have played so crucial a part in the advancement of neurophysiology and physiological psychology, and have found application to stuttering both yesterday and today. From Descartes onwards, reflex behaviour, which is involuntary and acts independently of consciousness, has been elaborated by a succession of notable scientists, not least of whom was Marshall Hall.[52]

Like his predecessors, Hall worked on decapitated animals. One experiment proved critical. Stimulating an intercostal nerve, he observed movement both in the turtle's fore and hind limbs, indicating that the nervous energy had travelled beyond the excited segment, and, moreover, in two directions. Since the spinal cord was generally conceived as being a string of semi-independent ganglia, this was a startling fact and implied that the cord was no mere corridor for conveying messages between brain and periphery, but was a through channel governed by its own vital laws.[53] Hall tried to convey this inherent dynamism by naming it the excito-motor or diastaltic nervous system. Its essential network lay within the spinal marrow and although separate nerves had yet to be demonstrated microscopically, Hall was certain of their existence. He consequently postulated an arc with three connections comprising: (1) incident or excitor nerves; (2) centric nerves of the true spinal marrow; and (3) reflex motor nerves.[54] These ideas were put before the Zoological Society of London at a meeting in November 1832,[55] the year he was elected a Fellow of the Royal Society.

Once this principle was accepted, there were no end of phenomena to which it might apply. The bodily sphincters and orifices were kept in equilibrium and regulated by a muscular tone maintained through the diastaltic system, and their relaxation or contraction during egestion, expulsion and so forth, were initiated by impulses mediated through that same system. Coughing, for example, could be interpreted as resulting not from mechanical action against parts adjacent to the laryngeal irritation, but from a neural arc passing along the sensory nerves via the spinal marrow back to the muscles. Only a restricted segment of cord was involved in so simple a reflex, but it could be triggered from farther afield, from the tongue, throat or gullet, in the case of swallowing.[56] There was, Hall asserted, no spot in the network that, once excited, would not tell upon the others: 'The entire system is naturally in a state of static tension, each part being in strict relation with *every* other', and this 'becomes dynamic force on the application of a stimulus'.[57] He drew a sharp distinction between this unconscious system and that of the cerebral hemispheres, concerned with willed movement, and consequently he conceived of no intermediary state.

The second phase of Hall's career followed the publication of his work in 1833. From then on, he devoted his time to applying these principles to diseases, resting his argument on two main facts. First, given the remote effects of stimuli, distant pathology could be responsible for a variety of symptoms. Thus, in childhood, dental, gastric or intestinal irritation might occasion squinting, crowing or convulsions; in adults, irritation of uterus, stomach or intestines might result in hysteria, epilepsy or asthma.[58] Secondly, since the neural arc has three parts, any one could be disordered. In dental or intestinal complaints, symptoms originated outside the spinal marrow and were called eccentric. If the marrow itself was morbid, disorders were classed centric. The excitation could also arise along the motor nerves themselves, as happened with certain tics.

Hall's interest in speech predated his animal experiments. On 3 January 1825, he read a paper to the Literary Society of Nottingham, his home town and the location of his first practice. The subject was articulatory mechanics and his remarks on stutterers were brief and limited to the observation that as they sang normally, they should be encouraged to speak in a free-flowing manner. Hall's references to stuttering continued to be short and brief, but gradually he saw the disorder as being governed by the simple principle that operated universally:

> *The Spinal or Diastaltic System* is the *Seat*, originally or secondarily, of *All Spasmodic* or *Convulsive Affections*. Disease of the encephalon may induce such affections by contact and *irritation*, or, though distant, by *counter-pressure*, affecting the spinal system. But, ultimately, *all spasm* is of this system.[59]

In 1836, Hall grouped stuttering with hysteria and chorea as one type of eccentric disease, intestinal irritation probably being its source, though it might sometimes be of centric origin.[60] The following year, when summarising the implications of stimulation to the spinal marrow within both the cord and medulla, Hall referred to the normal reflex activity that could follow upon nasal or palatal sensations and occasion sneezing or vomiting. He then stated that when such reflexes were morbidly augmented, diseases like tetanus, hydrophobia and stuttering could ensue.[61] By 1841, therefore, he was peculiarly prepared to participate in the debate aroused by stuttering surgery. His colleague, James Yearsley, had presented evidence that cures followed upon removal of uvula or tonsils. Hall took these reports seriously, asking himself the question: 'Is the uvula the excitor-regulator of articulation?', and further: 'Is it, in cases of stammering, unduly excitable?' Convincing analogies were to hand:

> Every voluntary act *combines* with itself an excito-motory action. The contact of an object with the palm of the hand, the sole of the foot, induces an additional muscular contraction beyond that of the original stimulus of volition. Articulation may be regulated in the same manner. A reflex arc between the uvula and the organs of articulation would not be more marvellous than many others. How extraordinary, for example, is the act of vomiting induced by irritation of the fauces![62]

So impressed was he by the uvula that he continued by questioning whether it or adjacent parts were not implicated 'in chorea . . . or in epilepsy itself!' Hall had touched on the mysteries of palatal action in his Nottingham paper. Now he was in a position to formulate more precise questions:

> What is the state and position of the uvula in articulation? The velum and, with it, the uvula are elevated and placed so as to close the posterior nares, when certain letters are pronounced. Are incident nerves, regulators of articulation, excited in this case? And are they unduly excited in stammering? And is stammering not only an undue *spinal* action (as I stated many years ago), but an undue *reflex* spinal action?[63]

In sketching these ideas to the Westminster Medical Society, Hall insisted that they were conjectural only. Because the uvula is raised during the articulation of many sounds, its elongation could not produce stuttering through irritation of the tongue. Possibly, however, a morbid excitability of its posterior surface might lead to dysfluency.[64]

This was by no means the extent of Hall's theory of disease. He appreciated that speech was essentially a voluntary act, readily upset by mental distress. In stuttering, he suggested that the unconscious reflex system took control, subverting the patient's will both over speech and respiration.[65] And since the will was involved, he later classed stuttering with chorea and Parkinson's disease, these maladies being similar in form if not in cause. The spinal centre was unduly excited and the stutterer, on wishing to communicate, finds 'the voluntary action of the organs of speech is carried to excess, by spinal or staltic action, or rendered abortive by emotion'.[66] Certain situations, therefore, served to enhance or inhibit the patient's muscular responses.

Hall explained the weakness of some muscles and the apparent excessive action of others through their 'irrito-contractility', a term he used to express the totality of neuro-muscular reactivity,[67] and which might be looked upon as the organic counterpart of the psychological state of sensitivity, so commonly ascribed to stutterers. This responsivity varied, not only from person to person, but between the various organs of a given individual; it was altered by circumstances affecting both the state of health and the constitutional disposition. Thus, a decaying tooth or constipated bowel would produce differing effects among individuals, and within the same person at different times. These effects could be modified by circumstances, which, for physical or psychological reasons, might alter the content and flow of blood. Hall believed that in muscles separated from the spinal marrow, irritability decreased, and in those separated from the brain, it increased. Basically, however, the paralysed muscle retained an inherent irritability which, though no longer responsive to the will, could be moved in stress or excitement because its connection with the emotional centre remained unsevered. This centre he placed in the medulla.

Aside from being postulated the centre of emotions, often so disturbed in stuttering, the medulla had other significance for speech pathology. Van Der Kolk's work revealed the central connections of the hypoglossal nerves and their morbidity in dysarthria. Earlier, however, Müller, whose own work on reflexes broadly supported Hall's,[68] was explaining the relationship between will and the medulla, which he conceived as the highest motor centre. Describing the motor, cerebral and spinal nerves as spread out in the medulla like the keys of a piano, he saw the will playing upon them, its influences travelling through outgoing nerve fibres like vibrations move along the length of a piece of elastic plucked at one spot.[69] Monro noted this analogy, which pertained to the third step in the speech chain and the one he considered at fault in stuttering, there being nothing wrong with the creation of ideas and the will, nor with the final stage of nervous action at the periphery.[70] Breathing irregularities might also be blamed on the medulla, whose role in respiration Legallois had demonstrated during 1812, and Flourens had subsequently elaborated after locating a specific vital node. Though the medulla was supposedly implicated in stuttering, the reasoning of commentators was vague[71] and some appear to have held their position gratuitously, while Müller, who might have expanded on this point, mentioned neither medullary action nor reflexes in his review of the problem.

In an age responsive to all manner of conjectures, it is significant that little was made of Hall's idea. At a stroke, he had provided a theoretical framework capable of accommodating the vicissitudes of stuttering, by showing how it could be self-perpetuating, and how the proximate, exciting and predisposing causes might interact. He himself did not discuss the question from this angle; his reference point was neurophysiological and his concern was with the application of his principles to general medicine rather than speech. He wrote no treatise on stuttering, yet his scattered remarks, and the experimental evidence adduced in their favour, should have excited interest. Certainly, some ideas became popular. 'You cannot go into a hospital or witness an interesting case', said Dr Sharpley, one of his first supporters, 'without the words "reflex function" or "excito-motor power", being used.' They were to become household words.[72] But frequently colleagues, most notably Charles Bell, eschewed reference to him. Amongst theorists of stuttering, some of Hall's notions were accepted, but often outside the context of the diastaltic system, and hence stripped of their force. Carpenter, initially an opponent of Hall's reflex system, came to acknowledge its merit and stated that the proximate cause of stuttering must be attributed to morbid centric or eccentric nervous action, more usually the former.[73] The same terminology was used much later by Abbotts.[74] In addition, Shuldham refers vaguely to 'spinal irritation' as a cause of stuttering, arguing, not unlike Hall, that there is associated muscular weakness and 'a weak muscle is an irritable one, and therefore the muscles involved in the production of speech are attacked with spasmodic action'.[75] Hence the value of fresh air and exercise.

Yearsley, as noted earlier, believed stuttering to be caused by stricture of the fauces and in explaining this as a reflex phenomenon he probably had Hall's ideas in mind. Lee, however, without mentioning Hall by name, denied that it might be based on the incident or reflex action of the spinal cord because, if so, the impediment would be permanent.[76] He therefore failed to take note of factors affecting the variability of responses in the excito-motor system. Bishop, for whom, like Yearsley, elocutionists were a thorn in the flesh, seems to have been well disposed towards Hall. Bishop attended to the effects of emotion upon the reflex system, particularly in relation to the heart and lungs. Because of the close connection in man between the voluntary and involuntary systems, it was possible for emotion to disrupt the reflexive mechanism and cause inspiration to become an irregular and conscious act. Disturbing repercussions in the cardio-vascular network may then interfere with voluntary actions and result in a speaker losing control over vocalisation,[77] as may occur both in dysphonia and stuttering.

A contemporary writer attributed neglect of Hall's work to prejudice within the Royal Society, which refused to publish his findings; to the prevailing interest in a new manifestation of humoralism; to the inherent difficulty of the subject matter; and because people often learned of it through biased secondary sources.[78] Modern biographers are inclined to blame Hall. He had a penetrating and versatile mind and his reformist views, ranging from abolition of flogging in the Army to increased safety of railway compartments, were presented in a forthright and fearless manner.[79] His own achievements were championed with equal vigour and defended with equal force. Many contemporaries kept their distance and their neglect or hostility only fomented his argumentative nature. Furthermore, it seems likely that they found the arrangement of his writings and his technical language unpalatable.[80]

Foreigners did not have to suffer this arrogance and Hall was well accepted in America and Europe. They also applied his principles to stuttering. Schulz placed the cause of the impediment in a disproportionately active excito-motory system, as did Lichtinger,[81] who isolated a cerebral from a spinal variety, the latter embracing centric and eccentric (reflex) forms.[82]

At home, Marshall Hall was not without friends. In 1846, the *Lancet* published a laudatory review of his *New Memoir*, with the judgement: 'We know of nothing so original, so diffusive, so developmental in its character, as the true spinal system.'[83] In the third section of the article, Hall is compared with Harvey and Bell. The reviewer ranks Harvey's discovery first, but states that Hall's was the most difficult, since the ground was less prepared.[84] A modern biographer has been unable to trace the source of these statements, usually attributed to Wakley,[85] but it was in print as being Tyler Smith.[86] At this time, he was largely responsible for editorial policy and had eagerly embraced Hall's interpretation of parturition as a reflex phenomenon, which particularly concerned him as founder of the London Obstetrical Society.[87] His book on parturition was dedicated to Marshall Hall; his treatise on stuttering, written under the pseudonym 'A Physician', was dedicated to James Yearsley, who, it should be noted, received support from Hall during the debate on stuttering surgery,[88] and was Smith's brother-in-law.[89] All three men were argumentative, and in the case of Smith and

Yearsley, this found an outlet in raillery against elocutionists. The *Lancet's* censure, directed particularly against Thomas Hunt, provides an example:

> A knowledge of the nervous system, of muscular action, and of the organs of voice and speech, are now so well understood, that stammering is no great mystery, and the principle treatment is so well known that the idea of keeping it a secret is absurd . . . After such men as CHARLES BELL, MARSHALL HALL, MULLER, and ARNOTT, have given their best attention to the pathology of stammering, and its means of relief, shall we sink to the HUNTS, the mere vocal posture-masters, for its treatment?[90]

These complacent words were most probably Tyler Smith's.

Granted that Smith did write the review of Hall's *Memoir*, it is pertinent to compare his thoughts on stuttering then, with those expressed previously in his book. In the *Lancet* he states:

> Speech is eminently aided by spinal action. The voluntary movements all produce fatigue when long continued. The amount of exertion of which the muscles of speech are capable without fatigue, is extraordinary, when their delicate organisation is considered.[91]

Stuttering provides a perfect illustration:

> As long as the vocal organs are at rest, as regards volition, there is no spasmodic action, but the moment volition, by contracting the laryngeal muscles, supplies the stimulus to the excitor nerves, the vocal and articulary muscles are thrown into violent spasm.[92]

Is the larynx now the excitor-regulator of speech? Was the uvula dropped on account of the disrepute incurred by stuttering surgery? Why should volition produce morbid action? And was this Smith's own interpretation? There is no mention of it in Hall's own writings. It seems that since the publication of his *Treatise*, Smith had shifted ground. Possibly his association with Marshall Hall was not of long standing, and although the *Treatise* was written in 1843, a year after he began investigating the connection between reflexes and parturition,[93] it may not have been long enough for him to develop their application to stuttering. In 1846, he was viewing it as an affection of the spinal system along with tics, squinting and wry neck,[94] but showing a likeness to chorea, which also could increase during voluntary movement.[95] Earlier, he had made much of chorea and the disharmonies between the voluntary and involuntary systems, as we shall see.

Imitation Versus Heredity

Victorians discussed both heredity and environment as a cause of stuttering, but rather than taking the holistic approach of seeing the organism-in-the-environment, they tended to oppose the two. The case for imitation, the most commonly cited environmental factor, was put by Thelwall early in the century:

> As for Hereditary Impediments! – what are these . . . but habits of imitation? . . . If little master hath a papa . . . that stammers . . . is it extraordinary, that the one (even before he can be aware that there is any other or better mode of speaking) should imitate this defect of the person from whom he is constantly aping almost every other action . . .[96]

More usually, the bad example came from school and *The Unspeakable* contains a characteristic situation. The young hero's troubles date from a meeting with his future teacher, the malevolent Mr Ogden. Instead of a handshake and verbal pleasantries, Charles is greeted by a spluttering man, whose hideously writhing expressions horrify yet fascinate him. As if compelled, the boy finds himself inadvertently mirroring Ogden's ungainly contortions.[97] Here the imitation is 'sympathetic' and unconscious, but stuttering could arise from deliberate mimicry or mocking.[98] It invited burlesque, but sometimes a participant found he had contracted more than he bargained for, and once habit took root the stutterer became his own model – the exciting cause to himself.[99] A stuttering teacher is plainly undesirable and Hunt says that Joseph Priestley left the schoolroom on that account.[100] From Priestley's *Memoirs*, however, it seems that his freethinking could be a reason for his failure to attract pupils. He attributed his own impediment to family inheritance. As a group, stutterers were particularly sensitive about being mimicked and could misinterpret a situation. Louis XIII was not alone in venting his ire upon someone he failed to recognise as a fellow sufferer.[101] And Prince Albert was probably not the only stammerer to be teased by his sister.[102]

Since today little is made of imitation in the genesis of stuttering, it is pertinent to enquire why Victorians gave it credence. Certainly, a *prima facie* case existed. Imitative power in children is undeniable, and stuttering was said to arise when the imitative faculty was most developed. Moreover, as 'contagion' in other spasmodic diseases spread through 'sympathetic imitation', then it probably did so with stuttering. Such analogical reasoning was popular but additional factors within the intellectual climate must also have fostered this line of thinking.

The power of imitation had certainly impressed thinkers. It had been discussed in relation to art, voluntary movement and the origins of man's sociability. Furthermore, Adam Smith accorded the allied notion of 'sympathy' or 'fellow-feeling' a central place in his moral philosophy. His writings were well known to Dugald Stewart, whose own analysis in *Elements of Philosophy of the Human Mind* came after that of language and before mesmerism. Mesmerism itself had vividly demonstrated how impressionable people can be. The French Academicians, unable to find any magnetic fluid, had condemned the phenomenon, but Stewart put the matter on a scientific footing by sifting the moral from physical agents, the former being conveyed through 'sympathetic imitation'.[103] Stewart's name appeared in numerous books on insanity and it seems likely that his ideas spread further afield, although in elocutionary circles he is mentioned only once, and then in connection with the 'suggestive power' which Cull equated with the capacity for associating images.[104]

Psychiatry may have had little to offer speech pathology but it was not bereft of a psychology and its place was taken by two indigenous philosophical schools, English and Scottish, that offered a theory of mental functioning. Stewart was in the latter tradition of faculty psychology and so, though admitting the force of associations, did not see the intellect as being totally passive. Along with the phrenologists, he conceived of it as having innate powers, 'original principles' or 'ultimate facts' of which imitation was one. Stewart used the word 'sympathetic' to depict the mimical powers as they influenced the bodily frame by a sort of identity with others, the will being almost in abeyance. He also distinguished between mimicry and acting, the former portraying idiosyncrasies of a given subject, the latter of a certain character stripped of individuality. Since the mimic uses no mirrors, Stewart postulated that the accuracy of his poses are gauged by some inner consciousness corresponding with that of his subject. Therefore, it is likely that something similar happens to everyone when confronted by strong expressions of emotion, which can excite corresponding feelings in others. These speculations must have struck a cord with elocutionists, who were pre-eminently concerned with model speech and whose thoughts were never far from the stage. In particular, the reflections on acting by Aaron Hill and Edmund Burke were noted by James Wright, possibly following Dugald Stewart's lead, as Wright had lectured to the Edinburgh Philosophical Association[105] and may have been familiar with Stewart's work. Burke was impressed by the way we tend to assimilate our features to those of others and in doing so share in their emotions. The great physiognomist, Campanella, became so adept at this that he 'was able to enter into the dispositions and thoughts of people, as if he had been changed into the very man'.[106] And habit aside, it was perhaps a similar identity with Lord Dundreary that caused Sothern to experience such difficulty speaking fluently off-stage and of adapting to new dramatic roles.[107]

James Wright, of Magdalen Hall,[108] Oxford, addressed his *Three Letters* to Sir Charles Bell, a Scot, whose own reflections on sympathy had been the subject of close examination.[109] With the 'contagion' of certain diseases and sympathy between bodily organs, physicians also had a good reason to consider the matter. Two were dogmatic about its relevance to stuttering. Poett saw '*contagio de visu*' as the one exciting cause[110] and Bartlett asserted that there were no cases which, by 'strict investigation', could not be attributed to imitation.[111] How strict his or other investigations were is hard to judge since, in England, Hunt alone produced figures[112] and these were cited in one journal only.[113] Overlooking this information, Shuldham contacted Coën, who had written an article 'On the Heredity and Psychical Contagiousness of Stammering' in *Allegemeine Wiener Medicinische Zeitung*.[114] For ease of comparison, the English and Viennese findings have been tabulated, and Coën's transposed into a percentage (Tables 5.1 and 5.2). Although using widely separated social groups, it is notable that both investigators reduce the role of imitation and roughly agree on the significance of heredity.

Finally, since hereditary impediments were considered incurable, speech correctionists had professional reasons for favouring imitation as a cause of stuttering. Dismissing physical transmission through tainted blood, Thelwall urged that instead of abandoning faulty speech to despair, it be approached with the confidence that melioration was possible. Rather than despairing, subsequent therapists were over-optimistic about what they could achieve.

There was some substance to the impression that stuttering ran in families and it is remarkable that three of the Darwins, so influential in shaping evolutionary theory and eugenics, suffered from the

Table 5.1: Causes of Stuttering in 200 Cases, After Hunt

Infantile infections, etc		7.5%
Fright or ill-treatment		5%
Imitation	voluntary	4%
	involuntary	9%
Inherited from	father	10%
	mother	5%
Unknown		49.5%

Source: Tabulated from James Hunt's *Stammering and Stuttering* (1870), p. 341.

Table 5.2: Causes of Stuttering in Coën's 67 Cases (Excluding the Eleven 'Stammerers')

Consequent upon scarlet fever (age ranges 5-16 years)	7.4%
Strong mental emotion	14.9%
Falls and other bodily injuries	26.9%
No assignable cause	50.8%
Of the above 67 cases, further causes operative:	
Imitation	4.5%
Heredity	16.4%

Source: Derived from figures in E. Shuldham's *Stammering and its Rational Treatment*, pp. 68-71.

complaint: Erasmus, his son and grandson, both named Charles, whose relationship was uncle and nephew.[115] Another grandson, Francis Galton, used pedigrees to prove the transmission of numerous abilities in his *Hereditary Genius* (1869), written at a time when various diseases, including deafness, were being familiarly linked. Eight years later, Goddard's study of the mentally and socially defective Jukes family in America served to confirm the long-standing fear in England that physical and mental handicaps were hereditary and associated with criminality, idiocy and depravity. More than once, 'stammering' was mentioned in this connection. Erasmus Darwin himself believed that if both parents suffered from a disease the family was doomed to extinction, but if one was free the offspring might escape, for otherwise the population would be riddled with epilepsy, gout and so forth.[116] Nevertheless, there was no point courting trouble and marriage to a stutterer was sometimes declined for fear the children would be similarly afflicted.[117]

Recognition of stuttering amongst relatives was nothing new, the Roman Balbus family being a case in point.[118] But though Victorians often remarked upon the tendency, evident in all spasmodic diseases, actual reports were few and sketchy. Beasley had a sister, niece and two or three cousins who suffered from the complaint;[119] an anonymous stutterer had a father and two children likewise affected;[120] six of Dodgson's sisters 'stammered';[121] and Henry Monro recorded three families, in two of which chorea or epilepsy were also present. One group was characterised by 'mobility', their activities being rapid, irregular and ill-sustained, while in another family, the father and three of the four boys were subject to stuttering, but the three girls were unaffected.[122] Describing the complaint as an unfortunate heirloom, Graves mentions a family in which three generations of males were involved,[123] and Abbotts' experience was similar.[124] However, Shuldham, based on information from Coën, provided the conflicting evidence so typical of this subject: four generations with indirect transmission through the female line (Table 5.3). This was as far as it went. There was no indication that whole counties stuttered,[125] and its reputed prevalence in certain regions was never attributed to heredity.

What conclusions were to be drawn from pedigrees, especially if

Table 5.3: Family Tree Known to Coën

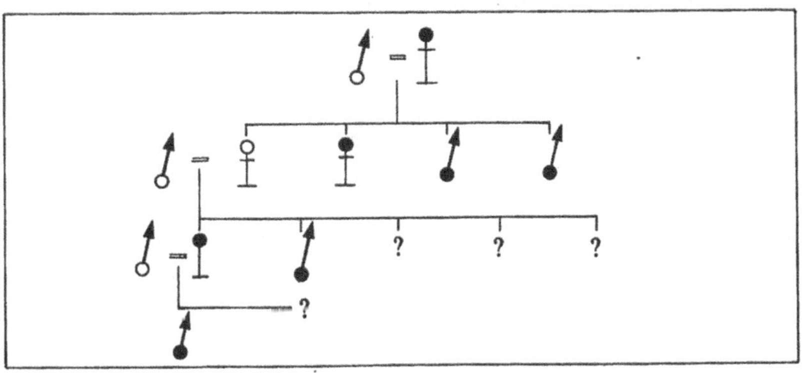

Note: Solid symbols – stutterers.

Source: Drawn from facts supplied in E. Shuldham's *Stammering and Its Rational Treatment*, p. 19.

stuttering were atavistic? The fact that it was 'known to run in families' convinced Cazalet 'that imitation alone may, and often does, produce the defect';[126] certainly more conclusive evidence for heredity would have been its presence in collateral branches of a family, having no contact with stuttering relatives.[127] However, though this was not forthcoming, under the influence of evolutionary theory even associationists were conceding that not all behaviour is learned: in place of innate ideas Bain put innate muscular movements. But what was being inherited? Tyler Smith suggested the imitative faculty.[128] Other writers mostly confined themselves to generalisations about inherent nervous sensitivity, the implication being that stuttering was not the inevitable consequence of circumstance. Monro, for example, postulated that it arose from 'a taint or defect ingrained in the individual from his first separation from the parent stock' and was congenital if not inherited.[129] By the end of the century there was still uncertainty over whether stutterers' nervousness reflected a neurological diathesis or a psychological reaction to their problem. Wyllie contended that it was common in children of 'neuropathic inheritance'.[130] The role of imitation was discounted neither by him nor Colman, who, lacking direct evidence of heredity, nevertheless believed that most stutterers had a neurotic family history and displayed neurotic tendencies.[131] This contention still lacks conclusive evidence.

Problems concerning the mechanism of transmission were rarely raised. If Charles Darwin found it 'unintelligible',[132] elocutionists had scant hope of establishing its operation in stuttering, and even today the matter is controversial. Experimentation in the eighteenth and nineteenth centuries centred largely on plant hybridisation and it was not until this century that the gene was named and found to act in a mendelian fashion. Twin studies and detailed pedigrees have now demonstrated that stuttering is unusually frequent in certain families and it is postulated that subtle neurological factors may underlie the impediment. A modern view is that it is 'something in the nature of a predisposition to faulty speech which is inherited', with certain environmental factors acting as a trigger.[133] We have therefore come full circle, the only difference being that contemporary students deny that imitation is a significant exciting cause.

Disharmonies

Like victims of Parkinsonism, doomed by some inner goad and halter to swing between festinant and frozen motion, conflict is of the essence amongst stutterers. However, their battle for equilibrium may entail surmounting a psychic vacillation, such as afflicted Sartre's uncle Joseph, who, 'trapped between the silence' of his father and the 'scolding' of his mother 'developed a stammer and spent the rest of his life struggling for words'.[134] Victorians may barely have glimpsed the psychodynamics of speech, but they did picture the stutterer as divided against himself in one of several ways, and these conjectures have affinity with the modern breakdown hypothesis, which centres on disorganisation.

Some saw discordancy within the oro-vocal structures. Others believed that the mind and/or brain failed to harmonise with the speech organs, but for Tyler Smith everything turned upon the relationship between voluntary and involuntary motion. And since stuttering spasms appeared only during a desire to speak, he ascribed blame to the voluntary system, in contrast to the view expressed some years before by Magendie. Through their independent but concurrent investigations, this French physiologist and Charles Bell did much to elucidate the function of the spinal nerve roots. The thoughts of both men also turned to stuttering around the same time, but here they were as much at sea as everyone else. Magendie believed that the spasmodic contractions, for which he could find no physiological reason, were understandable through reference to volition. Some articulatory muscles were fully under its control, others only incompletely so and, therefore, performed poorly at will. Drawing comparisons with gargling and swallowing, he states:

> in speaking we form the voice, we articulate, without knowing exactly what movements take place either in the larynx or in the mouth. There are numerous vocal phenomena of which the mechanism is yet far from being known to the physiologist. We will the end, and we attain it; that is all.[135]

Hunt pointed out that such automatic complex acts are governed by an 'organic intelligence', which for Magendie meant instinct, and it is 'this instinct which stutterers are in want of'.[136]

Before coming across Magendie's article, Lee believed he had expressed a similar opinion to the Westminster Medical Society though this seems questionable.[137] For him, fluency depended upon the harmonious interaction of the voluntary and involuntary systems. Speech is dependent on both, dexterity in the former being acquired with difficulty and conscious effort called for to master the latter. In either case, they are vulnerable to emotion, fatigue and debilitation, consonantal articulation being particularly unstable since it requires the concurrence of more voluntary muscles.[138]

Tyler Smith took issue with Magendie over his comparison of articulation with acts like swallowing, often present at birth and independent of learning; over his concept of voluntary action; and over the muscles this encompassed. It is not by knowing what muscles are moved that dexterity is acquired, but by 'gradual association' of the will and certain effects. Nevertheless, laryngeal movements 'are not the less voluntary on this account'. Smith conceived of nervous power as a sort of commodity that became 'trapped' in spasmodic muscles and was unable to continue its action. Often inappropriate muscles were stimulated by a volition that became misdirected along the nerves fanning out from the brain in a manner well portrayed by Müller's analogy.[139] Smith continued:

> This leads me to my view of stammering, which is that volition is, as it were, dispersed at the point where it excites the motor fibres, so that it excites a large number of them, or a different series than would be proper for the effect desired. As a consequence of this dispersion, other muscles contract besides those which are necessary, and by their contrary action put a stop to articulation, or prevent it for a time. An increase of the effort to speak usually adds to the severity of the impediment, and puts a still larger number of muscles in action, until, at length, the right chords happening to be struck, the stream of language flows on, till overtaken by a fresh clog of a similar description.[140]

Though this state could be provoked by emotion, paradoxically, sudden shock could upset the neural conflicts and restore harmony.

Not surprisingly, disunity was central to analyses by phrenologists, whose lead in localising an organ of language to the frontal lobes has been well documented.[141] They also responded promptly to the challenge of stuttering through Felix Voisin, a stutterer and court physician, judged to be the greatest authority on phrenology in France, if not the Continent.[142] Voisin published his *Du Bégaiement* in 1821, when his argument was based upon a fundamental phrenological tenet:

> . . . it is *the brain* that directs and combines all voluntary notions [*sic*], and consequently every disturbing cause, not local and

> not permanent, can affect the voluntary motions of speech only *through the medium of* the brain; and irregular action of the brain must thus be the indispensible antecedent or cause of the effect – stammering.[143]

Rejecting the traditional approach of speculating on the intellectual operations of the mind, Gall and his followers turned to those biological traits which differentiated species and individuals and were thus more accessible to his empirical method. Having isolated certain behavioural categories and correlated these with organs supposedly existing in the cerebrum,[144] it was conceived that symptoms of insanity resulted from over-excitement of a single or group of organs, which thus dominated the rest. Lack of 'co-operation among the active faculties' might also lead to:

> a *plurality*, instead of to a *unity*, of nervous impulses, and consequently to a *plurality*, instead of to a unity, of simultaneous muscular combinations; and the irregular plurality of purposes and of actions thence resulting constitutes exactly what is called stammering.[145]

This itself reflects:

> a conflict between the *desire* to speak well, the *fear* of speaking ill, or perhaps consciousness of a paucity or bad arrangement of the ideas which he is expected to communicate, or it may be a dearth of words in which to clothe them.[146]

Voisin's ideas reached British readers through Andrew Combe's extracts and comments, which also appeared in Robert Cox's *Selections,*[147] a book reviewed by the *Lancet*, where special note was taken of stuttering.[148] As Combe died in 1847, his nephews, James and Robert Cox(e), who edited the fourteenth edition of the *Principles*, must have been responsible for the passage on stuttering which appeared in that volume. Here it is argued that harmonious muscular activity is more easily disrupted in man, whose highly developed cerebrum confers greater flexibility and independence from instinctual behaviour. The penalty for such freedom is instability, since the automatic centres of the ganglia, medulla and cord have lost their autonomy and become responsive to misdirected or inadequate stimuli that may be set in train by excitement or conflicting emotions, like those liable to precede stuttering.[149]

The only explicit reference to phrenological organs was Cull's conjecture that stutterers' imitative faculty might be unrestrained[150] and another suggestion that they suffered from a deficiency in the organ of time.[151] The latter hypothesis was based upon Steele's theory that spoken language is subject to rhythmical pulsation,[152] the durations of which derive from a sense of timing.

One sympathising with the unproved doctrines of phrenology was the elder Poett, who was struck by the 'conformation' of stutterers' minds on two points: their anticipatory dread of hesitation and their 'hasty conception'.[153] Cull, however, argued against this because everyone produces ideas more speedily than words and stutterers as a group had no outstanding virtues, weaknesses or abilities. Indeed, his experience was that the 'cerebral organisation' varied considerably from patient to patient.[154] The hypothesis that stutterers' minds outstripped their physical capabilities was of ancient origin[155] and found a more recent proponent in the Frenchman, Rullier, who suggested that their speech organs were not commensurate with their lively imagination and intelligence. This 'exuberance of thought' and concomitant increase in 'cerebral irradiations' he likened to a 'fleet of horses in the chase, that left the muscles transfixed and trembling'.[156] In Britain, Borthwick thought this a plausible remote cause and supposed George Combe to have propounded it in his *Constitution of Man*.[157]

The ideas did not find favour with McCormac, who was more impressed by physical disharmonies and was the first British commentator to draw attention to the lack of accord between vocal and articulatory activity, especially when the stutterer was in a hurry.[158] The twofold or threefold division of the speech organs was referred to continuously in relation to the pathogenesis of stuttering, even into this century.[159]

The first man to popularise the idea was Sir Charles Bell, who, like Van Der Kolk, believed that complexity in the neural network bespoke complexity of function. The speech mechanism requires extraordinary co-ordination and he concludes:

> In a person who stutters, the imperfection is obviously in the power of *combination*, not in the defect of any single part. Whilst he cannot *combine* the murmur from the glottis with the action of the pharynx, he can speak in a whisper; that is, he can articulate the faint sound of aspiration, whilst he cannot at the same time vocalize the breath.[160]

As medical artist, anatomist, lecturer, physician and neurophysiologist, whose work on the spinal nerve roots was, like Hall's elucidation of reflexes, described as 'the greatest physiological discovery since Harvey's demonstration of the circulation of the blood',[161] Bell's reputation guaranteed that his views would be widely canvassed, even though they were based neither upon clinical experience nor intensive study. James Wright made much of them, his own contention being that it was the palate that was asynchronous.[162] Meanwhile, Tyler Smith ascribed stutterers' ease in whispering to the fact that as the glottis is then passive, only two neural combinations had to be mastered.[163]

By mid-century, one man to argue the case was Cazalet, who resolved stuttering into 'a simple expression – the want of due equilibrium between vocalisation and articulation'.[164] Poett cited this and Urling's views on causation, both of which he believed to be plagiarisms of his own, namely that the universal reason for stuttering was an endeavour to articulate without corresponding vocalisation, and this theory he claimed to be 'one of the many valuable scientific discoveries of modern times'. He postulated that both mechanisms failed in stage fright, but in stuttering the voice was at fault, with the result that the patient performed a dumb show rather like the bagpipe player who continues fingering his instrument once the bellows have collapsed.[165] Paget's emphasis was rather different. In applying 'stammering' to all those organs involved in sphincteral action, he surmised that the conflict lay between the expulsive muscles and those that must relax in order that this act be completed.[166]

Bristowe's interpretation reflects the growing influence of evolutionary theory upon neurology. He believed that those intricate neuro-muscular skills acquired last, and after laborious learning, were the most easily lost. Spasms might occur in writing or fingering the piano and when they affected speech, stuttering resulted. The articulators were the chief source of disruption, for, compared with the more instinctual breathing apparatus, their movements were highly complex and artificial.[167]

Within a decade, stuttering was again seen as an inco-ordination problem, this time in Wyllie's influential book, where yet another musical metaphor is invoked. Wyllie conceived that lack of promptitude in one speech organ relative to the other was responsible for hesitancy. Foreshadowing modern notions about laryngeal 'pre-setting reflexes', he argued that more usually the vocal mechanism lagged behind, the result being that vowels were not formed in time and the stutterer found himself dwelling upon consonants. He likened the violinist's bow-hand to the vocal mechanism and the string-hand to the oral, whose task was more complicated. The unpractised musician, in attempting to master the strings, was liable to forget that the bow also needed moving.[168]

What were the reasons for disharmony? According to Poett, mental energy was insufficient to permit the two sets of volitions to follow one another speedily and in proper sequence. Exhausted power was also signalled by repetitions, the patient reiterating the same syllable until irritability and excitability diminished and the mind regained the capacity to direct its volitions harmoniously. Poett believed that this 'true theory' admitted of no question since it could be demonstrated by artificial speech organs.[169] Wyllie blamed vocal delay on imperfect innervation, and articulatory spasms on an energy surcharge, which, when of sufficient magnitude, would stimulate contiguous nerves causing contractions in inappropriate muscles. This surcharge resulted from energy being deflected from one mechanism to another.[170] Other writers were still less precise. Inco-ordination was variously ascribed to the 'state' of nerves, 'weakness' of the nervous system, or a 'distraction' of its network. No one tackled the objection, put much earlier by McCormac, that an hypothesis of neural debility was difficult to square with the improvement in stuttering during old age, when the nervous system was enfeebled.[171]

A more thoughtful account came from Monro, who looked at both physical and mental disharmonies and helped popularise the idea that stuttering resulted from asynchrony of the oro-vocal mechanism. In debating whether the spasms of articulatory stuttering were primary or secondary, he favoured the latter view, arguing that they arise from the speaker's efforts to rectify a situation he did not understand by manipulating those muscles most under his conscious control. This inappropriate action was obviated in singing, when the mind focused upon the larynx. Thus, compared with the larynx, in ordinary speech the articulators were disproportionately energetic during stuttering, neural stimuli being unable to maintain both actions in equilibrium.[172] Furthermore, on account of congenital 'morbid irritability', the 'mental force' and 'physical motor power' were poorly matched. Homeostasis was precarious and available nervous power was apt to focus in one area, leaving others depleted. Behaviour followed suit, with simultaneous overactivity and paralysis.[173] This hypothesis, not dissimilar to the phrenologists', was an extension of Cullen's contention that states of 'excitement' and 'collapse' co-existed within the nervous system of insane patients. Their violence stemmed not from greater strength,[174] to be treated by depletory means, but from local irritability causing one centre, often the lower, to dominate. Hughlings Jackson embraced this concept, and, together with Darwin's ideas on evolution and Spencer's on dissolution, framed it into a comprehensive story of neurological breakdown, whereby the most recent skills disintegrated first and lower centres gained control. Applied to language, this shift of function from the complex and voluntary to the primitive and involuntary, left the patient with stereotyped and automatic utterance. Thus, in part, a theory of aphasia derived from one of stuttering.

Monro contended that stuttering children's nervous systems were congenitally depressed. Once movement was willed, the corresponding muscles, being relaxed and unfit for action, became tremulous and more irritable, until spasm supervened. Congenital weakness might disappear, but by this time emotional reactions would perpetuate the cerebro-spinal depression, particularly affecting the facial and respiratory nerves so indicative of one's mental state.[175] This line of thinking was not peculiar to Monro. Wright noted that some children were late talkers, their speech muscles being 'tardy' or 'sluggishly contrary'; if they were also intellectually bright, temperamentally sensitive and subjected to pressures, they would sooner or later stutter.[176]

The final arm of Monro's theory concerned the association of ideas which, being independent of physical and emotional factors, might operate in the absence of upsetting circumstances and after the congenital weakness was resolved. Pure habit remained. But by that time, it had acquired an independent existence.[177]

Associations and Habits

David Hartley's *Observations on Man* (1749), though not making its full impact for some half century,[178] ushered in a new era of associationism. It was also a divide between humoral and psycho-physiological interpretations of speech impediments. Previously, the interrelations of mental phenomena had been studied principally from an epistemological and pedagogic standpoint. Denying any specific distinction between sense and intellect, between animal and human life, English empiricists had considered the motions of mind as reflected in the simultaneity and sequences of images and feelings, designated by Locke 'association of ideas'. Extending the concept to muscular activity, thereby making it relevant to stuttering at two levels, Hartley presented the first comprehensive account of human behaviour based solely on this principle.[179]

As humoral theories went into eclipse, attention focused upon circumstances surrounding the moment of stuttering. This novel approach came from three eighteenth-century physicians, who were impressed by the power of imitation and interested in the muscular associations underlying stuttering: David Hartley, Erasmus Darwin and Alexander Crichton. Each was influenced by traditional English associational philosophy, but Crichton appears to follow the Scottish position on faculties. Though rarely acknowledged, the repeated reference to 'associations' by Victorian speech pathologists indicates that the ideas of Hartley, Darwin and Crichton were authoritative.

Hartley believed that through the interplay of sensation and movement, one conjured up the other and muscular actions flowed smoothly because a given motion tended to invoke the customary sequence. Stuttering arose when 'vibrations' to the mouth were disrupted, often by distressing circumstances. Pronunciation suffered and, once able to appreciate right from wrong, the child repeated as he searched for the correct sound. Hartley also considered the disorder's development and linguistic distribution:

> When the trick of stammering has once begun to take place in a few words, it will extend itself to more and more from very slight resemblances, and particularly to all the first words of sentences, because there the organs pass in an instant from inactivity to action; whereas the subsequent parts of words and sentences may follow the foregoing from association; just as, in repeating *memoriter*, one is most apt to hesitate at the first word in each sentence.[180]

This passage appeared in Rees' *Cyclopaedia*,[181] without acknowledgement, in an article possibly written by Joseph Watson, who certainly subscribed to Hartley's psychology.[182] The only other writer making explicit reference to the father of associationism was his namesake, A.M. Hartley, an elocutionist from Glasgow, who also made mention of Erasmus Darwin.[183]

Darwin, like Priestley, was a stutterer, a member of the Lunar Club and a populariser of associationism. One of his premisses was that: 'All animal motions which have occurred at the same time or in immediate succession, become so connected, that when one of them is reproduced, the other has a tendency to accompany or succeed it.'[184] This muscular connection he called *association*, the reciprocal stimulation of muscular and sensory motions being termed *catenation*. Speech impediments and the like arose when sensations, catenated with voluntary actions, were disrupted by feelings such as awe or bashfulness. With automatic connections severed, the patient fell back upon his will.[185] This rarely provided a solution, for what residual connections remained were liable to be clouded by the voluntary energy, especially if this were strong or engaged the attention.[186] In stuttering, disruption usually occurs between the initial consonant and following vowel,[187] the former being more voluntary:

> Hence when the mind of the stammerer is vehemently employed on some idea of ambition of shining, or fear of not succeeding, the associations of the motions of the muscles of articulation with each other become dissevered by this great exertion, and he endeavours in vain by voluntary efforts to rejoin the broken association. For this purpose he continues to repeat the first syllable . . . and strives in vain, by various distortions of countenance, to produce the next links, which are subject to association.[188]

Thus, whereas for David Hartley the repetitive symptom is an attempt to correct faulty articulation, for Darwin it is an effort to awaken habitual patterns. His idea, in principle, resembles modern discussions about stutterers' failure to initiate 'automatic serial responses' or 'dysautomaticity', which has been seen in the context of servo theory. Essentially, all skilled acts demanding 'motor planning' are liable to be upset through self-consciousness, on which account these conjectures have been classed as a form of the anticipatory struggle hypothesis.[189]

Rather than actually having articulated incorrectly, Crichton suggests that the child is uncertain how a sound should be said, and so:

> he then begins to pronounce in a different way, and the doubt again arises; he then returns back to the last pronounced syllable of the word, and repeats it, but upon coming to the letter the *doubt* again arises, and gives a different direction to the sensorial impression, and he again attempts to speak another letter. He cannot stop, for he is in the middle of a word, the pronunciation of which he has been accustomed to conclude, and he therefore continues to *struggle* with it, till at last, owing to some accidental causes, which it is not easy to discover, he accomplishes its proper utterance.[190]

It is noteworthy that Crichton, in particular, draws attention to doubt and struggle, two concepts that have preoccupied certain modern authors. Crichton, however, was primarily interested in the will and, looking at stuttering from this angle, he classed it as a disorder of volition, the will being uncertain rather than inconstant. A similar idea was later forwarded by Wyneken, in Germany, in contrast to Merkel, who postulated weakness of will.[191]

Crichton restricted doubt to pronunciation but Cull, applying the philosophy of 'suggestion' (the term preferred by Berkeley and Brown), extended it to stuttering itself, and thereby indicated how the complaint was self-augmenting:

1. memory of the hesitation
2. doubt regarding the present utterance, leading to:
3. another hesitation.[192]

Dread was commonly mentioned in connection with stuttering: Melville Bell,[193] Borthwick[194] and Gerdts all took note of its effects upon respiration. Gerdts was similarly explicit about its repercussions upon the psyche. Assuming there to be at least 100 faults a day, he states that after a number of years the child 'must have the thought "I shall stutter if I speak" firmly imprinted in his mind'.[195] Gerdts, and those of like persuasion, must therefore also be numbered as forerunners of the anticipatory struggle hypothesis.

Crichton was interested both in the will and forensic psychiatry and this led him to a novel and dynamic interpretation of bizarre behaviour, which he saw as invariably containing an inner logic – the madman always has a motive. As regards stuttering, this motive appears simply to have been conceived as an attempt to re-establish customary articulatory sequences and neither he, nor later Victorians, were tempted to speculate upon warped subconscious urges, such as are now postulated by the repressed need hypothesis.

Crichton envisaged two types of ideas: those that stayed in the mind and those having corporeal effects. The latter were initiated voluntarily, under sway of pleasure or pain. Action was determined by whether desire or aversion predominated and the will was free to the extent that it could deliberate. These ideas were further distinguished by their end product. Mental ideas, having only one term, cannot co-exist but they may compete:

> When two different shades of the same thought arise in quick succession, each of which necessarily has a tendency to affect the same set of nerves, the influence of the one is partially destroyed . . . and

> an incomplete bodily action takes place. If a sudden thought makes a person . . . imagine that there is a better expression for his thoughts than that which he is about to employ, the action is immediately interrupted, and he either stops, or stammers.[196]

Often arising from harsh discipline, Crichton saw it as ranging in severity from hesitancy to stuttering, a distinction not dissimilar to Wright's 'mental stammering' and 'stuttering'.

On the physical side, Crichton observed that one idea may have many terms, a whole train of action being common, and he asks: 'How the representation of a single letter in the mind is sufficient to produce such a complicated bodily effect?' Like Darwin, he believed that during learning each intention terminated in a single action, but eventually the will inhibits subsequent terms and, through a 'principle of concatenation', the sequence gradually sinks below consciousness. One wish is then enough to instigate the whole movement which can be combined with other such skills,[197] as when a person accompanies himself on the piano. This analysis of learning was mentioned throughout the nineteenth century stuttering literature, and credited to Neil Arnott, who, like Crichton, compared speech acquisition to the fingering of an instrument. Arnott noted that some acquired musical skills including speech by ear, whereas others needed intensive tuition if they were to pass muster. Stutterers, since they suffered from 'naturally weak or irregular association', came into the latter category.[198]

Habit was an integral part of association theory, since it was the legacy of past associations and the present evidence of their existence. The explanation of its mechanism went back to Aristotle and most psychologists accepted his three laws of contrast, similarity and closeness, whether in time, place, relation or society, some reducing all to a form of contiguity. Repetition was held responsible for the varying speed and strength of associations, and it was not until Thomas Brown's *Lectures*, containing nine secondary laws, that other factors received consideration. He pointed to the length, intensity, duration and recency of the connection. No one thought to analyse the growth of stuttering in such specific terms. The nearest attempt came from A.M. Hartley who illustrates with the word *mother*: 'the syllable *mo* is not organically more difficult to pronounce when joined to *ther*, than when alone', but the patient 'has been *habituated* to associate a *stammer* with the entire word' and second nature asserts her prerogative.[199] Nowadays, such words may be considered to be emotionally charged, but this factor was not explored by Victorians. Hartley's theory is expressed through a tortuous argument and derives from his namesake's remarks on laughter, crying and emotional lability in children. During these states they switch rapidly from pleasure to pain and concomitant diaphragmatic disruptions, if transferred to speech, occasion stuttering. Indeed, all behaviour patterns tend to widen their associations until the 'faintest resemblance of the original cause' is sufficient to excite them.[200] Once habitual, the secondary stage of stuttering had begun, according to Cazalet,[201] whose brief comments indicate a shift away from classifying stuttering anatomically.

Thomas Brown also maintained that a person's psycho-physical condition influenced the efficacy of associations and though no one explicitly applied this to stuttering, it was recognised that intense emotional states could initiate or fix the habit. Statistics were few (Tables 5.1 and 5.2) and less impressive than anecdotes. Thelwall tells of a teacher who forced his pupil under a horse's belly until 'convulsive terror produced a stammering that has afflicted him ever since', and of a Lancashire labourer suspending a young lad over a canal bridge 'till he was almost dead with terror and convulsive agitation'.[202] Then there was the hapless negro girl, whose stuttering commenced after being captured and shipped to Istanbul as a slave.[203] If one traumatic episode was enough to start the problem, constant fear of criticism and teasing could perpetuate associations, especially in the school room, when speech itself became the focus of nervousness. Paradoxically, emotion could also disrupt habitual patterns and facilitate unexpected eloquence, as Martin Tupper discovered on 18 June, while strolling through Lincoln's Inn Fields. On seeing the Duke of Wellington mobbed by a gang of reformers, he lept to the steps of Surgeon's Hall, and cried: 'Waterloo'. The effect was dramatic: 'That one word turned the tide of execrations into cheers' and the duke passed by him 'silently with a military salute'.[204]

Bodily states could likewise enhance or weaken the associational links and the best attempt to explain this was Monro's equilibrium theory. Over-reaction, signalling weakness rather than strength, predominates when health is delicate. In the two contrary conditions of fitness and exhaustion, stuttering improves. In the first instance, because good general tone keeps excesses in check; in the second, because nervous energy is spent, which accounts for why fluency may be regained towards evening.[205]

Associationism, as a primitive learning theory, was bound up with memory and the related subject of imagination. Aristotle noted its relationship with stuttering,[206] and Cull's developmental sequence has already been recorded. Bryan argued that the pronunciation of certain sounds was not inherently more difficult, as stutterers claimed, but only imagined to be so. Taking a wider view, Monro referred to the fatal power of imagination amongst primitives condemned by the Obey-man. Likewise stutterers have a morbid tendency to dwell upon certain words or situations, which they come to abhor, and this furnished Monro with another example of the correspondence between cerebral imbalance and mental pathology. In this case, equilibrium between reason and imagination is lost, partly because the patient is unable to comprehend so subtle a disorder, which, no longer within the ambit of reason, is abandoned to the free play of fanciful imagery. At this point, hesitation becomes stuttering.[207]

These accounts served to answer some questions, if the argument was that stuttering reflected a heightened imagination during puberty and its diminution with age. But it failed to explain why girls, in whom imagination was supposed to outstrip reason, were less affected; nor why it improved in the elderly, when habits are so fixed.

From the foregoing discussion two observations may be made. First, Victorian speech pathologists spoke less precisely than their immediate predecessors and were content to talk vaguely about 'associations' without specifying whether they meant ideas or movements, nor cogitating the sequence of events leading to the spasm. To some extent, this mirrors a general neglect of motion before Bain, but it is significant that Müller, who influenced Bain and derived his own ideas from Erasmus Darwin,[208] was as vague as his contemporaries on this point. Rooted in empiricist epistemology, associationism conceived the mind as highly malleable, its inner theatre totally determined by impinging impressions. Bain restored activity to knowledge through his emphasis on learning by doing, a fact that elocutionists implicitly recognised but failed to discuss, partly because their concern with the mechanics of speech production deflected attention from the actual learning process.

Secondly, it is apparent that eighteenth- and nineteenth-century thinkers began treading paths that are now well worn. This does not mean that contemporary ideas necessarily have any direct connection with the past, but rather that certain lines of enquiry have had a perennial attraction for investigators. Modern aetiological speculations have been placed into five groups.[209] Two of these, the perseverative theory and the repressed need hypothesis have no Victorian analogues. However, West's conception of stuttering as a miniscule convulsion bears resemblance to early discussions on spasms, though it is epilepsy rather than chorea upon which his theory pivots and which is examined from an organic rather than a symptomatic standpoint. Likewise, reflections upon speech discordancies and associations have aspects corresponding with the breakdown and anticipatory struggle hypotheses respectively. Moreover, there is a measure of agreement over the role of heredity in stuttering. Finally, though a far cry from Marshall Hall's conjecture about the uvula being the excito-regulator of articulation, modern theories analysing the complaint in terms of instrumental or operant conditioning[210] are traceable to him through the behaviourist school of psychology with its dependence on Pavlov's work, which was the experimental extension of Bain's marriage of reflexes and associationism. Current language may be different, but underlying it is a common orientation. While modern learning theorists speak of the 'environmental events and internal processes that influence the acquisition and extinction of stimulus-response relationships'[211] and 'reinforcements', Victorians looked to the exciting and predisposing causes responsible for the habit, and they provided anecdotes illustrating both these and the perpetuating causes.

Notes

1. Hunter and Macalpine, pp. 779-81, 1052-7.
2. Ibid., pp. 860-4.
3. Bacc. Med. Oxon., pp. v, 1, 2, 24, 27-8. Cf. Gerdts, pp. 53, 64.
4. Hunter and Macalpine, pp. 473-8.
5. Physician, p. 21.
6. MacDonald Critchley, 'The Beginnings of the National Hospital, Queen's Square (1859-1860)', *British Medical Journal*, 1 (1960), p. 1835 (1829-37).
7. John Syer Bristowe, *A Treatise on the Theory and Practice of Medicine* (London, Smith, Elder, & Co., 1876), pp. 945-50, 1002, 1005-9, 1053.
8. Blake, p. 4.
9. G.H. Brown (Compl.), *Lives of the Fellows of the Royal College of Physicians of London, 1826-1925* (London, The College, 1955), p. 92.
10. Bristowe (1880), pp. 94-197.
11. Henry Monro, *Remarks on Insanity* (London, John Churchill, 1851), p. 11. Possibly this admission was prompted by a review of his *On Stammering*, *London Medical Gazette*, 10 n.s. (1850), p. 30 (28-30).
12. *DNB*, vol. 13, p. 633.
13. Jones, pp. 153, 155.
14. Hunter and Macalpine, pp. 560-3.
15. Pershing, p. 777.
16. J.L.C.S. Van Der Kolk does not use the term 'dysarthria' but he makes some interesting observations on the neuro-anatomy of the brain stem serving articulation, see his *On the Minute Structure and Functions of the Spinal Cord*, trans. William Daniel Moore (London, New Sydenham Society, 1859), pp. 140-69.
17. Blake, p. 18.
18. *Mind, Breath*, p. 12.

19. Yearsley (1841), p. 5.
20. John Syer Bristowe, *Clinical Lectures and Essays on Diseases of the Nervous System* (London, Smith, Elder & Co., 1888), pp. 12-13.
21. Gerdts, pp. 11, 30, 40, 53, 64.
22. 'Stammering', *British Medical Journal*, 1 (1922), p. 666. Cf. 'Stammering', *British Medical Journal*, 1 (1922), p. 546.
23. See, for example, Isador H. Coriat, 'The Psychoanalytic Conception of Stammering', *The Nervous Child (N.Y.)*, 2 (1943), 167-71.
24. A. Bernard, p. 1.
25. Bristowe (1883), p. 843.
26. Hooper's *Medical Dictionary* (1820), pp. 602-16. Cf. Lennox Browne, *The Throat and its Diseases*, 2nd edn (London, Baillière, Tindall & Cox, 1887), p. 480.
27. William P. Alison, 'Of Spasmodic Disease' in *Outlines of Pathology and Practice of Medicine* (Edinburgh, William Blackwood & Sons, 1844), p. 698 (698-716).
28. *Garrison's History of Neurology*, rev. Lawrence C. McHenry (Springfield, Illinois, Charles C. Thomas, 1969), pp. 290-1.
29. Report of a memoir by M. Colombat, read to the French Academy of Medicine, 4 July 1843, 'New System for Curing Stammering', *Lancet*, 2 (1842-3), 746-7; Minute Philosopher, pp. 5-6; 'Stammering', *Lancet*, 1 (1878), 877-8.
30. McCormac, p. 13. Cf. H.R. Bramwell, 'An Anomaly in Stammering', letter to *Lancet*, 1 (1888), p. 257; Colman (1895), p. 1419. For an analogy with migraine see M.D., *British Medical Journal*, 2 (1893), p. 1311.
31. Blake, pp. 18-19. Cf. Kussmaul, p. 835.
32. Van Riper, pp. 49, 345. For modern approaches to tremor see ibid., pp. 130-2; S. Fibiger, 'Stuttering Explained as a Physiological Temor', *Speech Transmission Laboratory: Quarterly Progress and Status Reports*, 2-3, ed. G. Fant (Stockholm, Royal Institute of Technology, 1971), pp. 1-23.
33. McCormac, pp. 16, 56.
34. Romberg, pp. 321, 362-3.
35. Bristowe [1882], p. 1512, (1892), p. 1192. Cf. *The Nomenclature of Diseases drawn up by a Joint Committee appointed by the Royal College of Physicians of London*, 2nd edn (London, Harrison & Son, 1885), p. 27.
36. Rosenthal, pp. 113, 131, 133.
37. George Vivian Poore, 'Craft Palsies' in *A System of Medicine*, ed. Thomas Clifford Allbutt (London, Macmillan & Co., 1899), vol. 3, 17-18.
38. Robley Dunglison, *Medical Lexicon*, 15th edn (London, Trübner, 1857), p. 866.
39. Paget, p. 437; J. Paget, 'On Stammering with other Organs than those of Speech', *British Medical Journal*, 2 (1868), p. 149; discussed by Haward, p. 112. Cf. Bishop, p. 61.
40. Cited by Walter Houghton, in *The Victorian Frame of Mind* (New Haven, Yale UP, 1970), p. 226.
41. Rockey (1977), p. 89.
42. Kussmaul, pp. 787-8.
43. Poett jnr, pp. viii, 19-22, 32.
44. Dr Schultze, 'Stuttering occasioned by Worms' abstracted in *British and Foreign Medical Review*, 3 (1837), p. 231. See also: Abbotts, p. 47; E. Behnke [1893], p. 27; Physician, p. 33. Cf. Shuldham, p. 31.
45. Wyllie, pp. 408-9.
46. The sources of these views are too numerous to mention. Representative discussions are to be found in: Physician, pp. 11, 12, 15, 16, 21, 25-6, 31, 32-3, 40-1, 42, 43, 65; Bacc. Med. Oxon., pp. 16, 27, 28, 41, 43.

47. Metropolitan Free Hospital, 'Treatment of Stammering', *Provincial Medical and Surgical Journal*, 2 (1841), p. 91 (91-2).
48. Westminster Medical Society (1840-1a), 24-5.
49. Blake, p. 16.
50. Poett jnr, p. 25.
51. Editorial (1846b), p. 663.
52. Franklin Fearing, *Reflex Action* (New York, Hafner, 1964), pp. 1-14, 122-45.
53. Sir Geoffrey Jefferson, 'Marshall Hall, the Grasp Reflex and the Diastaltic Spinal Cord', in *Science, Medicine and History*, ed. E. Ashworth Underwood (London, Oxford UP, 1953), vol 2, p. 311 (302-20).
54. Marshall Hall, *New Memoir on the Nervous System* (London, Bäillière, 1843), p. 89.
55. These ideas were further developed in a paper read before the Royal Society on 2 June 1833, see Marshall Hall, 'On the Reflex Function of the Medulla Oblongata and Medulla Spinalis', *Philosophical Transactions of the Royal Society of London*, 123 (1833), 635-63. This became Memoir I of his *Memoirs on the Nervous System* (London, Sherwood, Gilbert, & Piper, 1837), pp. 1-40.
56. Hall, *New Memoir*, pp. 45-6.
57. Marshall Hall, *Synopsis of the Diastaltic Nervous System* (London, printers Joseph Mallet, [1852]), p. 13.
58. Hall, *New Memoir*, p. 63.
59. Hall, *Synopsis*, p. vii.
60. Marshall Hall, *Lectures on the Nervous System and its Diseases* (London, Sherwood, Gilbert, & Piper, 1836), p. 155.
61. Hall (1841), pp. 194-5.
62. Ibid., p. 195.
63. Ibid.
64. Westminster Medical Society (1840-1a), pp. 24-5.
65. Marshall Hall, 'Lectures on the Theory and Practice of Medicine', *Lancet*, 2 (1837-38), 71-2.
66. Hall, *Synopsis*, p. 60.
67. Marshall Hall, 'Irritability' in *The Cyclopaedia of Anatomy and Physiology*, ed. Robert Todd (London, Longman, 1839-47), vol. 3, 29-31.
68. Fearing, *Reflex Action*, pp. 141-5. Cf. Bishop (1851), p. 55.
69. Young, pp. 116-17.
70. Bacc. Med. Oxon., pp. 23-7.
71. Though only brief, some reasons are to be found in Copland, p. 1362. This article is notable for its lengthy bibliography. See also above p. 58.
72. Cited in a letter from George Webster to Marshall Hall, *Lancet*, 2 (1846), p. 200.
73. Carpenter, p. 352.
74. Abbotts, p. 46.
75. Shuldham, pp. 59, 60.
76. Lee, p. 23.
77. Bishop (1851), pp. 61-3. The text of this passage was first delivered to the Medical Society of London in a paper on 'Certain Derangements of the Voluntary and Automatic Functions relating to the Circulation of the Blood, Respiration, Voice, and Speech', *London Medical Gazette*, 6 n.s. (1848), 117-19. Cf. above pp. 97-8.
78. Book Reviews, *Lancet*, 2 (1846), 224-5.
79. Edwin Clarke, 'Marshall Hall' in *Dictionary of Scientific Biography*, ed. Charles Gillispie (New York, Charles Scribner's, 1972), vol. 6, p. 60 (58-61).
80. Jefferson in *Science, Medicine . . .*, pp. 309, 317.
81. Potter, pp. 55, 62, 72.

82. Report of Lichtinger's papers, *British and Foreign Medical Review*, 20 (1845), p. 556; Kussmaul, pp. 835, 836.
83. Book Reviews, *Lancet*, 2 (1846), p. 157 (154-7).
84. Book Reviews, *Lancet*, 2 (1846), pp. 245-6 (244-7).
85. Jefferson in *Science, Medicine . . .*, pp. 304, 317.
86. Charlotte Hall, *Memoirs of Marshall Hall* (London, Richard Bentley, 1861), p. xvi.
87. *DNB*, vol. 18, 575-6; Obituary, *Lancet*, 1 (1873), 825-6.
88. See below pp. 214-15.
89. See Richard Dawson, *The London and Provincial Directory Unmasked* (London, Hughes & Hughes, 1849), p. 4; Thomas Hunt's letter to *The Medical Times*, 14 (1846), p. 261 and the editorial comment to Yearsley's reply in the same volume, p. 282. All three men state that Smith was Yearsley's brother-in-law. The *DNB* says he was a son-in-law. As Yearsley and Smith were only ten years apart in age, and died within four years of each other, the former relationship seems the most probable.
90. Editorial (1846a), p. 558.
91. Reviews, *Lancet*, 2 (1846), p. 156.
92. Ibid.
93. W. Tyler Smith, *Parturition and the Principles and Practice of Obstetrics* (London, John Churchill, 1849), p. vii.
94. Reviews, *Lancet*, 2 (1846), pp. 186-9.
95. Reviews, *Lancet*, 2 (1846), p. 156.
96. Thelwall (1810), p. 59. Cf. Bartlett, pp. 44, 50-1.
97. *Unspeakable*, p. 20.
98. McCormac, pp. 37-8; Minute Philosopher, p. 4; Shuldham, p. 25; Wright (1835), pp. 22-3; Urling, p. 53. Cf. Blake, p. 8, who suggests that one Hebrew word for stuttering – *lah-gehg* – really means 'mocking'. It seems more likely, however, that this meaning is derived, since the root *lcg* connotes a gurgling sound in the throat and hence indistinct speech on this account.
99. Poett jnr, p. 32.
100. Hunt (1861), p. 149.
101. Hunt (1870), p. 236n. Cf. Shuldham, pp. 21-3; McCormac, p. 43; *Unspeakable*, p. 107.
102. Elizabeth Longford, *Victoria R.I.* (London, Pan Books, 1966), p. 214.
103. Hunter & Macalpine, pp. 640-1.
104. Cull (1835), pp. 29-30.
105. Wright (1839), p. 3.
106. Edmund Burke, *The Beautiful and the Sublime* (Oxford, 1796), pp. 142, 156.
107. Beasley (1905), p. 135.
108. Now Hertford College.
109. W.P. Alison, 'Observations on the Physiological Principle of Sympathy chiefly in reference to the peculiar doctrines of Mr. Charles Bell', *Transactions of the Medico-Chirurgical Society of Edinburgh*, 2 (1826), 165-228.
110. Poett jnr, p. 21.
111. Bartlett, p. 44. Cf. A.M. Bell (1900), p. 234.
112. Hunt (1870), p. 341.
113. Caleb, p. 147.
114. Shuldham, p. 18.
115. Krauss, *Erasmus Darwin*, pp. 40, 80-1; *The Autobiography of Charles Darwin*, ed. Francis Darwin (1892) (New York, Dover, 1958), p. 94.
116. E. Darwin, *Temple of Nature*, p. 45.
117. Poett snr (1833), pp. 32-3.
118. Luchsinger, *Folia Phoniatrica*, 22, p. 217.

119. Beasley (1885), p. 52.
120. XYZ, pp. 5-6.
121. 'Speech Impediments in the Dodgson Family', *Jabberwocky*, no. 3 (1970), p. 2.
122. Bacc. Med. Oxon., pp. 41-2; cf. Blake, p. 17.
123. Graves, p. 660.
124. Abbotts, p. 17.
125. Wright (1835), p. 24.
126. Cazalet, p. 15.
127. Physician, p. 13.
128. Ibid. Cf. Thelwall (1810), p. 123; Cull (1833), p. 20.
129. Bacc. Med. Oxon., p. 24. Cf. ibid., pp. 27-9, 31n; Monro, *Remarks*, p. 11.
130. Wyllie, pp. 22-3.
131. Colman (1899), pp. 450-1.
132. Hunt (1870), p. 284.
133. Beech and Fransella, pp. 24, 83-6, 103-4.
134. Jean-Paul Sartre, *Words* (1964) (Harmondsworth, Penguin Books, 1967), p. 12. Dr Sartre did not speak to his wife for 40 years and communicated by signs at meals.
135. Magendie, cited by Lee, pp. 8-9. Cf. Hunt (1870), p. 94; Physician, p. 29.
136. Hunt (1870), pp. 94-5.
137. Lee, p. 7. This was probably a reference to the meeting reported in the *Lancet*, 2 (1840-1), 77-8.
138. Ibid., pp. 9-10, 22.
139. Physician, pp. 21-31.
140. Ibid., pp. 24-5.
141. Young, pp. 134-43, 146, 147, 148-9.
142. 'Intelligence', *Phrenological Journal*, 5 n.s. (1842), p. 87.
143. Review of *Du Bégaiement* . . ., pp. 459-60.
144. Young, pp. 18-37.
145. Review of *Du Bégaiement* . . ., p. 460.
146. Ibid.
147. Robert Cox (ed.), *Selections from the Phrenological Journal* (Edinburgh, MacLachlan & Stewart, 1836), pp. 143-51, where Andrew Combe is named as the reviewer of Voisin's book.
148. Book Review, *Lancet*, 1 (1836-7), 107-8.
149. Combe, pp. 248-9. According to the *DNB* (vol. 4, 1341-2), his brother, Robert, also assisted in editing it.
150. Cull (1833), p. 20.
151. 'Observations on the Faculty by which we perceive and compare the divisions of Duration or Time', *Phrenological Journal*, 4 (1826-7), 516-17 (509-23).
152. Rockey (1977), p. 86.
153. Poett snr (1828), pp. 49-50.
154. Cull (1833), pp. 22-3.
155. Aristotle, *Problems*, 903b 23.
156. McCormac, pp. 65-9. Cf. Gerdts, p. 36; Kussmaul, p. 836.
157. Borthwick, pp. 48-9.
158. McCormac, p. 35.
159. See three articles in a controversy headed 'Stammering – What Is It?', *Lancet*, 1 (1922), pp. 960-1, 1130; 2 (1922), p. 54.
160. C. Bell, p. 317. Emphases added.
161. Neuberger, cited in *Garrison's History*, p. 189. Cf. ibid., p. 274.
162. See above p. 119.
163. Physician, pp. 26-7.

164. Cazalet, p. 17; Poett jnr, p. xxviii. Cf. Abbotts, p. 24; Bishop, p. 67; Hunt (1861), p. 139.
165. Poett jnr, pp. vi, xi-xxxvi, 13-16, 19. Cf. Urling, pp. 12-16, 19, 22-6, 29-30, 43-4, 46-7, 49, 51-3; Bacc. Med. Oxon., p. 5 on the bagpipe analogy.
166. Paget, p. 437. Cf. Kirkes' *Handbook*, p. 533.
167. Bristowe (1883), p. 844.
168. Wyllie, pp. 1-3, 18-20, 23.
169. Poett jnr, pp. 18-19.
170. Wyllie, pp. 2-3, 18-19.
171. McCormac, pp. 64-5. Cf. ibid., pp. 39-40.
172. Bacc. Med. Oxon., pp. 8, 36-7.
173. Monro, *Remarks*, pp. 10-19.
174. Ibid., 'A Syllabus of the Argument'.
175. Bacc. Med. Oxon., pp. 33-5.
176. Wright (1839), pp. 36-7.
177. Bacc. Med. Oxon., pp. 37-8.
178. W.B. Pillsbury, *The History of Psychology* (London, George Allen & Unwin, 1929), p. 97.
179. Howard Warren, *A History of Association Psychology* (London, Constable, 1921), pp. 5-8, 47, 56, 67-9.
180. D. Hartley, vol. 1, 260-1. Capitals omitted.
181. 'Stammering', *The Cyclopaedia*, ed. Abraham Rees (London, Longman, 1819, but probably written 1816), vol. 33. Cf. 'Larynx', vol. 20, giving an organic interpretation of stuttering.
182. Watson, *Instruction of the Deaf and Dumb*, pp. 3-4, 20-33.
183. A.M. Hartley, p. 30.
184. E. Darwin, vol. 1, p. 30.
185. Ibid., p. 189.
186. Ibid., pp. 192-3.
187. Ibid., vol 2, p. 505.
188. Ibid., vol. 1, p. 193.
189. Bloodstein, pp. 30-2, 34.
190. Crichton, vol. 2, p. 82. Emphases added.
191. Kussmaul, pp. 834, 837.
192. Cull (1835), pp. 31-2. Cf. Bloodstein, p. 183.
193. A.M. Bell (1900), p. 253.
194. Borthwick, pp. 23-4.
195. Gerdts, pp. 33, 39, 42, 61, 64.
196. Crichton, p. 79.
197. Ibid., pp. 74-8.
198. Arnott (1827), pp. 587-8.
199. A.M. Hartley, p. 55.
200. Ibid., p. 34.
201. Cazalet, p. 18.
202. Thelwall (1810), p. 55.
203. Hunt (1870), p. 353n.
204. Tupper, *My Life*, p. 66.
205. Bacc. Med. Oxon., pp. 42-3.
206. *Problems*, 903b 21.
207. Bacc. Med. Oxon., pp. 7, 29, 51-3.
208. Young, pp. 96n, 114-21.
209. Bloodstein, pp. 26-35.
210. Gene Brutten and Donald Shoemaker, 'A Two-Factor Learning Theory of Stuttering', in Travis' *Handbook*, pp. 1035-72.
211. Ibid., p. 1035.

6 THERAPEUTIC PRACTICES

There are few conditions 'in which so many contrarieties exist' as stuttering,[1] and no subject posed such barriers to lucid exposition.[2] Its cure was seen as problematic and straightforward;[3] possible, but improbable.[4] Kingsley, for example, believed it to be 'perfectly curable', though the possibility of finding a cure was 'literally worse than none'.[5] Over 20 years after two authorities had asserted that the remedy was simple,[6] *The Unspeakable* related a series of abortive cures that were not confined to its imaginary hero.

Lack of ingenuity was not the reason for uncured stutterers. By 1828, the disparate remedial fashions that are still associated with the disorder were already apparent, for Poett was prompted to write: 'Various means have, from time to time, been devised for the removal of Impediments of Speech; but, after floating for a short time on the tide of public favour, they all successively sunk into merited oblivion.'[7] Past failures, rather than provoking discouragement, acted as a spur. Their challenge led to the search for a trustworthy system. With Itard, McCormac asserted that 'thousands of years' had 'elapsed without any individual having ever been able to discover and communicate to the world any means by which this distressing affliction could be alleviated',[8] yet he felt confident of his own infallible cure. The numbers claiming to have elucidated stuttering suggests a steady climb along the road of inventive brilliance, from Broster's 'perfectly original discovery'[9] in 1825, judged second only to Jenner's in his time,[10] to Ball's 'great discovery' at the end of the century.[11] Much of this was bravura, for success in a *laissez-faire* economy often depended upon creating confidence. Practitioners were entrepreneurs, cognisant of the value of showmanship, and the individualism they embodied was reflected in their various systems. Many believed, with Chapman,[12] that the system was all, and this gave it an economic importance which fostered secrecy. But commitment to a system was not without its benefits, for the enthusiasm it generated provided the remedial programme with perhaps its most vital element.

In commending their individual systems to all in need, Victorian elocutionists were not entirely self-interested. Ideally, it was best to forestall stuttering by the judicious selection of household staff, whose speech should be distinct and slow, so that the child would have a fit model to imitate.[13] But if a problem developed, treatment should begin early, before habit took root. M'Minn even went so far as to suggest it start in the 'cradle', and he was probably right in thinking that this was an original proposal.[14] Contrary to popular and also some medical opinion, children were unlikely to outgrow it.[15] Given prompt attention, Beasley anticipated a 95 per cent cure rate.[16] Alexander Bell treated five-year-olds,[17] and Abbotts thought prognosis was most favourable between the ages of seven and sixteen, though he had worked with people over sixty.[18] However, probably most patients were teenagers or young adults, and since their problem was then more severe and their need most pressing, they were likely to have a greater degree of determination. Those to whom they looked for help varied considerably in educational background and philosophical outlook. Also varied were the price and length of cures, which might be effected through correspondence courses and through treatment in diversified locales, including residential institutions.

Practitioners

The multifarious factors provoking investigations into stuttering undoubtedly contributed to the intellectual range and growth of the discipline, but it did not lead to a balanced and unified group offering a uniform standard of treatment. The divisions were roughly threefold: stutterers and non-stutterers; medical men and elocutionists; quacks and bona fide therapists. Such fundamental divisions not only hindered mutual understanding, but made for positive friction. However, since the groups were not mutually exclusive, allegiances were not always predictable.

The best therapist, it was argued, was a former stutterer, who understood the anguish and was well placed to pass on personally tested advice. Certainly many practitioners on the Continent[19] and in America[20] were former stutterers. And, unlike today, this was true of Britain in the persons of Beasley, Bernard, Bryan, Borthwick, Caleb, M'Minn, Monro, Palmer, Solly, XYZ and Mr Julion.[21] Some would have felt with Kingsley that 'Every stammerer is to me a friend at once, by unity of sorrow: – after all, perhaps the most sacred unity on earth'.[22] This was in accord with *Balbus balbum rectius intelligit* – 'a stammerer understands a stammerer more correctly than any one else does' – said to be an old proverb,[23] probably deriving from the Latin saying in St Jerome's *Works*, namely, *balbum melius balbi verba cognoscere*.

Against this, Mason pointed out that the logical outcome was that physicians could only cure diseases to which they themselves had been subject. Further: 'It is not by means of the *feelings* that the cure of stammering is effected, but by a knowledge of the *nature of the infirmity*.'[24] Mason thus overlooks the fact that even the most ignorant and unscrupulous quack has had his successes.

Some physicians stuttered, but others entered the therapeutic arena believing their physiological knowledge conferred special insights. Physicians who appear to have engaged in speech treatment, at least for a period, were Abbotts, Abercrombie, Arnott, Blake, Bishop, Lewin, McCormac, Shuldham, the two Poetts, Yearsley, the anonymous XYZ,[25] and possibly Bartlett, Colman, Monro, Palmer, Tyler Smith and Wyllie. Aside from these specialist physicians, medical ideas on the management of stuttering were poor, and no dentists seem to have been consistently engaged in treatment.

Elocutionists were a more heterogenous group. Clergy, by virtue of their calling, had a special interest in speech and were directed to the relief of suffering. It is hard to gauge their numbers. Perhaps only a minority published treatises, but pastoral duties must have brought many into contact with sufferers, some anxious to join their ranks. Prayer was an obvious form of advice, though whether the 'fanatic' who 'pretended to effect a cure by prayer, and supernatural agency' was a cleric is not clear.[26] His pupils were duped, but Martin Tupper, a religious man who had beaten Gladstone for the theological prize at Christ Church, maintained that prayer had succeeded where the doctors failed.[27]

The Reverends Bryan, Cazalet, Chapman, D'Orsey, Evans, Plumptre, Sandlands and Foster were broadly in line with the new elocutionary movement, which placed high value on verbal excellence. Typical of this tradition in its later stages was Joe Edgar Foster whose manly presence, rich flexible voice, intellectual and highly emotional countenance and graceful, majestic gestures made him a most popular speaker.[28] Foster, a Cambridge graduate, was a pupil of François Delsarte, the teacher of vocal music and operatic acting in Paris, whose influence appears to have been much greater in America.[29] Paris was where Raymond Solly went to master his own problem by frequenting the Comédie Française and the Conservatoire de Déclamation and learning from the masters.[30] In England, as well as Browne and Behnke, elocution had theatrical and musical associations through classes offered by the Royal Academy of Music,[31] the history of which was written by Cazalet, also a Cambridge graduate and a man with considerable knowledge of instruments. The Rev. Sir Frederick Ouseley had been important to the Academy, and it was to him that Helmore's book on stuttering was dedicated, Helmore himself being choir master to the Prince Consort and a person particularly concerned with church music.

One man who nearly entered the Church was Thomas Hunt. This had been his intention while studying at Trinity College, Cambridge, but, after successfully assisting a fellow student, he decided to make the cure of stuttering his life's work and he left the university prematurely.[32] His system was perpetuated by his son, James, whose belief in the inferiority of negroes now makes him an unsympathetic figure. Nevertheless, his understanding of speech defectives was impressive and they were probably the chief source of his income. Hunt was a member of numerous societies, founding the Anthropological Society in 1863 and becoming its first president.[33] Cull shared his interest in ethnology, but Hunt's wide-ranging approach to man was accompanied by an equally broad view of speech and after his untimely death in 1869 no work of substance on stuttering appeared in Britain.

Another family who were as strong practically as theoretically were the Bells, in contrast to the Beasleys. Bernard Beasley senior, though he reports reading fairly widely, felt it of little value and placed greatest store by what he had learnt from curing himself and others.[34] Presumably this was genuinely fruitful, for he was called the 'greatest living authority' on the subject,[35] and it was noted that an 'African gentleman' travelled 5,000 miles to consult him.[36]

The distinction between charlatans and bona fide therapists is not so easily drawn, because allegiances and acceptable practices cut across the medico-elocutionary dichotomy. Freidson points out that nowadays the distinction between 'paramedical' and 'irregular' workers or 'quacks' is a sociological rather than a technical one, as the work each does may differ little.[37] The same might be said of lay and medical Victorian speech correctionists, as elocution was the therapeutic mainstay of both groups. Nevertheless, to some doctors all non-medical men were quacks. One quack cure, sold by a foreigner around 1835 in London, is reported as consisting 'of steaming the throat with aromatic herbs – the copious use of cathartics – of speaking with a piece of Indian-rubber under the tongue – and of learning the German language'.[38] Whatever the merits of this treatment programme, taken individually, some of these practices were favoured in orthodox circles. Moreover, as Kingsley pointed out, medical assistance could be worse than quackery, which he defined as 'catching at one phenomenon, and legislating exclusively for that, careless whether it was a symptom or an exciting cause'.[39] By this criterion, many verged on malpractice.

Misrepresentation also lies at the heart of quackery. A therapist might pose as a doctor,[40] sometimes after having purchased a foreign diploma,[41] and the registration clauses of the Medical Act seem not to have stopped this practice. A former patient of Abbotts styled himself variously 'doctor', 'reverend' and 'captain' whilst in Australia, and Abbotts likewise objected to an advertisement that ran: 'Stammering, and other defects of speech, cured in six lessons; consultation free; no mechanical appliance.'[42] Its author also turned his hand to singing, music and dancing instruction, which left Abbotts 'almost lost in admiration of the many qualities thus displayed in print'. He further objected to an advertiser who first claimed to have cured himself after 30 years' suffering, and later put it at 40 years. Possibly this was Beasley, as a similar discrepancy appears between two articles about him in *The Illustrated London News*. However outraged Abbotts might have been, it speaks relatively well if this was the worst advertising he could find. Advertisements obviously provided scope for misrepresentation, but if shameful claims appeared in print, they probably have not survived. Those available are reasonable statements of their authors' aims, such as that of Dr Altschul (Figure 6.1), who also advertised in the *Medical Directory* (1892, p. xxxiii) and was probably one of many who treated stutterers without writing on the subject. Altschul offered certain recovery, which itself smacked of charlatanism. But he was in good company, as the Bells guaranteed a cure, distinguishing themselves from quacks in that they did not require advance payment. Furthermore, their ability to mitigate the problem was suspiciously quick – three lessons. Nevertheless, they abhorred charlatans, whom they identified as those charging large fees, irrespective of results, for a system that was unscientific and secret.[43]

Covert practice has long been condemned and recently quackery and the selling of a secret remedy have been equated.[44] By this yardstick, the Hunts, Beasleys and Broster stand condemned. Their position, however, was not unprecedented. Braidwood kept his deaf teaching methods secret, as did Henry Baker, who also took stutterers, and placed pupils under a penalty bond of £100.[45] The Hunts exacted no oath of allegiance[46] and James maintained that his experience was the only secret, that is, the application of quite unmysterious principles. As Thomas Hunt put it in his wrangle with the *Lancet*:

> It is true that I have required my pupils not to divulge the method – a precaution its simplicity and the ineffectual attempts to pirate and

Figure 6.1: Dr Altschul's Advertisement

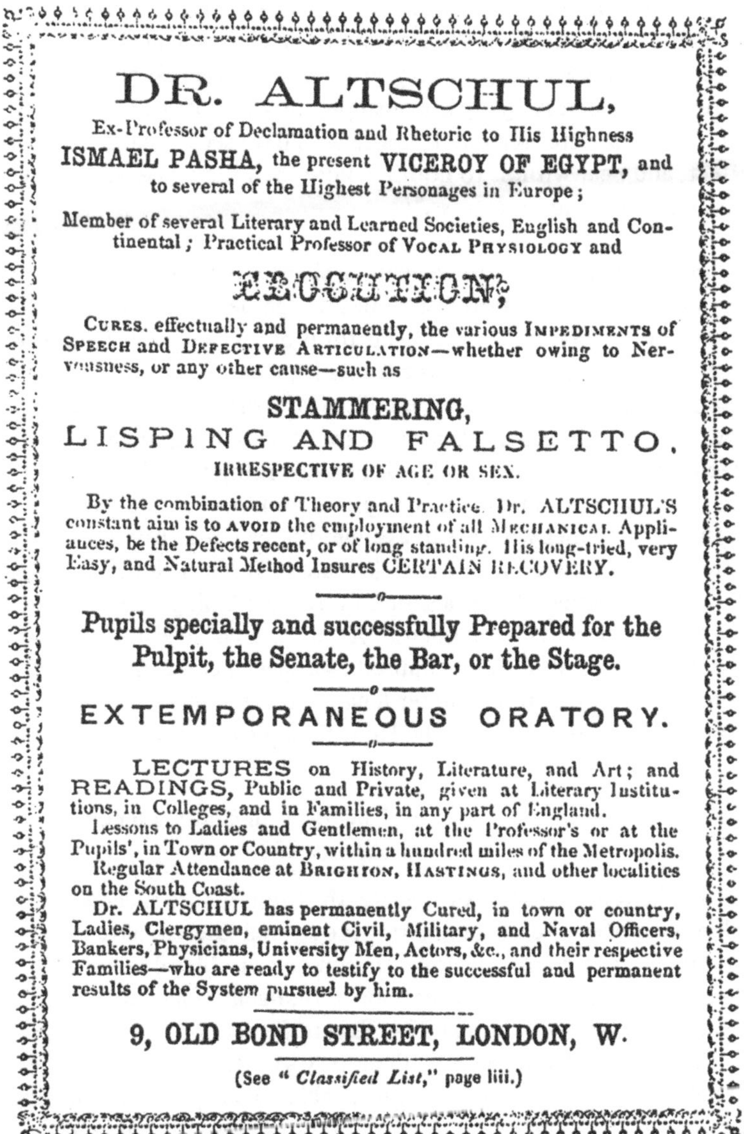

DR. ALTSCHUL,

Ex-Professor of Declamation and Rhetoric to His Highness
ISMAEL PASHA, the present VICEROY OF EGYPT, and
to several of the Highest Personages in Europe;

Member of several Literary and Learned Societies, English and Continental; Practical Professor of VOCAL PHYSIOLOGY and

ELOCUTION;

CURES, effectually and permanently, the various IMPEDIMENTS of SPEECH and DEFECTIVE ARTICULATION—whether owing to Nervousness, or any other cause—such as

STAMMERING,
LISPING AND FALSETTO,
IRRESPECTIVE OF AGE OR SEX.

By the combination of Theory and Practice, Dr. ALTSCHUL'S constant aim is to AVOID the employment of all MECHANICAL Appliances, be the Defects recent, or of long standing. His long-tried, very Easy, and Natural Method Insures CERTAIN RECOVERY.

Pupils specially and successfully Prepared for the Pulpit, the Senate, the Bar, or the Stage.

EXTEMPORANEOUS ORATORY.

LECTURES on History, Literature, and Art; and READINGS, Public and Private, given at Literary Institutions, in Colleges, and in Families, in any part of England.

Lessons to Ladies and Gentlemen, at the Professor's or at the Pupils', in Town or Country, within a hundred miles of the Metropolis.

Regular Attendance at BRIGHTON, HASTINGS, and other localities on the South Coast.

Dr. ALTSCHUL has permanently Cured, in town or country, Ladies, Clergymen, eminent Civil, Military, and Naval Officers, Bankers, Physicians, University Men, Actors, &c., and their respective Families—who are ready to testify to the successful and permanent results of the System pursued by him.

9, OLD BOND STREET, LONDON, W.

(See "*Classified List*," page liii.)

Source: Reproduced from John Johnson Collection, New Bodleian Library, Oxford.

> practise it suggested, for the sake of self-preservation; but in the rigid sense of the words, secret means there never were any, and never was secret less guarded. Hundreds of the relatives of pupils, medical gentlemen, and intelligent individuals of all classes, have been constantly invited to witness my process; and to speak of 'a disreputable secresy' [*sic*] is a misrepresentation of the case. How can that be a secret remedy to those who have seen it carried into effect, and bear witness to nothing more than they have seen – the whole process and its success.[47]

Thus, an important reason for remaining silent was to prevent a genuine system from falling into disrepute through being misapplied by ignorant or dishonest individuals. This form of secrecy protected both therapist and patient, and with the Hunts it proved fully justified.[48]

Thomas Hunt died in 1851, aged 49, after a short illness. He left a widow and eight children,[49] the eldest son, James, being then only eighteen. In these circumstances, it is not surprising that the practice was in disarray. First, one of the daughters took over and it was not until 1854 that James was free to assume full responsibility. By this time, the family's good name was in jeopardy. Thomas Hunt's London rooms had been situated over a shop run by a Mr Urling, the landlord and a trader in lace and baby-linen.[50] After Thomas' death, Urling saw an opportunity for establishing himself as a speech correctionist. To this end, he made use of his former tenant's correspondence, which promoted a sharp rebuke from the Hunt family's lawyers:

> 14, New Boswell Court, Lincoln's Inn,
> 7th April, 1852.
>
> Sir, – The representative of the late Mr. Hunt, whose success and celebrity in the cure of stammering are so well known, have instructed us to communicate with you on your illegal conduct in advertising yourself as the successor to that gentleman, and in opening the letters to him at 224, Regent Street.
>
> You must be fully aware of the injury you are inflicting on the late Mr. Hunt's family by the unjustifiable course you are following; for you *not only open letters which do not belong to you*, and assume a position you are not entitled to, but *actually used the testimonials of the late Mr. Hunt*.
>
> We shall wait a reasonable time before resorting to the legal proceedings we have determined upon, to give you an opportunity

to enter into sòme explanation of your past conduct, and enable you to guarantee that it shall not be repeated.

We are, Sir,
Yours obediently,
HARRISON & LEWIS.[51]

Mr. G.F. Urling, Sen.

This letter may have curtailed Urling's activities, but it did not end them. In 1858, he published a book which contained his own version of the episode. He claimed to have become involved with stuttering through an acquaintance with a friend of the elder Hunt. On Hunt's death, being under the impression that members of the family were unable to continue the work and fearing that the 'germ of truth' might be lost, he 'took up the challenge' and ultimately went on to supersede Hunt's ideas, as well as to reject his system of secrecy. He maintained that his new method was so good that he had had only one failure, a young nobleman aged thirteen who left for Eton after only two weeks of treatment, expressing his dissatisfaction through a letter. In Urling's view, he had been lured away before the remedy was complete by a 'mystic' who 'spread tidings' of his incapacity.[52] The patient's father was probably the peer who found Urling's knowledge 'superficial' and who turned to James Hunt with success, which led the latter to conclude that 'to fit a child with a lace cap, and to cure it of stammering, are quite different accomplishments'.[53]

The Hunts were not alone in their quarrel with Urling. Poett felt aggrieved because he believed Urling to have purloined his ideas. Taking the lines attributed to Virgil:

Versiculos feci,
Tulit alter honoris

he brought them up to date with:

Dr. Poett wrote a book,
Another all the honour took.[54]

Probably even more galling was the fact that members of his own profession should have encouraged Urling to write the book, reviewing it favourably[55] without revealing its source. Asserting priority for his book, which, written in 1858, he imagined to be 'the first to break through the secret quackery' of the previous 30 years, he felt chagrined that others had ignored his name 'as a myth that had no existence', and asked: 'am I not justified in taking the present very moderate course for vindicating my right to the labours of my own brain?'[56] Quoting two chapters as proof, Poett made a similar charge against Cazalet,[57] who was credited by the *Lancet* with taking the 'affliction out of the hands of quacks'.[58] However laudable Poett may have believed his stand against secrecy to be, it was not without ambiguity. First, he was well disposed towards the Hunts, whom he did not view as a threat to his own priority claim, even though he and Thomas began practising in the same year. And secondly, he overlooked his own father's secrecy.[59]

Those charged with quackery were frequently denounced as 'mystics' or 'empirics'. In antiquity, the latter word denoted a sect of physicians who followed experience and were opposed to the rationalists' opinion that illness must be treated only by those who understood its origin. Gradually, the best of both systems merged. But by the nineteenth century, the word had acquired criminal associations and 'instead of signifying one who learns by the experience of others', it often implied one 'unable to profit by his own'[60] – hardly a fair judgement of Beasley or the Hunts. But others felt that misleading or ill-advised practice did not amount to quackery: there had to be some outrageous deception, some oath of secrecy, some guarantee of cure, or some extortionate fee. To this might be added, the promise of a quick, if not immediate, cure.

Duration and Costs of Cure

Most writers agreed that prognosis depended upon the severity of stuttering, the patient's age and assiduity, and the therapeutic circumstances. For example, while regular lessons were common practice, Poett believed that eradication of the fault necessitated living in or near an institution for some time. Understandably, there was wide latitude in the projected periods of cure, but, with their public image in mind, most therapists would have wanted to emphasise the minimum rather than the maximum time likely to be involved. Thelwall tells of a particularly diligent girl whose problem resolved after only a dozen lessons.[61] It is not difficult to elicit fluent speech, even from the worst stutterer, in a much shorter time, and hence the quack was well placed to impress patient and audience by effecting a rapid metamorphosis with the minumum of effort, to collect his fee with impunity and leave, attributing any backsliding to the patient's negligence. Such party tricks, however, were not confined to reprehensible individuals. William Hall reported that the malady could be rectified in 'one minute's time',[62] and both the Bells and Hunts indicated that relief could be obtained quickly. This inspired confidence in patient and referring doctor. The physician Sir James Eyer was suitably impressed by one of Thomas Hunt's sessions. 'In half an hour', reported Eyer of a severe stutterer, 'he spoke with as much ease and freedom as any youth of his age would do, in whom no impediment had ever existed.'[63] Hunt then accurately predicted the cure would take eight lessons. Hunt himself was under no illusions that the fluency produced in 20 minutes was a cure; complete mastery was the work of time[64] and depended upon motivation. James suggested that after a residential stay of one month, further advice might be necessary to prevent relapses.[65] In Beasley's institutions the period of residency varied from a week to over a year,[66] while the Bells found patients establishing new habits in twelve to sixty lessons.[67] Madame Behnke usually obtained a favourable outcome in three months, but this was reduced to a fortnight in the case of doctors, because they could 'see at once the physiological principles' underlying her exercises.[68] By adhering to a simple rule of closing the teeth and inspiring deeply, another sufferer conquered his problem in six months.[69]

The situation was rather different for those seeking help through the written word. Some of the less technical books were designed for such people and contained warnings, encouragement and general advice. They were not, however, intended to replace personal instruction and might be looked upon as a form of advertisement. Despite giving preeminence to their system, few practitioners were prepared to minimise the value of personal contact. In Beasley's view, young patients needed constant supervision and a few months' practical teaching was more efficiacious than years of reading. The latter was like trying to master boxing, billiards and so forth from a book.[70] M'Minn likewise refused to treat by correspondence, but was prepared to make good any omissions in his book on receipt of a stamped envelope.[71] The main risk was that patients might misinterpret instructions; also they could be inappropriate to their case. Whilst a good adjunct to treatment, written advice should therefore be individually adapted.[72] To this end, Abbotts sent out a questionnaire,[73] and XYZ called for a description of the difficult sounds, requesting 5s in postage stamps by way of remuneration.[74] His instructions, however, failed to impress at least one recipient, who described them as 'trashy extracts from elocutionary works'.[75] Abbotts, after 15 years' experience with correspondence courses, had had such good results that he frequently recommended them in preference to other forms of treatment for those living distant from London.[76] But perhaps the greatest enthusiast for such treatment was Mason, who in 1876 established what he believed to be the first Manual of Instruction.[77] This was based on the Natural System, known as far away as India.[78] The main claims for such a course was that it encouraged self-reliance, was as successful as personal supervision and might even be quicker, and was available to all.[79]

A.M. Hartley believed that the distinction between those who professed to cure stuttering in a few days or hours and those that believed them was that the former were 'Knaves, and the latter *fools*; and deserved to be *fleeced*' of exorbitant sums.[80] He mentioned no figure, but records of charges are available. One man paid £20 for a silver plate,[81] and a former sufferer, Walter Yearsley, was expected to pay £25 for a mechanical device and a few lessons,[82] more than five times the price of some silver watches.[83] The Bates' appliances sold for $35 in America,[84] but their price in England was not stated (Figure 8.1, p. 233). By comparison, Butterfield's Alphabetic Speculum was cheap.[85]

A medical degree was no reliable guide to the uninitiated. Yearsley charged ten guineas for excising the uvula with a pair of scissors,[86] though for one patient whose father was a naval surgeon only two guineas were required.[87] The improvement following such a procedure might be long enough to encourage payment, but when one patient declined to pay, Yearsley took him to court. Yet the *Lancet* maligned Thomas Hunt for reaping 'tolerably abundant harvests' from his flourishing practice. 'I instruct many pupils to acquire a natural, instead of a painful and obstructed mastery over that [vocal] organ', he retorted, and so 'I really cannot be persuaded that it is creditable to impeach our fair earnings, and abuse us by calling names.'[88] The difficulty with stutterers was that they required continuous attention, and this physicians were unlikely to provide, since, unless their charges were exorbitant, they could be employed more lucratively in other ways, which was Hartley's explanation for their poor success.[89] Nevertheless, it is clear that many of them looked upon elocutionists as a threat to their livelihood.

Not everyone specified fees in their publications and patients were sometimes invited to write for information, when obviously their circumstances were taken into consideration. The most detailed list of charges was provided by Thelwall and based on his contention that training a child's faculties was a more responsible occupation than teaching him to dance or play the piano. He charged resident pupils £250 p.a. and non-residents 70 guineas for a quarterly course of instruction, which brought in a handsome income during his heyday.[90] By mid-century, the Napoleonic wars were over, the cost of living had dropped by almost half,[91] and elocutionists were commonplace. Nevertheless, their fees remained at much the same level. James Hunt charged 25 guineas at the beginning and the same again at the end of an unspecified period of treatment, with minor defects costing about ten guineas for twelve lessons.[92] The latter fee was what Melville Bell asked of stutterers, the rate being a guinea for individual lessons.[93] XYZ offered instruction at 10s 6d a visit, any Tuesday or Thursday.[94]

The most suspect fee was the flat sum, exacted irrespective of a patient's condition or response to treatment. Probably of this type, and having substance in reality, was the secret cure offered to Monckton for 100 guineas by a gentleman practising on an island 90 miles from London.[95] There was certainly no fiction about the Reverend Dr Joseph Beaumont. Before curing himself and becoming an impressive orator, this Wesleyan preacher spent 'some time' with Thelwall, and subsequently agreed to pay 100 guineas for the guidance of Mr Broster.[96] It has been said that Broster was a quack,[97] but some respectability accrues to him as he was reportedly one of the most successful curers in the country and was called to treat Dugald Stewart after a paralysis[98] that left him with a 'stammer'.[99] This metaphysician and others in his social class were in a position to pay, but many stutterers seeking help were young men aspiring to the professions, who would have been unable to contemplate Broster's rates if they came from a middle-class family with £250 a year. Even if supplemented with an apprenticeship, like David Copperfield's for £90 annually, they would still have had to look elsewhere. And if, like the impecunious Micawber, they had struck hard times and were forced to match expenditure to an income of £20, they would have had to forego any thought of speech lessons unless fortunate enough to be one of those whom Broster[100] and others treated gratuitously, amongst whom was Bernard Beasley, who gave one tenth of his time freely.[101] In addition to his tuition fee, Broster asked an extra 5 guineas a week for full board and lodging,[102] 2 guineas more than James Hunt and XYZ were asking some 30 years later. This in itself was a guinea more than a respectable London family expected to receive from paying guests visiting the Great Exhibition.[103] No doubt their facilities fell far short of Broster's, but as these are not recorded, direct comparisons are difficult.

Erasmus Darwin had prescribed a stay in France for his eight-year-old son Charles, thinking that speaking another language would relieve his stuttering; in fact, he simply acquired fluency in French.[104] Others thought foreign travel also beneficial.[105] Those wanting more specific assistance during their European tour could apply to Gerdts, a practitioner of 25 years' standing. Unlike the publications of his more famous Continental colleagues, Gerdts' book appeared in English; it ran into several editions and was reviewed and advertised in British journals.[106] Before embarking, prospective clients could consult referees in England, such as Lady Isabel Cust, of 99 Onslow Square. Once assured, they could leave for Bingen-on-Rhine where they would be fed and housed for £25 a month in advance. For this they received:

> a room with a splendid view
> morning coffee, butter, bread and 2 eggs
> 11½ o'clock, lunch
> 1¼ o'clock, a good dinner
> 5½ o'clock, coffee with butter and bread
> 9 o'clock, a good supper

to which was added a daily bottle of good wine. Tuition was extra and entailed six to seven hours work a day for a recommended minimum period of twelve weeks.[107] Herein lies the main difference between contemporary and nineteenth-century practice, which principally served the affluent classes who frequently received intensive therapy, often in a residential setting.

Venues

Because deaf education and remedial elocution both aim to improve communication in the verbally handicapped, they have sometimes been confused or identified. It was not unusual for teachers to tackle both, and it is likely that certain acoustically normal non-verbal children found themselves in deaf schools, if not mental homes. Even stutterers, whose hearing was not in question, had received help from teachers of the deaf like John Wallis and Henry Baker. And in Europe, Franz Gall and Jean Itard were two notable examples of physicians connected with deaf asylums, in Vienna and Paris respectively, as well as being amongst the earliest nineteenth-century speech pathologists. Further research is necessary before there can be any certainty over Continental practices, but it seems that several of the principal contributors to speech correction were teachers of the deaf, and that both remedial classes and teacher training programmes for stuttering often took place within deaf schools.[108] In Britain, by contrast, association between the two professions was limited. Joseph Watson dealt briefly with speech correction in his *Instruction of the Deaf and Dumb*, and Alexander Graham Bell was affiliated with Susanna Hull's deaf school in Kensington. However, Bell's interest in deafness did not flower until he reached America. Significantly, other connections in London show European influences. E.J. Seltman, situated at 66 Victoria Street, adopted a German system for curing stuttering that had found favour with speech correctionists at Swedish government institutes for the deaf and dumb.[109] Meanwhile, William Van Praagh, who was familiar with Continental writings, also assisted stutterers. A Dutch teacher of the deaf, he was sent to England during 1863 in response to a request for guidance by Baroness Mayer de Rothschild. His abilities led to a staff appointment at the Central London Throat and Ear Hospital and directorship of the Association for the Oral Instruction of the Deaf and Dumb, attached to which was the first college for teacher training of the deaf in the English-speaking world.[110] It is noteworthy that later, when formal training programmes for speech therapy were first established, they were not associated with deaf institutions.

To what extent Thelwall was responsible for this position is hard to gauge, but he did exclude two categories from his own institute: the deaf and severely defective individuals. To conjecture, it seems likely that Thelwall was merely explicating a principle latent within the new elocutionary movement, which was essentially normative in orientation and held perfection as an ideal. As much of the impetus for speech correction in Britain derived from this source, we have a possible explanation for why stuttering classes were rarely located in deaf schools or hospital clinics.

Thelwall's establishment was probably the first to specialise in assisting speech defectives, but its activities were not limited either to such pupils or to speech correction. Indeed, its clientele was as varied as its education was liberal. Thelwall began in Liverpool in 1805, but within six months he had moved to London where he had various addresses over the next 30 years and where he was assisted by members of his family.[111]

A rather different centre was the Kensington College of Elocution headed by Joe Edgar Foster. Records of the College appear to be lost, but it would be interesting to know whether it was connected with Dr Thompson's school at Kensington, where James Wright succeeded John Walker as elocutionist. This was probably the school founded by Alexander Longmore in 1761 at Bullingham House and subsequently run by Dr Robert Thompson and family until after 1817.[112] Walker may well have been free to lecture there, as his own establishment, the Walker–Usher school at Kensington Gravel-pits closed in 1770. Thompson's school was principally for normal speakers, but Wright may have treated some of his defective speakers there. In addition, he attended noble families; visited schools, amongst which was Eagle House, Brook Green, where Martin Tupper had been a pupil; and he ran his own establishment, first at Arundel House, Balham Hill and then at Grove Hall in Clapham.[113] Butterfield's work at Eton is the only other record of speech correction being carried out in regular schools.[114]

In some instances, private institutions seem to have been little more than the family house opened to a few, the bulk of the practice being non-residential and involving occasional attendance at pupils' residences. The Bells, for example, seem to have operated principally from their professional rooms in three capitals: Dublin, Edinburgh and London.[115]

The main objection to residential care was that it provoked morbid attention to speech[116] and provided ready models for a sufferer's imitative proclivities, which caused Blake to state that it was 'open to the gravest question' whether 'the promiscuous herding together' of stutterers should be sanctioned.[117] It was also liable to produce hot-house plants,[118] but despite believing that the afflicted needed sheltering from cradle to grave, Monro disputed that schools would be generally beneficial. He believed that adults should find a profession which made few calls upon speech,[119] but this was hardly better than the 'negative' cure they themselves might achieve by avoiding situations where stuttering seemed inevitable.[120] On the other hand, youngsters rarely possessed enough self-discipline to adhere unerringly to therapeutic rules,[121] and their removal from taunting school fellows could only bring benefit. In an institution, the stutterer might learn about his own defect through watching others, and those with mild problems would appreciate the consequences of neglect.[122] Residential care would provide a sanctuary, a tolerant and understanding atmosphere,[123] through support from fellow sufferers and staff. But the moral treatment they received was far more embracing and extended to their whole milieu. What stutterers needed as much as tongue-twisters and recitations was a new outlook on life. Recreation was as much the answer for the frightened child as for the adult wearied by social failure, professional inadequacy and perhaps ill-health. So important was moral treatment that Dr Warren, whose publication was well received in Britain, believed that it alone was sufficient to effect a cure. However, he had reservations about treatment being carried on away from home as he thought that the patient was more liable to relapse once he resumed his old associations.[124]

The changing concept of causes in psychiatry was underscored in Pinel's *Traité médico-philosophique sur l'aliénation mentale* of 1801,[125] where he introduced the term 'moral' treatment. The connotations of this word were broad, having little to do with ethics, but signifying zeal, hope, reason, confidence, a certain life-style and inner meaning,[126] and the disentangling of confusions and errors. But even before Pinel, humane Englishmen had appreciated the value of an open door policy, ventilation, exercise and stimulating activities, and the shift from madhouse to asylum was exemplified in Samuel Tuke's Retreat, a small Quaker foundation in York. Some progressive institutes of this kind still had occasion to resort to the rotary chair, cold douche, dark room and straitjacket, and their basic therapeutic principles often rested on gaining ascendency over the patient, albeit only through 'getting his eye'.[127] Nevertheless, these were unfortunate necessities and the main emphasis was liberal. The ideal milieu for moral treatment was described by Browne, a psychiatrist and phrenologist:

> Conceive a spacious building resembling the palace of a peer, airy, and elevated, and elegant, surrounded by extensive and swelling grounds and gardens. The interior is fitted up with galleries, and workshops, and music-rooms. The sun and air are allowed to enter at every window, the view of the shrubberies and fields . . . is unobstructed . . . all is clean, quiet and attractive. The inmates all seem to be actuated by the common impulse of enjoyment, all are busy, and delighted by being so.[128]

Brampton Park (Figure 6.2), one of Beasley's institutions for nearly 20 years, matched this description in almost every detail.

Brampton Park, with its history reaching back to the middle ages, was a mid-seventeenth-century house, rebuilt around 1820 by Lady Olivia Sparrow. Through her daughter's marriage to the Duke of Manchester, it passed into ducal hands.[129] Beasley leased the property in 1889 for £300 p.a. For his purposes, it could not have been more

Figure 6.2: Brampton Park

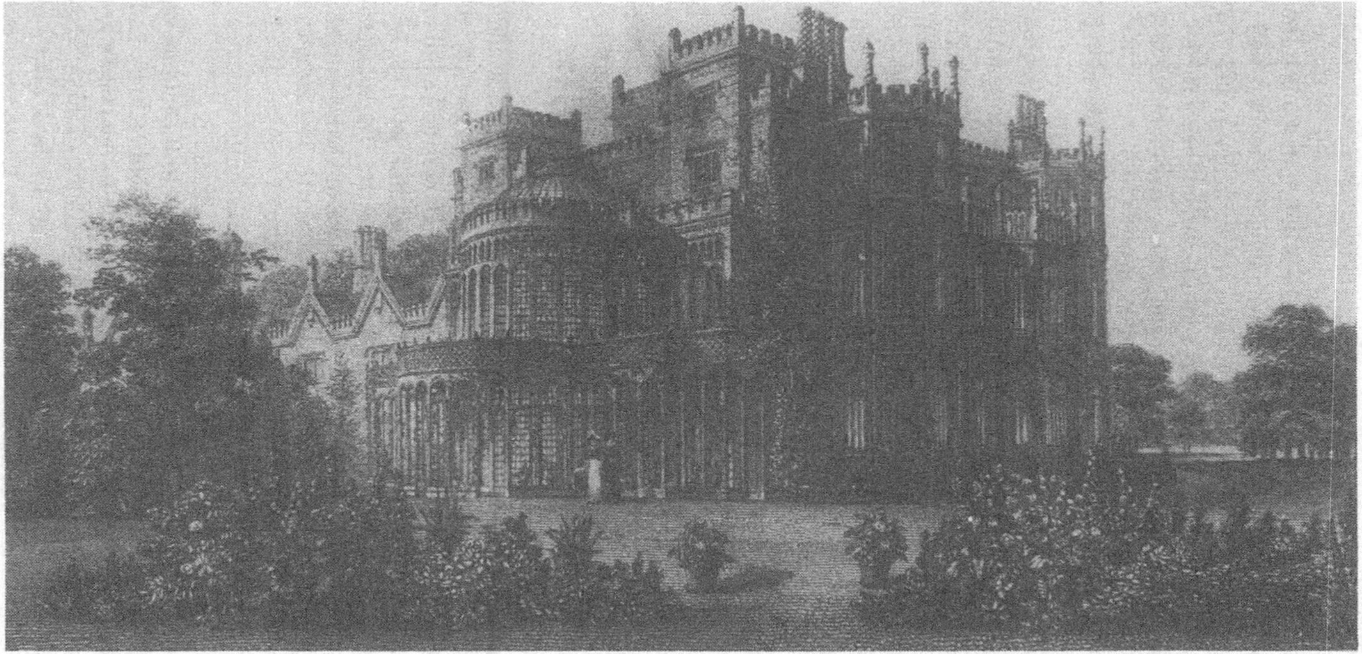

Source: From a drawing by W. Finley (published by Rockham, Strand, 1823) in the Huntingdon Local History Collection.

ideal as he subscribed to the tenet of muscular Christianity – *mens sana in corpore sano* – and he quoted Kingsley on this subject.[130] Close to the Cambridgeshire hounds, Brampton Park had facilities for numerous other outdoor sports,[131] not least shooting, for which he paid extra rent. Beasley himself was an excellent shot, having previously been a rifle manufacturer and a member of the English Eight for the First Elcho Challenge Shield at Wimbledon, a match commemorated in verse.[132]

Beasley, a freemason of the Socrates lodge,[133] also exploited the other potentialities of his residence to the full. One important feature was a theatre seating 40 people. The cathartic value of drama had been fully appreciated by the Greeks, and Shakespeare used it to stir guilty emotions in the play within *Hamlet*. By the late eighteenth century, the therapeutic effects of acting had been recognised by Johann Reil, who endeavoured to relieve mental conflicts by appropriately staged situations or specially written plays, and to this end, he recommended that every asylum have a theatre, as well as offer music therapy.[134] In England, Joseph Cox tried to shift his patients' faulty thinking through the vivid impressions created by 'pious frauds'. His deceptions included an array of theatrical effects from thunder to phosphorescent signs, and an actor might appear representing some archetypal figure.[135] Since World War II, psychodrama has been popularised by the Morenos in North America and occasionally used with stutterers, who often have less hesitancy on stage. Such was this situation with Mrs Inchbald, whose impediment 'drove her from company', yet 'seemed no bar to her becoming an actress' since 'stage declamation, being a raised and artificial thing afforded more time for enunciation'.[136]

Beasley made use of two forms of drama. First, the stutterer was put to the test in mock trials and other simulated situations.[137] But much of Beasley's effort went into theatrical productions, such as his *Julius Caesar*, which was a feature of his Speech Days, when patients would also demonstrate their fluency in lectures, recitations and speeches, achieving what once seemed impossible.[138] So perfect was their articulation that the *Westminster Budget* said Brampton Park resembled an elocution academy rather than an institute for stutterers.[139] Several notables provided the sense of occasion, amongst them the Earl of Sandwich and the Duke of Manchester.

Academic pursuits were not neglected. Tutors were Oxford and Cambridge graduates[140] and the hours of study on a par with Eton and Harrow, but Beasley's educational philosophy precluded cramming. Pupils could be prepared for university, and arrangements made for students or public schoolboys to attend in their vacations.[141]

Before moving to Huntingdon, Beasley spent ten years in Green Bank House, set in only 30 acres near Birmingham.[142] In 1907, Beasley junior had removed to Birkdale, Lancashire, where he may have met Walter Yearsley, by then running government approved classes for stutterers in local schools. Yearsley refers to a well-known specialist of 25 years' standing offering him a partnership,[143] and he also praised Beasley senior, whose experience he put at 5,000 stutterers.[144] Another report, however, numbers his patients at 1,500.[145] But whatever the case, the institute ran into financial difficulties,[146] and Beasley intended leaving for Maidenhead.[147] He never went. Brampton Park was gutted by fire in January 1907[148] and within a fortnight Beasley was dead.

Beasley also had a London establishment, in Brondesbury, run by his son-in-law Mr Ketley. This arrangement was similar to the Hunts', who complemented their rooms in town with seaside residences. Thomas Hunt was originally a Dorsetshire squire and his summer retreat was situated on Swanage Bay from whence patients could take walks to the delightful family farmhouse in Godlingstone, once an appanage of Corfe Castle.[149] James, however, favoured Hastings, where he and the Reverend H.F. Rivers ran an establishment called Ore House,[150] one of their pupils during 1859 being Charles Dodgson.[151] Rivers was married to Hunt's sister, Elizabeth, and one wonders what effect this environment had on their young son, William Halse Rivers, who developed a stutter.[152] Much later, he was to have a tangential connection with another branch of speech pathology through his association with Henry Head. While at Cambridge, William occupied the first British post in experimental psychology, but many of his interests were anthropological, possibly fostered by the numerous texts he inherited from Hunt,[153] whose death was soon followed by the family's departure from Ore House.[154] Thus ended an institute which, like many enlightened private insane asylums, was unable to survive its proprietor. But despite Hunt's reputation, even this house was obviously little known, for a surgeon writing to the *Lancet* enquiring about help with his stuttering,[155] received the reply that it knew of no institutions offering relief.[156] Those in existence were, therefore, rather dim lights on a dark scene.

Physicians also made a practice of opening their homes to stutterers. Shorthouse stayed with Mr Bishop for some months,[157] and Poett thought the homes of married physicians ideal for children of the upper classes, and he exhorted his colleagues to interest themselves in the complaint.[158] James Yearsley's treatment, however, may have been administered in the Orthophonic Institute to which he refers.[159] Possibly this was a branch of his Ear Institute in Sackville Street, Piccadilly, the first Ear, Nose and Throat Hospital in the world, founded in 1838.[160]

Another medical establishment was the Hospital for Affections of Speech, founded in 1884[161] and situated in Woburn Chambers, 22 Henrietta Street, Covent Garden. The building, owned by the Duke of Bedford, had architectural merit,[162] but as it was designed for professional rooms the 'hospital' possibly comprised only a suite. It was staffed by Dr William Abbotts, whose name is associated with hay-fever, plus two medical officers, who were joined by a dental surgeon, which suggests that some patients had structural anomalies. Outpatient attendance is given as 850 or upwards per year, though whether this represents patients or visits is not stated. Six former patients of Abbotts sat on the management committee, but the venture lasted for only about a decade. Nevertheless, the concept is remarkable and foreshadows the contemporary call for some national diagnostic clinic. It also indicates the gradual shift from private educational establishments to a hospital setting, a shift further exemplified in the Behnkes' practice, carried on partly at Guy's and the London hospitals.

There was no sign of financial support for these services, or even interest in government circles. This contrasts sharply with the deaf, mentally handicapped, crippled and epileptics, who were variously the object of legislation, philanthropy and a Royal Commission.[163] Given the state of diagnosis, however, it is likely that in practice some severe speech defectives were affected by this legislation, but it was not until the 1944 Education Act that they were ensured of education appropriate to their problems. This Act enabled a grant to be given to Moor House, a special school for such children and only the second of its kind in the world.[164] Stutterers were in need of therapeutic rather than educational facilities, but their needs were not officially recognised until 1905 to 1906, and then only in the North of England and Scotland.[165] For this, Walter Yearsley takes some credit, but much of the impetus came from Leon Berquand, whom Arnold Bennett had consulted in Paris and whom he followed to Aberdeen.[166] Berquand had already established classes on the Continent, where services and support for speech disorders appear to have been greater. Space does not permit an account of these, which embraced investigatory commissions, the training of teachers, the establishment of professional bodies, as well as the founding of institutes and classes in elementary schools, so that some free treatment was available.[167]

This disregard for stutterers by the British government was not an isolated anomaly, but reflected its general disinclination to enter the field of education or give support to science. Remedial elocution may further have suffered in Britain because it was not associated with education for the deaf. Gerdts, in Germany, suggested that their connection was detrimental to stutterers,[168] and this may have been so therapeutically. Administratively, however, the reverse was possibly true, as society felt an obligation to cater for the deaf. Schoolfield may be right that American speech pathology was retarded by the Bells' preoccupation with deafness and the telephone;[169] in Britain a liaison with deaf education might have hastened official recognition of speech problems as it appeared to do elsewhere.

British treatment centres for stuttering, then, were relatively short-lived organisations, dispensing some charity, but run principally for the livelihood of their proprietors. They were spread unevenly over the country and, outside the family, little training was offered. Visits to schools and hospitals were minimal. This was markedly different from the Continent and the difference between the two areas is reflected in the fact that the International Association of Logopaedics and Phoniatrics, with its nerve centres in Berlin and Vienna,[170] was established roughly a decade before the British formed the Remedial Section of the Association of Teachers of Speech and Drama and the Society of Speech Therapists, and two decades before these organisations amalgamated to form the College of Speech Therapists in 1945. In the absence of any such body, Victorians relied upon their entrepreneurial spirit to publicise and promote services for stutterers.

Notes

1. Physician, p. 9.
2. XYZ, p. 3.
3. Bryan, *Stammering*, p. iii.
4. A. Hartley, p. 53.
5. *Charles Kingsley* (1901), vol. 3, p. 267; Minute Philosopher, p. 7.
6. Arnott (1827), p. 561; McCormac, p. x.
7. Poett snr (1828), pp. 10-11.
8. McCormac, p. v.
9. A Pupil, 'Lines Addressed to John Broster, F.A.S.E.' *(Blackwood's) Edinburgh Monthly Magazine*, 18 (1825), p. 731 (730-1).
10. A Pupil, 'Broster's System for the Cure of Impediments of Speech', *London Magazine and Review*, 2 n.s. (1825), p. 533 (533-6).

11. Ball, p. 5.
12. James Chapman, *The Music, or Melody and Rhythmus of Language* (Edinburgh, Michael Anderson, 1818), p. xxiv.
13. Wright (1835), p. 26. Cf. quotation from Sheridan in Gray, pp. 17-18.
14. M'Minn, p. 32.
15. Abbotts, p. 52; Beasley (1905), pp. 28-9; Bryan, *Stammering*, p. vii; Shuldham, p. 10; [Mason] (1885), p. 11; Alex J.D. D'Orsey, 'Stammering and Stuttering', letter *British Medical Journal*, 1 (1885), p. 1322. Cf. A. Bell, pp. 56-8.
16. Beasley (1885), p. 46.
17. A. Bell, p. 12.
18. Abbotts, pp. 51, 55.
19. Astrié, Becqueral, Chégoin, Guillaume, Rullier, Serres d'Alais, Voisin, Coën, Gerdts, Lindt, Merkel and Wyneken. Also the writer of: 'Remarks on Stammering, by a Sufferer', *Medico-Chirurgical Review*, 33 n.s. (1840), 489-91.
20. Hammond and Warren.
21. Wright (1843), pp. 52-3 refers to Mr Julion of Lambeth. Possibly this was the M. Jullien who arranged vocal and instrumental music concerts.
22. Cited by Potter, p. 40.
23. M'Minn, p. 2.
24. Mason (1884), p. 9n.
25. XYZ, pp. 4, 15. This writer, medically trained and living at 11 Russel St, North Brixton, was possibly William King. A man by that name is listed in the *Post Office Directory* (1857) as a chemist, and in *Kelly's Directory* (1859) as a surgeon. No one at that address appears in the *Medical Register*.
26. A. Bell, pp. 46-7.
27. Tupper, *My Life*, p. 73; Hudson, *Tupper*, pp. 14-15, 20.
28. 'The Rev. J. Edgar Foster', *Elocutionist*, 2 (1883), p. 62.
29. Claude Shaver, 'Steele MacKaye and the Delsartian Tradition' in *History of Speech Education in America*, ed. Karl Wallace (New York, Appleton-Century-Crofts, 1954), pp. 202-18.
30. J.R. Solly, *Acting and the Art of Speech at the Paris Conservatoire. Hints on Reading, Reciting, Acting and the Cure of Stammering* (Birmingham, Charles Cooper & Co. and London, Elliot Stock, 1891).
31. Letter dated 2 March 1976 from the Librarian, Royal Academy of Music. See also *British Medical Journal*, 1 (1888), p. 278 where a doctor recommends instructions to stutterers contained in the Appendix of *Grammar of Elocution* by John Millard, who was professor of Declamation at the Royal College of Music.
32. *DNB*, vol. 10, p. 280.
33. Ibid., pp. 266-7.
34. Beasley (1885), pp. 12, 30-1.
35. *Illustrated London News*, 89 (1886), p. 560; 'Brampton Park', *Illustrated London News*, 95 (1889), p. 837. Cf. Walter Clarke, *Stammering* (London, [1907]), p. 2; W. Yearsley, pp. 81-2.
36. Beasley (1905), p. 57.
37. Freidson, p. 49.
38. Cull (1835), p. 9.
39. Minute Philosopher, pp. 7, 8.
40. Beasley (1885), p. 10.
41. Abbotts, pp. 10-12. Cf. ibid., p. 50.
42. Ibid., p. 11n.
43. A.M. Bell [1853], pp. 27-48; A. Bell, pp. 12, 14-16.
44. A. Dickson Wright, 'Quacks through the Ages', *Pharmaceutical Journal*, 124, 4th s. (1957), p. 44.

45. Ruth Bender, *The Conquest of Deafness* (Cleveland, Western Reserve UP, 1960), pp. 65, 72-3, 75, 106, 112, 117, 124.
46. *Unspeakable*, p. 145.
47. T. Hunt, p. 504. Cf. Urling, p. 78.
48. Minute Philosopher, p. 10.
49. 'Obituary . . . Thomas Hunt', *Illustrated London News*, 19 (1851), p. 238.
50. *Unspeakable*, pp. 140, 145.
51. Poett jnr, pp. x-xi.
52. Urling, notice, pp. 6-8, 62-3.
53. Hunt (1854), p. 67. Cf. Thelwall (1810), pp. 82-3.
54. Poett jnr, p. xxi.
55. For reviews of Urling's *Vocal Gymnastics* see: *Lancet*, 2 (1857), p. 224, *Dublin Journal of Medical Science*, 24 (1857), p. v.
56. Poett jnr, pp. xviii-xix.
57. Ibid., pp. xxv-xxvi.
58. Review of Cazalet's *Stammering, Lancet*, 1 (1857), p. 246.
59. Poett snr (1828), pp. 58-9.
60. 'Ancient and Modern Empirics', *London Medical Gazette*, 2 n.s. (1838-39), 815-16.
61. Thelwall (1810), pp. 64-6.
62. W.W. Hall, *Popular Cyclopaedia* (London, Simpkin & Marshall and Glasgow, Thomas D. Morison, 1892), p. 211; W.W. Hall, *How to Live Long* (London, Sampson Low, Marston, Low & Searle, 1875), p. 166.
63. James Eyer, 'Cure of Stammering, – No. IX', testimonial letter reprinted in *Lancet*, 1 (1846), 557-8.
64. 'Notes on London by an Outside Barbarian' subsection 'Stammering', *Chambers's Edinburgh Journal*, 7 (1847), p. 233.
65. Hunt (1863), pp. 194-5.
66. Beasley (1885), pp. 37-8.
67. A.M. Bell [1853], pp. 37, 45-8.
68. R. Behnke, p. 324. Cf. n.a., *Lancet*, 2 (1891), p. 362.
69. Correspondent, 'The Cure of Stammering', *Lancet*, 1 (1869), p. 484.
70. Beasley (1885), pp. 32-3, 34-7; Gerdts, pp. 5, 16.
71. M'Minn, pp. 3, 56. Cf. Hunt (1870), p. 299.
72. Cull (1833), p. 24.
73. Abbotts, p. 58.
74. XYZ, p. 16.
75. *Unspeakable*, p. 139.
76. Abbotts, pp. 57-8.
77. [Mason] (1883), p. 152.
78. [Mason] (1882), p. 90.
79. Mason (1884), pp. 3, 4.
80. A.M. Hartley, p. 31.
81. Abbotts, p. 49.
82. Walter Yearsley, *Stammering* (Accrington, J. Broadley, 1909), p. 6.
83. Advertisement, *Literary Gazette*, no. 1532 (1846), p. 508.
84. Potter, p. 93.
85. See below p. 228.
86. J.F. Symonds, 'Ten Guineas for Clipping the Uvula', letter to *Lancet*, 2 (1840-1), p. 594.
87. W. Egan, 'Uvula-Snipping for Stammering', letter to *Lancet*, 2 (1840-1), 637-8.
88. Editorial (1846a), p. 557; T. Hunt, pp. 503-4.
89. A. Hartley, p. 57.

90. Rockey (1979), p. 172.
91. John Burnett, *A History of the Cost of Living* (Harmondsworth, Penguin, 1969), pp. 190, 196-205.
92. Hunt (1858), p. 13.
93. Firth, p. 117.
94. XYZ, p. 14.
95. *Unspeakable*, pp. 89, 90, 106-7.
96. Urling, pp. 3-4. Cf. R-P., 'Stammering', letter to *British Medical Journal*, 1 (1888), p. 55, where Broster's fee is put at 300 guineas.
97. Potter, p. 46.
98. Physician, pp. 36, 64.
99. After the third edition of his *Treatise* and Broca's paper on language disorders, Hunt modified his terminology, and in *Stammering* (1870, p. 69) he said that Stewart was aphasic.
100. 'Notice respecting Mr Broster's newly discovered system for the removal of impediments of speech and defective articulation', *(Blackwood's) Edinburgh Monthly Magazine*, 17 (1825), 46-7; Broster, p. 7. Cf. Abbotts, p. 50.
101. Blathwayt, p. 575.
102. Urling, p. 4.
103. Advertisement, *Illustrated London News*, 19 (1851), p. 152.
104. C. Darwin in *Erasmus Darwin*, p. 81. Cf. Bartlett, pp. 65, 66, 69; Blake, pp. 17, 21; Coote, p. 612; McCormac, p. 80; Thelwall (1812), p. viii. Dr Blake specifically recommended French 'as it is a language demanding great lip play, very defective in most cases', see: letter, *Lancet*, 1 (1891), p. 123.
105. *Unspeakable*, pp. 123-4.
106. *Elocutionist*, 2 (1883), pp. 46, 52, 58, 66-7, 70, 80, 82, 95. See also: *Journal of Laryngology and Rhinology*, 2 (1888), p. 185 where a book by Gerdts entitled *The Cause of Stuttering and Natural Cure* (1887) is reviewed.
107. Gerdts, pp. 30, 31, 46, 65, 77.
108. Eldridge, pp. 39, 43-4, 51; Potter, p. 66.
109. Seltman, *Physique*, 1, p. 140. Seltman, whose views received medical approval, was possibly following Denhardt's system, see correspondence *British Medical Journal*, 1 (1886), p. 431; 2 (1892), p. 1210; *Lancet*, 2 (1891), p. 362,
110. Bender, *The Conquest of Deafness*, p. 145; correspondence in *British Medical Journal*, 1 (1888), p. 569; 1 (1894), p. 504; 2 (1897), p. 1547; *Lancet*, 2 (1873), p. 797; 2 (1895), p. 1620.
111. Rockey (1979), pp. 171, 173.
112. Information from Mrs P.K. Pratt, Borough Librarian, Kensington Central Library, London, W.8. Letter dated 2 March 1976.
113. Wright (1839), pp. 26-7, 45, 52; Wright (1843), pp. viii, 9, 55.
114. See above pp. 30, 44n81.
115. A. Bell, p. 12; A.M. Bell [1853], pp. 12-13, advertisement.
116. Bacc. Med. Oxon., p. 17.
117. Blake, p. 3.
118. M'Minn, p. 23.
119. Bacc. Med. Oxon., p. 59.
120. Borthwick, pp. 38-9.
121. Poett jnr, pp. viii, 32-3.
122. Hunt (1863), pp. 221-2.
123. M'Minn, pp. 29-30.
124. *H–T* (1860), p. 335; Hunt (1870), p. 111; *British and Foreign Medical Review*, 6 (1838), 253-4, where an extract appears from Dr Edward Warren's *On the Cure of Stammering by Moral Means*, which probably relates to his 'Remarks on Stammering', *American Journal of the Medical Sciences*, 21 (1837), 75-99, reprinted in *Journal of Communication Disorders*, 10 (1977), 159-79.

125. English translation – 1806.

126. S. Bockhoven, 'Moral Treatment in American Psychiatry', *Journal of Nervous and Mental Disease*, 124 (1956), 172-3 (167-94).

127. Walk, pp. 807-37; Bynum, pp. 318-28.

128. W.A.F. Browne, *What Asylums Are, Were and Ought to Be* (Edinburgh, A. & C. Black, London, Longman, 1837), p. 229.

129. *The Victoria History of the Counties of England. Huntingdonshire* (London, St Catherine's Press, 1936), vol. 3, 12-13.

130. Beasley (1885), pp. 55-8; Helmore, pp. 62-4; Shuldham, pp. 60-2. The association between education, health and gymnastics was widespread and of long standing, see the writings of Gretchen Finney, e.g. 'Vocal Exercise and Nineteenth-Century Hygiene in France', *Clio Medica*, 12 (1977), 147-71. Stutterers were thought to benefit both from the improved health derived from general, respiratory and vocal exercise, and from the specific didactic training to which the latter could be adapted. It was suggested that a healthy voice meant a healthy body (Holmes, p. 99) and Swedish gymnastics and dumb-bells were particularly recommended. Moreover, sports could develop moral fibre. See below, pp. 192, 197n52, 226-8, 236n10; Colman (1895), p. 1420; Haward, p. 112; Hunt (1870), pp. 147, 170; Sandlands, p. 72; Yearsley (1843-4), p. 290.

131. Beasley (1905), advertisement, inside front cover.

132. 'The Battle of Wimbledon', *Punch*, 43 (1862), p. 23.

133. 'Death of Mr. Beasley', *Hunts. Post*, 16 February 1907; 'Death of Mr. B. Beesley [*sic*]', *Hunts. County News*, 16 February 1907.

134. Harms, pp. 806-7.

135. Walk, p. 824.

136. James Boaden (ed.), *Memoirs of Mrs. Inchbald* (London, Richard Bentley, 1833), vol. 1, 5-7.

137. Blathwayt, p. 578.

138. Beasley (1905), pp. 55-8.

139. Cited in ibid., pp. 58-9.

140. Blathwayt, p. 578.

141. Beasley (1905), advertisement.

142. Beasley (1885), pp. 39-47.

143. W. Yearsley, *Stammering*, p. 6.

144. W. Yearsley, *Self-Cure*, p. 82.

145. Blathwayt, p. 579.

146. Item dated 18 December 1906, Letter Books, *Manchester Papers*, deposited in the Huntingdonshire County Record Office, from whom permission to examine them was kindly given; letter to creditor, dated 2 March 1907, from the duke's agent. Beasley's will, however, shows effects worth £2,800.

147. Letter to Mr Cooke from Beasley, 12 January 1907. *Manchester Papers*.

148. Reported in: *Daily Mail*, 25 January 1907, *Hunts. County News*, 26 January 1907, *Hunts. Post*, 26 January 1907.

149. *Unspeakable*, pp. 153-4.

150. Hunt (1870), pp. 369-70.

151. Katherine Rivers, *Memoirs of Lewis Carroll*, an undated and unpaginated issue of *Library Research News*. For the most recent account of Dodgson and his speech problem, see Morton N. Cohen (ed.), *The Letters of Lewis Carroll* (London, Macmillan, New York, Oxford UP, forthcoming 1979), vol. 1.

152. Reginald Pound, *Arnold Bennett* (London, William Heineman, 1952), p. 31.

153. B.J. Mack, 'W.H.R. Rivers: The Contexts of Social Anthropology', (Oxford Univ. D. Phil. thesis, 1975), pp. 21, 27.

154. The establishment closed in the latter half of 1872. Information from the

Area Librarian, East Sussex County Council.

155. A Country Surgeon, letter to *Lancet*, 1 (1869), p. 420. Cf. Letters to: *Lancet*, 2 (1890), p. 1066; 1 (1896), p. 748; 2 (1897), pp. 1433, 1509; *British Medical Journal*, 1 (1881), p. 218; 1 (1883), p. 750, 2, pp. 1103, 1269; 2 (1884), pp. 596, 644; 1 (1885), p. 874; 1 (1886), pp. 278, 374, 431, 669, 2, pp. 800, 959; 1 (1887), pp. 250, 697; 2 (1890), pp. 992, 1048; 2 (1891), p. 223; 1 (1894), pp. 426-7; 1 (1899), p. 771.

156. 'Notes . . . Answers . . .', *Lancet*, 1 (1869), p. 518. Cf. 'Instruction in Schools for Stammerers', *Lancet*, 2 (1886), p. 413, which indicates that school children in Brunswick received some organised help.

157. *Life . . . of . . . Shorthouse*, vol. 1, p. 15.

158. Poett jnr, pp. 33, 34. Cf. *Household Words*, pp. 467-8.

159. Yearsley, *Statement*, p. 5.

160. R. Scott Stevenson, 'A Hundred Years of Otology: from Yearsley to Lempert', *Medical Press*, 238 (1957), 596-7 (596-602). Cf. Yearsley (1841), p. 31.

161. The hospital is not listed in the London Medical Directories before 1886, so 1874, given as the date of its founding in *The London Medical Directory* (1886), p. 333, is probably a misprint. Though it does not appear in the *Directory* after 1891, Abbotts was still referring to it in 1894.

162. *Building News*, 4 (1858), pp. 186, 187, 190; *Survey of London*, 36 (1970), 237-8.

163. Pritchard, pp. 62-3, 95-114, 151-8, 196, 222-7; Jones, pp. 185-7, 191-7, 288-9. For a list of deaf schools and classes see A. Farrar, *Arnold on the Education of the Deaf*, 2nd edn (London, National College of Teachers of the Deaf, 1923), pp. 90-1.

164. Silvia Hudson Smith, 'Moor House School', *Speech*, 11 (1947), 16-18.

165. Sykes, *Growth and Development of Speech Therapy*, p. 7; *Manchester Education Committee Annual Report, 1905-6*, pp. 46, 153-4; *Report of the Liverpool Education Committee for the year 1907-8*, p. 67.

166. Pound, *Bennett*, p. 165.

167. Eldridge, pp. 39, 51-2; Hartwell, p. 101. Note attached to the Manchester copy of Chervin's *Du Bégaiement considéré comme vice de prononciation* (Paris, (1867); *Rapport présenté à la Société d'Education de Lyon Par une Commission . . . composée de M. Le Dr. Desgranges . . . instituée par M. le Senateur Prefet du Rhône pour l'examen de la Méthode Curative de Bégaiement de M. Chervin Aîné, Lyon, 1866*, p. 21; 'The Cure of Stammering', *British Medical Journal*, 2 (1872), 333-4; 'The Treatment of Stammering', *British Medical Journal*, 2 (1874), p. 376; 'Stammering', *Lancet*, 2 (1874), p. 461; Advertisement, *The Voice* (1879), p. 144 cited by Schoolfield, p. 116.

168. Gerdts, p. 10.

169. Schoolfield, p. 116.

170. J. Perelló, *The History of International Association of Logopedics and Phoniatrics. I.A.L.P. 1924-76* (Barcelona, Editorial Augusta), p. 14.

7 MEDICINE AND SURGERY

It behoved those classifying stuttering as a disease to find a medical remedy and one obvious course was to improve patients' vitality. No one disputed Yearsley's statement that stuttering 'sympathises in an extraordinary degree with the state of the general health',[1] nor with the need to stimulate circulation and lungs by exercise. This could be aided by curing disease conditions and by diet directed towards rectifying digestive troubles. Critics had said that most treatises on stuttering contained 'about as much value as the current pamplets on balneology',[2] a popular subject in mid-century when spas were still fashionable. Edwin Lee, in fact, had kept Englishmen informed on Continental developments through his various publications on hydrotherapy and watering places and it is not surprising that some should have commended cold sponging to stutterers.[3] Sea-bathing was also considered beneficial,[4] but a warm salt bath would substitute.[5] With all this, elocutionists had no quarrel. For M'Minn, a perfect cure depended upon perfect health[6] and Madame Behnke believed the removal of obstructions to breathing should precede elocution.[7] Indeed, there was implicit agreement with Bishop's contention that patients should be assisted in acquiring voluntary control simultaneously over their mental and vocal functions. The most rational approach came from Shuldham, who said it was 'for the medical man to find out any disorders of the health, and to rectify them' and 'for the elocutionist to discover the disorders of speech, and by elocutionary help to rectify them'.[8] But several of his colleagues were unwilling to surrender control and the arguments on both sides continued. While 'rhetorical lessons' were powerless against lung adhesions, affectations of the cranial nerves[9] and other derangements of the nervous system,[10] the record had shown that medical men had not treatment within their 'power'.[11] For those wishing to arrogate stuttering to themselves, this was an uncomfortable fact and must partly account for the profession's extraordinary response to surgical treatment. In the absence of a psychiatric specialty, what were the alternatives? Drugs and local remedies were hardly panaceas, neither were electricity and mesmerism. Moreover, the latter were not confined to the medical profession, even though it produced the chief pioneers and authorities. This left surgery, which initially looked as if it might send elocutionists scurrying and finally yield the problem into medical hands.

Drugs and Local Treatments

Although Mason advised stutterers to take nothing but '*courage, advice,* and *pains*',[12] elocutionists generally condoned the use of drugs, which they and physicians saw principally as an adjunct to therapy. The rationale for such treatment was rarely explained, but can be deduced from causal theories and the medicines administered. It was reasoned that a stutterer's system needed depleting and building up, so calling for anti-phlogistic measures and tonics. These were not viewed as contradictory: Yearsley recommended both purgatives and tonics for 'facial' and 'choreal' stuttering.[13] There was also a case for bracing the muscles, nerves and circulation, yet most patients needed relaxing. Were excitants or anti-spasmodicants, stimulants or sedatives required? The drugs prescribed were those currently popular, especially for nervous disorders. Several had variable actions, depending upon their strength. Gelseminum, for example, had analgesic, hypnotic and anti-phlogistic properties, whereas arsenic was an anti-spasmodicant and restorative, especially to the respirators.[14]

Purgings had been a therapeutic mainstay of humoral medicine and there was reason for their use amongst stutterers. James Hamilton had found them beneficial in tetanus, hysteria and chorea and his *Observations on the Utility and Administration of Purgative Medicines in several Diseases* (1805) was influential. Anthelmintics counteracted worms and other irritants initiating the distant reflexes said to underlie various spasmodic affections. Furthermore, their depletory action reduced plethora and had been manifestly successful in Bostock's widely reported case[15] of a young lad who had been placed on a strict diet and given jalap and calomel, followed by Epsom salts, whenever his stuttering returned.

Much less popular was bleeding, but local or general blood-letting was occasionally recommended.[16] Though stutterers had been temporarily relieved by leeching, Poett did not endorse the practice.[17] Nor did Alexander Bell condone blistering, a patient of his having been treated with a collar of Spanish Flies at a public hospital.[18] Blistering was a treatment inherited from humoral medicine; it was used by Mercurialis for balbuties and found effective in loosening Samuel Johnson's tongue following his stroke. Its modern advocates were James Yearsley and Tyler Smith.[19] Yearsley's objection to elocutionists was that they interpreted stuttering as one complaint requiring one remedy. His approach was flexible, varying with the site of the spasm. Those unfortunate enough to be laryngeal stutterers had moxa or tartaremetic ointment applied to the hyoid bone (Figure 2.1, n23, p. 55), a treatment used in epilepsy and chorea and designed to produce an eschar, blister or irritation.[20] Along with surgery, it was a practice Wright strongly denounced in his *The Stutterer's Friend*, a publication directed specifically against Yearsley and Tyler Smith.[21]

Emetics were mentioned, but they failed to rank with purgatives, which were rivalled in popularity by restoratives, particularly tonics. Broster reputedly placed great store by diet,[22] and recommendations ranged from plain food[23] to vegetarianism[24] and meat eating,[25] with Kingsley cautioning against all 'hot slops'.[26] Stutterers themselves were amongst the many who bore witness to the efficacy of tonics: a dose of strychnine enabled M'Minn to 'face the music',[27] whilst the combination of tonic and alternative had assisted Bernard, who was the only one to provide a formula:

> ℞ Liq. Arsenicalis (Fowler's), mxxx;
> Liq. Strychniæ, mxlviij;
> Aqua Menthæ Pip., ad℥iij
> One teaspoonful twice daily after meals[28]

Interestingly, the speech pathologist who probably knew most about drugs, Samuel Potter, had little to say about them in connection with stuttering.[29] In England, those giving them most attention were Shuldham and the younger Poett.

Drugs and emotions affect individuals differently, those with languid muscles finding fluency in anger or under the effect of stimulants.[30] Similarly, alcohol could produce what was sometimes called 'stammering' or it might promote fluency and loquacity. But despite their sedative effects, alcohol and tobacco were frowned upon. Drinking was not a problem, at least in Mason's practice and smoking was rarely excessive (Table 3.1, p. 79), so abstinence would not have proved difficult.

Sedatives may have general effects or be specific to one of the systems. Gerdts administered a special tincture for diaphragmatic cramps,[31] whereas others valued drugs beneficial with epilepsy, chorea and 'nerves'.[32] Those specifically mentioned were stramonium, hyoscyamus, belladonna, ignatia, valerian and opium,[33] but a critical note was sounded by Shuldham, who warned that the soothing effects of chlorate hydrate, bromide of ammonium and bromide of potassium were outweighed by their depressive action.

Lotions and potions are the speciality of mountebanks but their activity seems to have been minimal over the century. The only bizarre treatment, highly valued by the patient, was licking mustard.[34] It was not stated whether this served to stimulate salivation, so often reduced in fear,[35] though not in Abbotts' patients, who were prescribed astringents and gargle for the opposite condition.[36] The quack medicaments mentioned earlier (p. 169) were little different from those prescribed by many doctors. And, in fact, Victorians had to look to earlier times for a dubious remedy:

> An Admirable Confect, which assuredly Cures Stuttering or Stammering in Children or grown Persons, tho' never so bad, causing them to speak distinct and free, without any trouble or difficulty; it remedies all manner of Impediments in the Speech, or disorders of the Voice of any kind, proceeding from what Cause soever, rendering those Persons capable of speaking easily, free, and with a clear Voice, who before were not able to utter a Sentence without Hesitation; its stupendious Effects, in so quickly and infallibly curing Stuttering, Stammering and all disorders of the Voice and difficulty in delivery of the Speech are really Wonderful.[37]

This was sold at Mr Osborn's Toyshop for 2s 6d a pot along with elixirs for consumption, snuff for purging headache and a chymical secret to rectify vapours in women. If this was a more disreputable remedy than those known to Victorians, then they were not too badly off, since it probably amounted to little more than a throat lozenge.

Electricity and Hypnotism

During the eighteenth century there emerged two phenomena having medical applications and a tenuous connection through their association with magnetism: electricity and mesmerism. The association proved more verbal than real, for the forces exerted were quite different. Being poorly understood and exciting remarkable effects, their therapeutic boundaries were ill-defined and their proponents not always orthodox physicians. However, it was by no means unusual for those contributing to some branch of speech pathology to have written about one or the other – Bequerel, Benedict, Bristowe, Duchenne, Féré, Braid, Edwin Lee, John Ashburner and Edgar Foster – though this did not entail an application to stuttering.

Electricity was first used medically in 1743-4 by Krüger of Halle, and some 20 years later apparatuses for generating this static or frictional form was installed in several London hospitals. Meanwhile, Galvani had demonstrated electricity in animal tissue, which led Volta to the battery and the 'pile' bearing his name.[38] The direct current which they discovered laid the foundations for experimental electrophysiology. It also was used as a general panacea for nervous and muscular disorders until about 1830, when the induced current of 'faradisation' was introduced, and this is what 'electrotherapy' usually signified. After 1888, electricity was employed in diathermy and in this century, through electro-encephalography, it has revealed much about neurological disorders, though not stuttering.

Having proved efficacious with both vocal and nervous problems, it was hardly surprising that electricity should be tried on stutterers. For functional aphonia its benefits were reputedly unequalled,[39] possibly because an hysterical element was frequently present, and writers on stuttering often obscured their argument by bringing vocal problems or paralysis into this part of their discussion.[40] To elicit voice, the current was initially applied externally, but Duncan Gibb introduced British doctors to direct stimulation of the cords.[41] As stutterers' muscles were reputedly weak, either through debility or disuse, galvanism provided a ready stimulant, while its sedative properties could soothe the system. As an antispastic remedy it was popular for chorea and those spasmodic affections[42] that had been classed with stuttering.

The first detailed account of galvanism and stuttering appeared during the debate on surgery, when an 'operation' using specially designed 'elegant little instruments' was devised for removing the tip of the coccyx so that a needle might be inserted into its cancellated bone. On wishing to speak, the patient somehow connected this needle to the wire from a small galvanic battery resembling a hunting watch. The current, travelling up his vertebral column and through the fauces, kept his palate 'distended like a sail' and his uvula 'floating upon its stream like a pennant'. Appropriately, the eminent observers were 'electrified' by his perfectly regulated voice and the intention was to patent the 'truly philanthropic discovery'. No such record seems to exist, probably because its real worth was soon apparent: the lad thus 'cruelly victimised' was soon worse than ever.[43]

Within a decade, the *Lancet* was again raising the subject, this time in connection with a query over whether there was an effective cure of stuttering. With a preface that the complaint had unfortunately been left to unprincipled quacks, the writer suggested that the deficient nervous energy of lingual stuttering might be rectified by a stream of electricity through the tongue.[44] His method, however, was not favoured by another correspondent, who recommended a two-pronged approach: general and local. First, the 'fluid' should be applied to the whole system by holding the ends of the conductors in the hands whilst the machine was fully active. Secondly, the conductors should be placed at the nape of the neck and upper chest. After five or six sittings lasting fifteen minutes for each procedure, the time should be doubled and, in severe cases, repeated daily for weeks. Horne believed that past failures were due to insufficient treatment and inefficient apparatus, the primary and secondary coils being too small.[45]

Whether this advice was heeded is not known as those using electro-therapy rarely described their technique. On the Continent, the treatment was used by Coën, coupled with elocution, where the system needed bracing. It was also used by Rosenthal – who galvanised the head, larynx and hypoglossal nerve[46] – and by Klencke. Evidently unaware of other work, Potter, in America, thought static electricity worth trying and suggested that the patient sit on an insulated stool for 15 to 20 minutes daily while being charged with franklinic electricity, then back in vogue.[47] In England, possibly under the influence of Duncan Gibb, the remedy was tried by James Hunt[48] and also by Bristowe,[49] of the Bristowe-Smart coil, who went into great detail on its application in nervous diseases. Klencke and Hunt found it benefits transitory, but Althaus thought the continuous current a useful adjunct when response to didactic treatment was slow.[50]

For Blake, attributing stuttering to weak external pterygoid muscles, electricity provided an obvious solution. He used electro-cautery for the nasal inflammations that could aggravate stuttering, and he 'educated' the muscles by combining a faradic-gentle secondary current with a voltaic current of one milliampere, which was gradually raised to two, through an electrode placed behind the soft palate and a wetted disc on the malar bone of the same side, a 'commutator' preventing injury. Reinforcement was provided by a trained masseuse who, with an electrode on his arm in contact with one on the patient's neck, stimulated the respiratory muscles by effleurage, petrissage and tapottement.[51] Like Coën, he supplemented the treatment with Ling's exercises, an approach also favoured by Shuldham.[52]

Much less was said about hypnotism, partly because its application to neurotic conditions awaited Bernheim's work of 1884, and because the British Medical Association's disapproval was not removed until

1890. But as stutterers were supposedly impressionable, their disorder being duè to auto-suggestion[53] or 'contagion', it was reasonable that this proclivity be turned to therapeutic advantage. To a limited extent, it was used by various people: one patient was told that he was under the mesmeric influence of a 'professor' who took his fee and disappeared;[54] Arnold Bennett later tried the auto-suggestive psychotherapeutics of Couéism;[55] Walter Yearsley consulted two professional hypnotists;[56] and stutterers must have learnt something about personal magnetism and thought transference from Foster, since these were subjects that he offered to resident pupils at his vicarage in Ipswich.[57] Amongst physicians, Kingsbury reported one success[58] and Tuckey, with experience of twelve patients, extolled its value with children and considered it the best remedy for young adults.[59]

Dugald Stewart had prepared the ground for differentiating between the physical and moral agents associated with animal magnetism. The distinction was further elaborated by James Braid, a Manchester surgeon, who separated mesmerism, supposedly dependent upon magnetic fluid, from braidism, which recognised the neurophysiological laws actually operative.[60] In this natural state of heightened sensibility, which Braid called 'neuropnology', later termed 'hypnotism', patients were therapeutically receptive, and amongst the many conditions he claimed to have alleviated were deafness and aphonia.[61] Significantly, stuttering was not one of them. His investigations into mesmeric phenomena began in November 1841, just when the controversy over surgery for stutterers was dying down.

Operations

The preceding months had witnessed an unprecedented interest in stuttering, reflected in the journal coverage which was far in excess of the space given the subject over the previous half century. Dozens of items appeared in print: some treatises, technical reports, notices and comments, many abstracts from foreign journals. The early months were marked by a naive optimism amongst certain surgeons, who, theoretically confident of the analogies they were drawing and readily convinced by patients' post-operative performance, believed they were on the threshold of a new and dramatic cure.

The seeds had been sown ten years earlier when Professor Stromeyer, of Hanover, had relieved *clubfoot* by dividing the Achilles tendon. The operation was of long-standing but his technique made it a viable remedy that was widely adopted. One of those to benefit and later champion the operation was Dr William Little, who himself suffered from talipes of the left foot and had undergone Stromeyer's treatment. Whilst in Germany, he took the opportunity to call upon another colleague, Frederick Dieffenbach, one of the most active operators. In Little's opinion, he was 'justly celebrated for the dexterity of his operations'[62] and James Yearsley conceded that he had 'perhaps enriched the field of medical surgery more than any other living surgeon'.[63] His award of the Legion of Honour indicates the estimation in which he was held by Frenchmen. Apparently, so impressed was Dieffenbach by Little's new found mobility that he embraced clubfoot surgery 'with the whole ardour of this genius'.

Discounting undoubted abuses, there is no question that many benefited from surgical intervention: tenotomy represented a significant advance in orthopaedic treatment. But if cripples could be cured, there was hope for those suffering other contortions. The surgeons' imagination had been fired. Stromeyer began sectioning wry necks whilst Jules Gueron, in France, was attracting attention by his division of back muscles for spinal distortions. Then, seven years after the first talipes operation, Stromeyer proposed another – for squinting,[64] also called strabismus after the Greek geographer Strabo. Neither Stromeyer nor other protagonists in the ensuing priority squabble seems to have realised that the idea itself was not new. Symmetry may be achieved by trying to balance opposing muscles, either by cutting the stronger of the pair, or by interfering with its innervation. The former notion had been aired in America around 1813,[65] the same time that Charles Bell had contemplated sectioning the nerve.[66] Not wishing to experiment on humans and unable to locate a cross-eyed monkey during a London-wide search, Bell resorted to severing the facial nerve in a normal animal, which, unexpectedly, 'began to grimace with redoubled energy, but entirely on one side of his visage, the other remaining quite motionless'.[67] The expression resembled that of a distinguished actor who, Bell realised, was not endowed with extraordinary ability to control each side of his face independently, but suffered a palsy that later bore his name.

Dieffenbach, as bold as he was dextrous, carried out squinting operations towards the end of 1839. Popular acclaim followed and soon this disfiguring condition was thought to be 'under the absolute control of surgical skill'.[68] 'There is not', said Mr Phillip Bennett Lucas of the Metropolitan Free Hospital, 'a single operation in surgery which has met with so much success, or has been so extensively adopted within a short time, as the one first performed[[69]] by Professor Dieffenbach for the cure of Strabismus.'[70] With such triumphs to hand, further experimentation was inevitable and drooping lids, short sight and fixed stares were obvious targets for the ocular surgeons. Meantime, Dieffenbach was casting around for other, perhaps more intractable, conditions on whch to focus his skill. And so, a year almost to the day after the Académie des Sciences first heard of his squinting surgery, it received notification of an even more sensational operation, this time upon the *tongue*.[71]

Emboldened by the ease and apparent success of the ocular cures, Dieffenbach and others were well disposed to apply their techniques elsewhere. A suitable situation presented itself in the form of a patient with an inward turned eye and nystagmus, who also happened to stutter. The strabismus was convulsive, both it and the speech fluctuating in severity. Dieffenbach was quick to postulate an analogy between the two conditions and hindsight provided all the confirmation he required: stuttering and squinting had co-existed in several previous patients.[72] This was quite feasible. Indeed, such associations were age old and reached back into literature, Dante recording:

> there came to me in a dream a stuttering crone,
> squint-eyed, clubfooted, both her hands deformed,
> and her complexion like a whitewashed stone.[73]

Victorians sought an explanation for the concomitance. It could be attributed to distant dental irritations.[74] Alternatively, spasmodic affections like squinting might compound the picture,[75] or stuttering might arise from the extraneous muscular movements provoked by a patient's endeavours to overcome the spasm,[76] an interpretation approaching a modern view.[77] The association was also taken seriously earlier this century, when it was almost suggested that the two conditions formed part of a syndrome.[78]

Dieffenbach was further encouraged by his accomplishments with spasmodic facial contortions, which were possibly Bell's palsy. In fact, history repeated itself: Stromeyer was the first to conceive of dividing the facial muscles and Dieffenbach was the first to do so.[79] The analogy he drew was between the palsied face and the muscular contraction of clubfoot, 'which takes place at the expense of their paralysed opponents'. By severing muscles responsible for lifting the lid, he was able to facilitate eye closure on the affected side, with marked improvement in physiognomy.[80] The reasoning behind stuttering surgery was similar:

squinting had been called 'club-foot of the eye'[81] and stammering was viewed as squinting of the mouth. As Mr Lucas said:

> When the remarkable success attendant upon the division of the muscles of the human eye in strabismus was placed beyond all doubt, it was rational to suppose that the application of a similar operation to the muscles of the tongue in cases of stammer, where that organ presented deviations from its natural form, or was bound down or otherwise limited in its accustomed mobility, would be also attended with as happy results.[82]

Undoubtedly, some of the patients operated upon had oral anomalies which, if not actually of causal significance, were thought to be so, whilst others had neurological handicaps.[83] Misdiagnosis was aggravated by the terminological latitude of the word 'stammering' and Dieffenbach, although referring to the distinguished work of Schulthess, failed to adopt his verbal distinctions. Moreover, since many of the surgeons' previous experience of verbal defect was with cleft palate, they were disposed to a mechanical view. Analogy is central to advances in knowledge, its usefulness depending upon whether the examples taken for comparison have consistency and substance. Metaphor is unlikely to lead scientists aright, but if the conditions in question are poorly understood, its presence may not be recognised. It was realised that the two conditions were not directly comparable, but given the prevailing muscular theory of squinting and the surgeons' poor grasp of speech pathology, the analogy drawn was simplistic rather than ridiculous.

Dieffenbach's first operation took place on 7 January 1841 and by the end of the month he had carried out another 16. Though not all cases were prefectly cured, he felt confident enough to publish his results. To forestall any priority controversy,[84] he immediately notified the *Medicinische Zeitung* and within the month he had informed the French Academy and the Hufeland Medical Society, and had written his *Memoir*. This was soon translated, in part and fully, by Franz[85] and Travers respectively. A review of the latter also included descriptions of his operative methods,[86] as did reports from Lee[87] and Amussat,[88] another article taken from the French being published under Dieffenbach's own name.[89] The general public, too, were quick to receive news of what was afoot.[90]

Meanwhile surgery had become the treatment of choice for squinting. Numerous operations were performed[91] in Germany, France and even England, where surgery was not so much in vogue and medical treatment said to excel.[92] As the prevailing touchstone for prestige seemed to be novelty rather than good sense, it was inevitable that a priority wrangle should develop. No sooner had the dispute between Bennett Lucas and Franz died down over who introduced Dieffenbach's squint operation to Britain,[93] than a similar battle over stuttering surgery began. Reports reached Britain that Amussat had contemplated the operation before hearing of the German work;[94] and Velpeau pointed out that he had been publicly advocating palatal surgery as early as 1837, on account of stutterers' high vaulted palates, but he had desisted because the peculiarity was not universal. However, when he became aware of Dieffenbach's activities, though still in ignorance of the method used, Velpeau decided to test his new hypothesis and to reserve his 'right of priority' over surgery of the genio-glossi muscles (Figure 2.1, n21, p. 55). Despite this, he conceded that the palm probably went to a M. Thierry, who had operated on a child some years before. This was presumably during the 1820s, since the patient was a young man when Velpeau heard of him.[95] Whether this preceded the American operations is not clear; evidently Malebouche stated the Mrs Leigh had proposed surgery and that this was carried out many years before the fashion developed in Europe.[96] England could also field an early operator in Joseph Poett senior, who employed surgery infrequently but 'when required', on which occasions the cure was 'instantaneous'.[97] What this entailed is not stated, but we know that Martin Tupper was a patient of his,[98] and it is safe to assume that he and the 'Dr. P.' who planned operations on the tongue and lips were one and the same.[99] Tupper's father, a doctor, prevented this just in time and there are no other clues to Poett's surgical activities.

In 1841, the British protagonists in the priority debate were Yearsley and Braid. Yearsley was an innovator by temperament, but although a student of Itard's, he did not emphasise the functional aspect of stuttering. On receiving the Continental news, he wasted no time in recording that his own, less radical operation, had preceded Dieffenbach's by one month.[100] This prompted the Scot, James Braid, to press his own claim on the basis of operations carried out in September 1840.[101]

There seem to have been seven British operators,[102] comparable with the German[103] and fewer than the French.[104] But wherever, some of the greatest names in surgery were involved, one being Alexander Lizars, who had held the Chair of Surgery at Edinburgh University since 1831. Lizars was well suited to hazardous operations; earlier, he had been associated with Robert Liston at the Royal Infirmary and both men epitomised the intrepid qualities of contemporary Edinburgh surgeons.[105] The two differed, however, on the value of the knife to stutterers.

Whereas Lizars practised on cadavers and Franz read early reports in the original German, Bennett Lucas, sometime President of the Harveian Society, seems to have embarked on this surgical adventure on the basis of newspaper reports, never previously having considered the matter. Nevertheless, he quickly deplored the fact that medicine had left 'uncultivated an extensive field, in which . . . the empiric has not been slow to exhibit himself as an apparently scientific and assiduous labourer'.[106] So once again elocutionists were under attack, this time from a surgeon whose own standards were highly questionable. Rashness, in fact, was a characteristic of Bennett Lucas; so given was he to prevailing fads that he became embroiled in railway speculation, then rampant, and was forced to flee to France.[107]

In the days before anaesthetics and antiseptics, the range and type of operation possible was limited and hence, also, the scope for novelty and genuine originality. Danger and pain attended many procedures and called for surgeons of mettle and patients with great fortitude. Desperation was often the ground from which fortitude blossomed and professional ambition may well have given many operators the drive to tackle their more dangerous or unpleasant assignments. The former was true of Frau Doenau, mother of Dieffenbach's first patient, whose worry over her 13-year-old son's inarticulateness disposed her to clutch at straws. So severe were his contortions that Dieffenbach made another comparison: 'The species of fear and horror which some stammerers have at the pronunciation of certain sounds seems to be analogous to the agitation and agony occasioned by the sight of water in cases of hydrophobia, and might, not unaptly, be termed phonophobia.'[108] Although coming close to admitting the presence of psychic forces, Dieffenbach did not hesitate to recommend lingual surgery. In fact, his theoretical position was ambiguous for while it was logical to shorten the tongue so that its tip assumed the position supposedly ideal for speech,[109] the main purpose of Dieffenbach's efforts was to interrupt the 'nervous influence' underlying spasm, not least in the vocal cords. Mention of this area may reflect his contact with Müller, who followed Arnott, examined the excised fibres and, along with Romberg, observed the operations.[110]

To forestall a charge of prejudice and narrow perspective, Dieffenbach tried three surgical approaches: cutting through the root of the tongue from beneath, either subcutaneously or by severing the skin, and excising a portion from the upper part (Figure 7.1).[111] Though more severe, the latter method, subsequently described as 'glossotomy'[112] or 'glossectomy'[113] had the advantage of lifting the tongue tip (Figure 7.2). He rejected shortening the tongue by amputating its tip because this would not interrupt the 'abnormal nervous influence'.[114] Dieffenbach fully recognised other possibilities for experimentation and anticipated 'a vast field for the discovery of modifications' to his operations.[115] How right he was! One popular variation was to insert the knife into the flesh beneath the tongue (Figure 7.3). As already noted in chapter 4, Amussat and Boyer were agreed 'that stuttering, like squinting, depends on a deviation of the tongue and contraction of certain muscles, which prevent it from striking the *palate* freely'. To counteract this, division of the genio-glossi muscles was indicated.[116] After cutting round the muscles inside the jaw bone,[117] Amussat found that scarring was liable to restrict the tongue's new freedom of movement, and so he would reopen the wound and insert charpie between its free edges.[118] Paradoxically, whereas Dieffenbach operated to reduce tongue length, Baudens believed that spasm and shortening were the problem. But to elevate the tip the answer was much the same and consequently, as success depended upon total division of the fibres, he severed them near the jaw to a depth of one inch and when the spasms radiated to the neck, he extended the section to the genio-hyoid muscles (Figure 2.1, n22, p. 55). Variations along these lines were also practised by Petrequin,[119] Velpeau[120] and Froriep,[121] as well as Bennett Lucas, and probably Braid, in England.

A modification considered even safer by Bonnet was to approach the muscles through a small puncture under the chin, thereby minimising bleeding and inflammation.[122] Though this operation was described in English during April,[123] Lizars did not refer to it when recounting his own very similar technique, apparently developed independently. In his case report, Lizars noted that the patient's tongue was shorter than usual, but he made no effort to justify the treatment, and one gets the impression that his chief interest was to test a new surgical technique.[124]

Another radical measure was to section the nerves causing spasm. Interrupting the laryngeal innervation had long been mooted and rejected by Arnott[125] and Cull.[126] But Phillips turned his attention elsewhere, believing that Dieffenbach's success resulted from having inadvertently severed the lingual nerve.[127] Simply cutting this would be a more straightforward and logical procedure, given that the 'nervous influence' needed changing. The idea also occurred to Dieffenbach's book reviewer[128] and to Dr Clutterbuck,[129] but it was dismissed by

Figure 7.1: Horizontal Division of the Tongue With Excision of a Wedge-shaped Portion

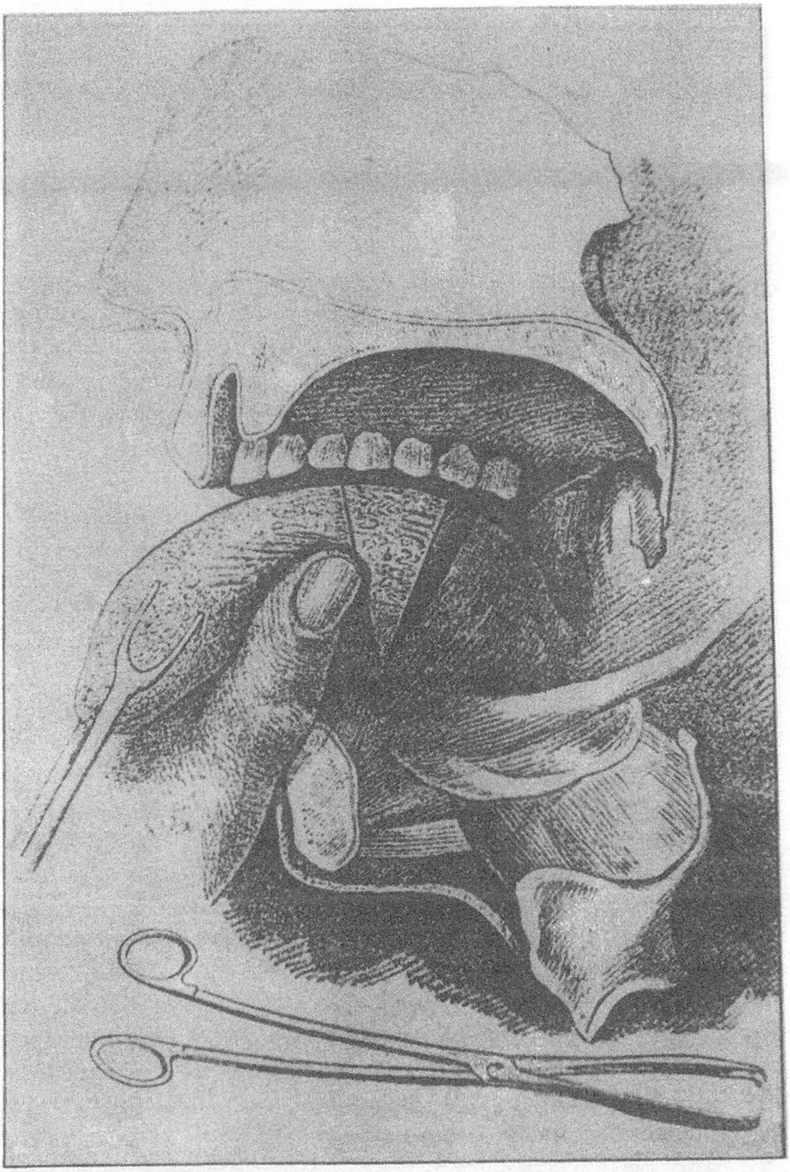

Source: J. Dieffenbach's, *Memoir*, plate 1.

Figure 7.2: View of the Tongue After a Wedge-shaped Portion Had Been Removed

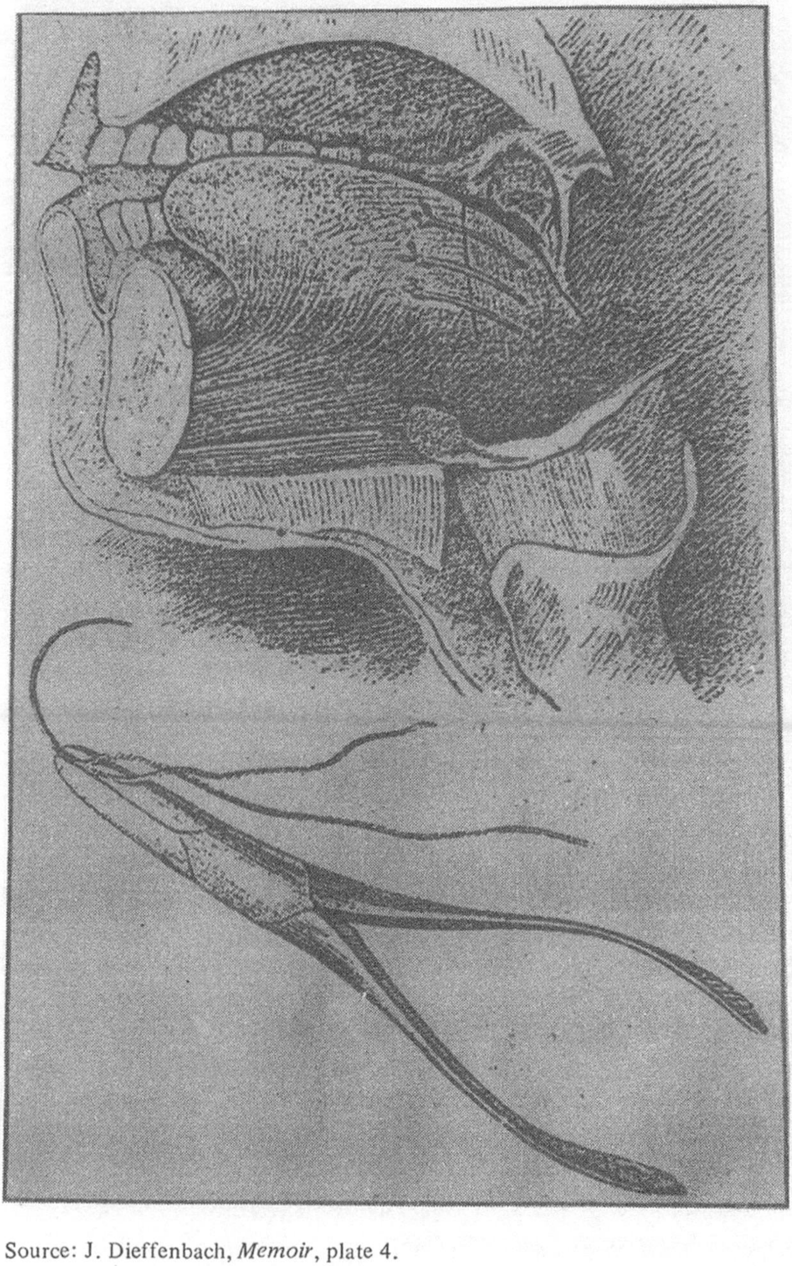

Source: J. Dieffenbach, *Memoir*, plate 4.

Figure 7.3: A Sublingual Operation

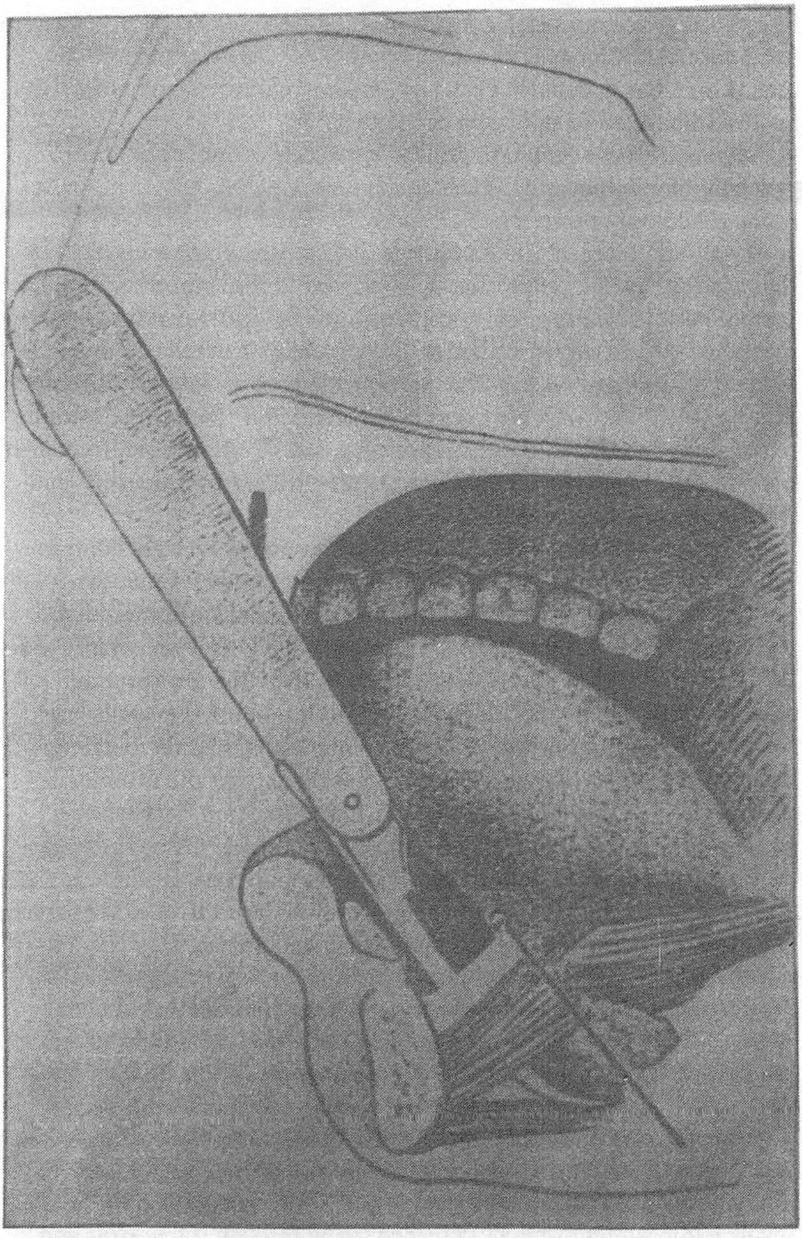

Source: C. Phillips, *De la Ténotomie*, plate 12.

Yearsley, who stated that nothing but paralysis of the laryngeal and lingual muscles would result.[130] In view of Müller's belief that the hypoglossal was responsible for all tongue movement, Yearsley's concern was reasonable, but was not shared by Phillips, whose experiments made him 'conspicuous' in Paris and evidently contributed to him being made a Chevalier of the Legion of Honour.[131]

No such glories accrued to British operators, whose surgery was generally more moderate, Tyler Smith reporting that only two glossectomies had been performed in London.[132] Franz[133] and Lucas[134] certainly did one each. The advantage of also using minor surgery was that variety enabled treatment to be tailored to the symptom. Braid prescribed tonsillectomy for obstruction to the glottal passage and he amputated the uvula when its length supposedly irritated the epiglottis.[135] Lucas used words like 'stammer doctor' as an articulation test for apical sounds. When patients failed, division of the tongue lowering muscles was indicated. Depending on the case,[136] he selected from eight operations,[137] and, in fact, believed that he had carried out every one that had been recommended.[138]

Yearsley's eightfold classificatory system similarly enabled him to tailor treatment to symptoms. He had adopted surgery when two patients suffering from both an ear infection and a stutter regained fluency after aural operations.[139] Though initially believing that it was difficult to prescribe specific operations because the disorder could not be easily classified,[140] he later changed his mind. The uvula was removed in gutteral stuttering and, proudly claiming to be the doctor who used tonsillectomy the most frequently in cases of stuttering or deafness,[141] he extirpated the tonsils, too, if infected.[142] When the oro-nasal orifice needed widening, he removed tissue from the velum and sectioned the palatine arches.[143] Further, he placed a seton in the fraenum or lip for lingual and labial stuttering respectively. The former substituted for cutting the fraenum, which had the unfortunate consequence of reducing the oro-nasal aperture, once the tongue was no longer anchored forwards. With tissue removal, glossectomy had the reverse effect, Yearsley attributing the operation's success to the enlarged aperture it caused.[144] Despite his theories, Yearsley's practices were often inconsistent. In one place he suggests that erratic tongue movements were modified not by the seton as such, but by the accompanying soreness,[145] it being observed by several people that healing and a relapse of speech often coincided.[146] Yet in a patient whose uvula had been removed, he threaded string through the nostrils and mouth, not to introduce a principle of discomfort, but to raise the soft palate mechanically.[147] He also employed acupuncture, without giving reasons.[148]

Those maligning surgeons frequently charged them with quackery, and operations such as the foregoing reveal the narrow line between orthodoxy and malpractice. Doctors who had been opposed to wholesale squint-cutting were in the forefront of what was designated a 'new specimen of charlatanism'.[149] In France, Gerdy attributed the mania for tenotomies to 'the mercantile spirit of the day' which pervaded Europe and was, he said, a 'shameful charlatanism, whose only aim was gold'.[150] Similar sentiments were expressed by the Society of Medicine at Brussells, which, in applauding a Dr Zoude's critical memoir on stuttering surgery, warned that '... "the insatiable desire for notoriety and temporary success often makes a man work almost entirely for his own profit, when he is pretending that all that he does is for the progress of science" '.[151] The various manifestations of quackery tended to proliferate endlessly, causing one writer to liken them to the hydra of mythology, the *Lancet* no sooner having succeeded in striking off one head of the 'seven-headed monster' than another appeared in its place.[152]

The imputation of quackery arose, not only because of these financial motives and the dubious theoretical basis of the treatment, but because of its consequences, which ranged from the uncomfortable to the fatal. Gradually publications started listing them: sore throat and nasal speech,[153] temporary blunting of taste,[154] abscesses,[155] difficulty swallowing,[156] shooting pain from the wound to behind the ear lobe[157] and tumescence of the salivary glands requiring reduction by leeches.[158] Worse still were the fatalities, stemming from infection, asphyxia and haemorrhage. Velpeau lost a patient through 'purulent absorption'.[159] Another Frenchman reputedly died after a severed fraenum permitted the tongue to roll back and suffocate him.[160] In addition, there were probably several deaths from blood loss. Dieffenbach, well aware of this danger,[161] was not wholly responsible for the demise of a Jewish medical student, since the young man 'escaped' from hospital and, after a long journey home, imprudently tore out the stitches. The local surgeon's efforts to control the bleeding proved ineffectual, as did Dieffenbach's personal intervention the next day.[162] In a similar position, Guersant resorted to cautery, compression and alum,[163] and even comtemplated ligating the lingual arteries.[164] Finally, after losing a twelve-year-old boy through haemorrhage, he warned: 'If the success of this operation so loudly proclaimed, induces patients too easily to submit to it, they will here find a salutary check to their enthusiasm ...'[165]

If not imprudent, Continental surgeons were certainly unlucky. The worst that seems to have happened in this country was severe haemorrhage in one of Braid's outpatients. A 19-mile horse-ride is not the ideal way to recuperate from such an operation, and the bleeding began after the man's arrival home and was controlled by the local physician only with the greatest difficulty.[166]

Creditably, doctors in England anticipated tragic consequences before the first deaths were announced. Indeed, Bartlett, despite considering surgeons 'peculiarly fitted' to treat stutterers, outlined the dangers inherent in oral surgery before 1841.[167] Then, early that year, one writer feared that fatalities might result from unskilled people being tempted to operate with inadequate knowledge;[168] another pointed to the risk both of haemorrhage[169] and of losing the tongue. The latter could come about either through ulceration, sloughing,[170] or by the tongue being torn out accidently, when severed at its base. This particular calamity was apparently avoided, but its possibility was raised in connection with Fowler's book on Persia, a country in which tongue removal was the fate of criminals. As there was no severe detriment to speech, the editor of the *Literary Gazette*, a staunch supporter of Thomas Hunt, suggested that the Persian method might be 'more humane and efficacious' than the recent practices of surgeons. And 'though it must be rather inconvenient to be without a tongue for other purposes (were it only for licking the lips), we would advise Mr. Hunt, who cures stammering without cutting or maiming at all, to look to his laurels . . . '[171]

It was the severity of Dieffenbach's operation that particularly alarmed reviewers of his *Memoir*. One said that such experimentation would be 'most unwarrantable' in British hospitals;[172] another went further, describing it as 'one of the greatest outrages upon modern surgery';[173] and a third stated:

> Having overcome the muscular errors of the eye, he now gives forth that he is also master of those of the tongue, – not by an operation at once simple and scientific, as in the former case, – but by a cruel mutilation, difficult to both parties in execution, not unlikely to prove wholly destructive to the organ, dangerous even to life itself, founded on an unphilosophic assumption of an unstable theory, unsupported by the result of practical experiment, and altogether unworthy of the present position of surgery – seeming rather as if empirically revived from amidst the barbarities of the dark ages.[174]

If mutilation was involved, then it was suggested that operations would be in breach of Lord Ellenborough's Act,[175] which served to protect the public against excesses of this kind, though not against minor measures like tonsillectomy.[176]

This Act had a long history. In England, the putting out of eyes and severing of tongues had been carried out by private persons to a sufficient extent that during the middle ages it became necessary to control the practice by law. Various other bills relating to mayhem followed, one of the more important being the Coventry or Maiming Act of 1670, which was reframed by Lord Ellenborough more than a century later. The new Act bearing his name made it a capital offence, amongst other things, to cut or maim with a sharp instrument. The critics of stuttering surgery were evidently unaware that this Act, along with 56 others, had been repealed in 1828 and replaced by Peel's 'Offences against the Person Bill'. This law, however, was in the same spirit as those it replaced and was aimed at preventing wounding with malicious intent, hardly a motive attributable to the surgeons, however ill-advised their treatment.

Other detractors had recourse to parody and sarcasm. In an allusion to Yearsley, it was suggested that his physiology was learnt from the 'Society for the Confusion of Useful Knowledge'.[177] Few doubted that some stutterers had become fluent following surgery, but was this due to it? While blood loss itself might have been salutary, most accredited the improvement to moral impressions. Dr Chowne believed that, given the patient's confidence, mesmerism would be equally effective. And Dr Thomson suggested that, if operations had to be done, then 'a curious little figure' be carved on the surface of the tongue. It was also said that cures might be had by snipping off the tip of the nose,[178] or boring a hole in the palate.[179] Even primates might benefit from such manoeuvres: monkeys having speech organs like man, would be ideal subjects for experimentation. One writer recommended that Yearsley try excising their uvulae, adding – 'Perhaps it might improve their chattering: who knows but in his hands it might make them talk?'[180]

Other attitudes to surgery may be gauged from the number of operations that actually took place and the period over which they were carried out. Yearsley was still talking about minor procedures in 1843, but by late 1841 radical surgery was on the wane in England, if not already abandoned. Hence the British were censorious of reports that Continental operations continued. In 1844 Petrequin was again cutting round jaw muscles,[181] and the following year Dieffenbach was still recommending surgery, if only in 'the most obstinate cases' unresponsive to other measures.[182]

Continental commitment was likewise reflected in the extent of surgery. By 1845, Dieffenbach had performed about 80 operations,[183] his pace comparable with Bonnet's namely, 42 sections of the lingual muscles by July 1841. French enthusiasm was evident in the first four months when 200 stutterers had been treated,[184] 33 by Amussat, whose total reached at least 85,[185] this presumably excluding the 55 tongue-tie operations credited to him.[186] In England, minor surgery prevailed. Braid saw 'scores' of people, more than could be accounted for by the local population[187] and Yearsley chalked up 300 operations in a four-month period.[188] The extent of lingual surgery is less clear, but Lucas' complement of radical operations was around 18.[189] Taken together with Lizars' operation and an unspecified number by Braid, we may assume that in Britain this surgery was applied to fewer than 50 patients and possibly half that number.

The appeal of surgery was that it offered a quick and near miraculous cure, and miracles were what was needed. The vicious circle of disappointments, hopes and renewed failure engendered wishful thinking and imprudence:

> There is, in the human mind, a love for novelty and a predilection for the marvellous . . . It is not surprising therefore that the love of the marvellous should extend to objects that respect health, when so many flattering promises (however fallacious) are held up to the desponding invalid, whose weakness leads him to credulity and his distempered imagination to hope and confidence.[190]

Such was the position of many stutterers. But perhaps their hope was justified, as miracles seemed to be happening. It was no exaggeration, said Yearsley, 'that some patients have sat down before me *dumb*, and, after the operation, have gone away speaking freely'.[191] Similarly, Lucas' clinical judgement was vindicted when a patient excelled himself with the word 'hippopotamus'.[192] Sometime before, Frederick Doenau had impressed a member of the Berlin Medical Association with his prompt articulation of 'preobadschenskoy',[193] which tempted a British critic to remark that if this meant 'very bad surgery', as it looked, then the boy should be encouraged in his laudable remarks.[194] Scepticism of Dieffenbach, however, was not new. An assessment of Phillips' book *The Surgery of Dieffenbach*, written in 1840, acknowledged the Prussian's originality, but observed: 'an impression is also left on the mind of the reader that he is deficient in carefully distinguishing those cases in which operation will be really beneficial, and that he excels more as a skilful manipulator than a sound surgeon'.[195] A similar verdict could be passed on the disciples of stuttering surgery.

But just what were the results? There were two ways of finding out: observation of the surgery and investigation of testimonials. As if he were running a side-show, Yearsley issued invitations to his operations and exhibition of patients, that extended to the general press.[196] Large numbers might be present at a time[197] and witnesses soon exceeded 500.[198] So, however sharply critics might speak, many notable colleagues gave the remedy some credence. Most were impressed. *The Times* reported that Yearsley had proved the value of surgery 'beyond the possibility of doubt',[199] and the *Athenaeum's* representatives believed that the audience had caught Yearsley's own conviction, which would have weighed with them 'had we never observed how far more apt a number of persons are to be gulled than a few – they confuse each other, and foment each other's warmth of imagination', a confusion which spread to the patients,[200] who 'stammered out that they were better'.[201] A more impartial judgement was that at best they were only marginally improved.

However self-deluded, Yearsley was exonerated from any charge of wilful deception.[202] Indeed, he was always most open about his actions and testimonials. These testimonials Poett decided to check and when he announced that they were often inaccurate, Yearsley accused him of bribing the patients and so confusing them that their speech broke down. Endeavouring to establish the truth, the *Lancet* directly compared information supplied by the two men. Sometimes there was broad agreement, but two documents from a George Butler containing entirely contradictory statements led the *Lancet* to conclude that one was a forgery.[203] The truth may have been that the patient's speech relapsed. Yearsley conceded that this could happen, but he stoutly maintained that he had not misrepresented the facts at the time of writing, and he obtained another affidavit from Butler to this effect.[204] Poett's position in all this was somewhat hypocritical. No word was breathed of his own operations and the fifth edition of the book where they had been mentioned was retitled and directed against surgery.[205]

Much of the debate took place at meetings of the London and Westminster Medical Societies, and was then reported in the leading professional journals. Similar debates occurred in Paris, where interest was intense. When Amussat first presented his cases to the Académie de Médicine uproar ensued, which one British critic described as 'an *emeute* of the most disgraceful nature'.[206] The consequence was that a vast gathering attended the next meeting.[207] Reactions in London were more muted, though there was much excitement.[208] Discussions were obviously lively, but decorum prevailed.

The controversy finally resolved into a battle between Yearsley and all comers, and often turned on petty matters. His address to the Westminster Medical Society was a case in point. Those opposed to surgery criticised the Society for 'inviting' him to speak. The Society countered by saying he had only been 'permitted'.[209] Always quick in self-defence, Yearsley insisted that since he made no request, the question of permission did not arise.[210] Then his claim to originality was questioned: there was nothing new in amputating tonsils and uvulae.[211] This he conceded, but it did not negate his own contribution, which was to show that such surgery could help stutterers, as well as the hard-of-hearing.[212]

After six months, Yearsley felt badly treated. He resented the support supposedly given by the *Lancet* to 'stammering schoolmasters' and others,[213] and he suggested that their hostility stemmed from 'rivalry'.[214] In particular, he resented the *Lancet* printing a letter from Thomas Hunt in which surgeons were described as 'slashers'.[215] He could not continue to do battle with elocutionists, various correspondents *and* the editor of the *Lancet*; time would reveal that he had never distorted facts, maimed patients nor deluded himself. Meanwhile, he would continue to operate when stuttering was associated with 'disorganisation of the throat'.[216] Moreover, to avoid 'tampering' with his patients by 'unfair espionage', he had resolved to withhold their addresses and provide information only to people whose enquiries were free from malice.[217] The next dispute was with Robert Liston, who supported Hunt and condemned the 'unwarrantable incisions' that had left palates 'horribly mutilated'. Inferring that these remarks were aimed at him, Yearsley wrote to Liston for clarification and when no reply was forthcoming, he took the matter to the Royal College of Surgeons, which declined to intervene.[218]

But Yearsley was not without friends. Marshall Hall took his findings seriously,[219] and entrusted his own son to his care, with beneficial results to his hearing and articulation.[220] Others thought either that surgery was appropriate in certain instances, or should be give a fair trial. Greatest support, however, came from the anonymous writer whose book was dedicated to Yearsley:

> In looking round for a name to which the following pages may . . . be inscribed, none comes more prominently before, or appears more worthy of distinction, than your own.
>
> . . . The treatment of this grievous infirmity has been tacitly

> consigned to the domain of the empiric. You have led the way to a more just appreciation of its importance, and for this, independent of the valuable results of your investigations, you are entitled to the gratitude of mankind. To you belongs the merit of having first called in the aid of surgery in the treatment of stammering . . . yours are the only operations now performed in this country.[221]

The author, who considered his own experience second only to Yearsley's and Colombat's, adopted a pseudonym to show that he wrote from benevolence, not ambition. However, since he was Tyler Smith, Yearsley's brother-in-law, his opinions were far from impartial, which could explain the favourable report he gave on 200 of the patients Yearsley operated upon for defective speech.[222]

The two did not give up easily and the *Lancet's* tune changed five years later, when Tyler Smith was at the helm and in a position to settle old scores. Thomas Hunt's letters were no longer acceptable, because: 'A professional man can only give fair play to an honest equal. Quacks of all kinds are, according to our code, without the pale; and no more deserve mercy or quarter, than do reptiles or beasts of prey.'[223] Smith believed that all midwives were a mistake,[224] and he felt similarly about elocutionists. However wrong operations might be, the medical profession should not give any support to Hunt and thereby elevate 'this empiric into a judge of surgery.'[225] Such dissension placed patients in an unenviable position. It was a 'species of treason against all social law' to cure without a diploma and by implication to seek help from the unqualified.[226] The dilemma facing stutterers was clear: should they follow the advice of a respected physician, who may be wrong, or heed the warnings of an empiric, who may be right? One suggestion was that they consult their doctor, who himself might be guided by Lee's book.[227]

Elocutionists returned fire. In addition to the *Literary Gazette*, Thomas Hunt found *The Medical Times* receptive to his letters.[228] Bishop was also under attack, for although he held no brief for operations,[229] he epitomised some medical attitudes:

> Having thus narrowed the field, and taken, as it were, lawful possession of it, he proceeds at once most furiously to assail all trespassers upon his valuable property. Any one who has not taken out a medical degree for cultivating the flowers of speech that grow on these premises, and can only be reared by F.R.C.S.'s, is stigmatized as an empiric, an imposter, and heaven knows what else –

> so wicked and perilous it is to provoke the jealousy or interfere with the interests of the Lancet-armed proprietors of the soil . . . As teachers of elocution and schoolmasters have . . . ventured to intermeddle with the province of surgery; he proclaims, that none but he, and such as he, so trained and so gifted, are fit to be trusted with what has hitherto been the office of these parties, namely, the management of the voice in speaking . . .[230]

It was difficult for the elocutionists to defend themselves in positive terms since however well qualified they might be, the fact remained that they were not physicians.

In addition to Hunt and Wright, the Bells also spoke out forcibly against surgery. Alexander senior's denunciation was contained in a poem on the tongue, which ran into 72 pages and included several verses on surgery:

> Mark how th' obstructed tongue gets fluency:
> The stutt'ring patient's seated in a chair,
> And thus made handy for the gory man.
> One who could drink hot blood stands by with dish
> To catch in time the rushing, purple stream.
> The 'little member's' tam'd for once; press'd down,
> Like raving madman bound within his cell,
> That thus the cunning man may see his way
> To cut and come again – to cut again.
> He stares into the ill-assorted mouth; –
> His eyes examine well the prostrate tongue; –
> The coast is clear; in cabman's phrase – 'all's right.'
> Presto! Whack, whack! – Behold the stammer's gone.

and further:

> The sanguinary work goes on: the parts
> which the Creator wisely form'd for speech
> Are hack'd and mangled with a frantic zeal;
> The fragments of the lacerated mouths
> Are shewn in triumph to the wond'ring crowd,
> Who marvel much that superfluities
> In man's construction are but now expos'd,
> And only for the first time science-prun'd![231]

In time, the surgical treatment of stuttering became an embarrassing memory to the medical profession. Little mention was made of it after 1846 and by the end of the century Wyllie described the episode as one of the most melancholy in surgical history.[232] Strangely, however, it still found a place in a contemporary American orthopaedic text,[233] and now, phoenix-like it rises again, suitably dressed for the next times. In 1968, Stevenson wryly noted that the ghost of Dieffenbach would be interested in reports that stuttering had ceased after a frontal lobe operation and puzzled that no new cure had been announced.[234] But his perplexity would have been short-lived, for within five years it was being suggested that though 'oro-pharyngeal surgery turned out to be useless', neuro-surgery 'may have opened a new avenue to the understanding and treatment of the disease'.[235] No doubt this would have amazed John Bristowe, whose own neurological and medical enquiries proved fruitless, and who was forced to conclude that the only methods of real efficacy were educational ones.[236]

Notes

1. Yearsley (1843-4), p. 289.
2. Kussmaul, p. 828; Wyllie, p. 32; M'Minn, p. 5.
3. Franz (1840-1b), p. 815; Pershing, p. 779; Shuldham, pp. 62, 72, who approved of Coën's water cure.
4. Abbotts, p. 28; Romberg, p. 364; Philip Foster, 'Stammering and its Treatment', letter to *Lancet*, 2 (1894), p. 598. Cf. Thelwall (1810), p. 70.
5. Poett jnr, pp. 48, 49. Cf. Palmer, p. 70, who favours a 'shower-bath'.
6. M'Minn, p. 32.
7. R. Behnke, p. 324. Cf. E. Behnke [1893], p. 22; D'Orsey, *British Medical Journal*, 1 (1885), p. 1322.
8. Shuldham, p. 36. Cf. Foster [1885], p. 22, who seems to take certain of his ideas from Shuldham.
9. Blake, p. 5.
10. Poett snr (1833), pp. 64-5.
11. A. Hartley, p. 57.
12. Mason (1884), p. 5.
13. Yearsley (1843-4), p. 293.
14. For a contemporary understanding of drugs' actions, see A.G. Burness and F.J. Mavor, *The Specific Action of Drugs on the Healthy System* (London, Baillière, Tindall & Cox, 1874), pp. x, 7-8; Sam'l O.L. Potter, *A Handbook of Materia Medica, Pharmacy and Therapeutics*, 8th edn (London, Rebman, 1901), pp. 31, 39, 55, 61.
15. Bostock, pp. 72-7 reported in: *Lancet*, 1 (1830-1), 217-18, *London Medical Gazette*, 7 (1830-1), 176-7, *Medico-Chirurgical Review*, 14 n.s. (1830-1), 209-10.
16. Romberg, p. 364.
17. Poett jnr, pp. 40, 42, 43, 49.
18. A. Bell, p. 47.

19. Physician, pp. 43, 44.
20. Yearsley (1843-4), pp. 289, 291.
21. Wright (1843), pp. 25, 38.
22. Physician, p. 36.
23. Foster [1900], p. 20. Cf. Philip Foster, *Lancet*, 2 (1894), p. 598. Philip, a doctor in Leeds, was probably the brother of J. Edgar, see Foster [1885], p. 3.
24. Bostock, p. 74.
25. Franz (1840-1b), p. 815.
26. Minute Philosopher, p. 11.
27. M'Minn, p. 27.
28. A. Bernard, p. 7.
29. Potter, *Materia Medica*, p. 844; Potter, *Speech*, pp. 90-1.
30. Borthwick, p. 34.
31. Gerdts, p. 44. According to Appelt, p. 38, this consisted of rectified alcohol, peppermint oil and chloroform.
32. Haward, p. 112; Shuldham, pp. 63-6. Cf. Foster [1885], pp. 22-3. Apart from Foster's comments on drugs, which, 'resting on doubtful empiricism' might therefore 'be excised with advantage', a generally favourable report was given to his book by the *Lancet*, 2 (1885), p. 257.
33. Poett jnr, p. 49.
34. Borthwick, p. 51.
35. Forshaw, p. 4.
36. Abbotts, pp. 26, 34-5.
37. Advertisement, *Spectator*, nos. cxxii, cxli, clvix, clxxiv, ccclvi (1711), noted by Cazalet, p. 11n and Hunt (1870), p. 305n.
38. Garrison's *History*, pp. 124-7, 138, 279.
39. G.D. Powell, *The Practice of Medical Electricity*, 2nd edn (Dublin, Fannin, 1872), p. 107.
40. Abbotts, p. 30; Bishop (1851), pp. 64-5; Foster (1885), p. 23; McCormac, p. 52. Cf. Lee, p. 6n.
41. George Duncan Gibb, *The Laryngoscope in Diseases of the Throat*, 2nd edn (London, John Churchill, 1867), p. 109.
42. Powell, *Practice of Medical Electricity*, p. 175.
43. Correspondent, 'New Operation for Stammering', *Lancet*, 2 (1840-1), p. 240.
44. Medicus, *Lancet*, 1 (1848), p. 84.
45. J.H. Horne, 'Treatment of Lingual Stuttering by Galvanism', *Lancet*, 1 (1848), p. 163. Cf. Ronald Daniel, 'A Case of "Phonic Spasm" successfully Treated by Electricity', *Lancet*, 1 (1896), 288-9. The patient was said to be suffering from 'stammering of the vocal cords'.
46. Rosenthal, p. 134. Cf. ibid., pp. 120, 124, 130; Kussmaul, p. 840.
47. Potter, pp. 91-2. Cf. ibid., pp. 65, 68, 105.
48. Hunt (1870), pp. 318-19.
49. Potter, p. 68.
50. Julius Althaus, *On the Medical Use of Galvanisation and Faradisation*, new edn (London, J. Churchill & Sons, 1870), pp. 30, 37-8.
51. Blake, *Lip Chorea*, pp. 14-16, 21; Blake, *Lancet*, 1 (1891), p. 123.
52. Shuldham, p. 72.
53. Albert Moll, *Hypnotism* (London, Walter Scott, 1890), pp. 58, 205, 225, 243, 315-16.
54. Beasley (1885), p. 10.
55. Pound, *Bennett*, p. 30.
56. W. Yearsley, p. 18.
57. J. Edgar Foster, *Practical Lessons in Hypnotism* (London, Stationer's Hall, 1900), inside back cover.

58. G.C. Kingsbury, *The Practice of Hypnotic Suggestion* (Bristol, John Wright and London, Simpkin, 1891), pp. 177-8.

59. C. Lloyd Rickey, *Treatment by Hypnotism and Suggestion; or, Psycho-Therapeutics*, 4th edn (London, Baillière, Tindall & Cox, 1900), pp. 159, 182-3, 184. On the Continent, hypnotism was mentioned favourably in Dr Ferdinand Gruenbaum's *Eklärung des Stotterns, dessen Heilung und Verhüntung* (Leipzig, 1897), according to a report in the *British Medical Journal*, 2 (1897), 655-6.

60. F.A. Volgyesia, 'The Discovery of Medical Hypnotism', *British Journal of Medical Hypnotism*, 7 (1955), 2-13, 25-34; Hunter and Macalpine, pp. 640-1, 906-10.

61. C.A.S. Wink, 'The Life and Work of James Braid (1795-1860) with special reference to hypnotism as an orthodox medical procedure' (Oxford Univ. B. Litt. thesis, 1969), p. 81.

62. W.J. Little, *A Treatise on the Nature of Club-Foot and Analogous Distortions* (London, W. Jeffs, 1839), p. xi n.

63. James Yearsley, letter *Lancet*, 2 (1840-1), p. 589.

64. Lee, p. 70.

65. 'Origin of the Operation for Strabismus', *British and Foreign Medical Review*, 12 (1841), p. 564. The report concerns an American student to whom an operation on the internal rectus muscle was recommended during 1812-13. He was keen to undergo surgery but his father forbade it, fearing the eye might turn to the opposite side. This proved to be a problem with the operations. Cf. 'Surgical Treatment of Stammering well known to the Ancients', *Medico-Chirurgical Review*, 37 n.s. (1842), 198-201. The operation described was merely cutting the fraenum and the 'stammerers' chiefly children with delayed speech.

66. John Bell, 'The Bells of Edinburgh', *Surgery*, 38 (1955), p. 801 (794-805).

67. DuBois D'Amiens, cited in ibid.

68. 'On the treatment of Strabismus by the Division of the Muscles of the Eye', *Provincial Medical and Surgical Journal*, 3 (1841-2), p. 5 (5-7).

69. This is questionable.

70. Review of Lucas' *Practical Treatise on the Cure of Strabismus* (1840), *Provincial Medical and Surgical Journal*, 1 (1840-1), 83-4.

71. Lee, pp. 41-2.

72. Dieffenbach, p. 8.

73. Dante, *Purgatorio*, Canto XIX, 7-9. (trans. John Ciardi).

74. Ashburner, pp. 84, 160. Cf. Frank Blake, 'Stammering a Reflex Symptom', *St. Louis Courier of Medicine*, 13 (1885), p. 278.

75. Romberg, p. 363.

76. Physician, p. 25.

77. Bloodstein, 'Physiological Concomitants' in *Handbook*, p. 13.

78. W.S. Inman, 'An inquiry into the origin of Squint, Left-Handedness and Stammer', *Lancet*, 2 (1924), 211-5.

79. Franz (1840-1b), p. 816.

80. J.F. Dieffenbach, 'Treatment of Facial Hemiplegia, by division of the muscles on the opposite side of the face', *London Medical Gazette*, 2 n.s. (1841-2), 574-5.

81. Jules Guerin 'On the Operations for Strabismus, claims of M. Guerin', *British and Foreign Medical Review*, 10 (1840), 572-3.

82. Lucas (1841c), p. 248.

83. See Dieffenbach's patient Carl Stephen, *Memoir*, pp. 18-20. Cf. Lucas' patient above p. 133.

84. 'Notice respecting the Operation for Stammering', *British and Foreign Medical Review*, 12 (1841), p. 257.

85. Franz (1840-1a), pp. 921-2. Paper reprinted in: *Medico-Chirurgical Review*,

34 n.s. (1840-1), 552-6; *London and Edinburgh Monthly Journal of Medical Science*, 1 (1841), 299-303 (pagination corrected as appeared to be erroneous in the volume consulted). This and other surgical papers also reported in W. Braithwaite (ed.), *The Retrospect of Practical Medicine and Surgery* (1841), vol. 3, 80-7.

86. Review of four recent publications . . . , pp. 210-12. Cf. Review of Dieffenbach's *Memoir*, pp. 372-5; 'Dieffenbach on the Cure of Stammering by Operation, with Remarks', *Medico-Chirurgical Review*, 35 n.s. (1841), 206-9; Review, *Lancet*, 2 (1840-1), 20-2.

87. Lee, pp. 38-41.

88. Amussat (1841), pp. 293-4.

89. J.F. Dieffenbach, 'On the Cure of Stammering by a New Operation', *Provincial Medical and Surgical Journal*, 1 (1840-1), 402-5.

90. Item in 'Miscellanea', *Athenaeum*, no. 694 (1841), p. 141; John von Horn, 'Operation for the Cure of Stammering' letter to *Lancet*, 2 (1840-1), p. 15 (15-16).

91. The count for individual surgeons ran into hundreds, see contemporary medical journals for 1840-1.

92. 'French and English Surgery' containing a letter from E. Lee to the *Gazette Médicale, London Medical Gazette*, 16 (1834-5), 395-6 (394-6). Cf. E. Lee, 'Surgical Letters from Paris, No. 1', *London Medical Gazette*, 2 n.s. (1840-1), p. 37 (36-8).

93. Numerous letters with claims and counter-claims. See: *Lancet*, *London Medical Gazette* and *Provincial Medical and Surgical Journal* for 1840-1, where most of the assertions appear.

94. Academy of Medicine (1841), p. 135.

95. Ibid; 'M. Velpeau . . .', pp. 196-7.

96. Hunt (1870), p. 209.

97. Poett snr (1828), p. 57.

98. Poett snr (1833), p. 15.

99. Tupper, *My Life*, p. 73.

100. James Yearsley, 'Stammering', letter to *London Medical Gazette*, 1 n.s. (1840-1), 919-20.

101. Braid (1841), pp. 360-2; Braid (1840-1), p. 116.

102. Braid, Franz, Lizars, Lucas, Yearsley. In addition Lee operated, probably in France (*Stammering*, p. 58) and Bishop (1851, p. 46) refers to a Dr Scott.

103. Claessen, Dieffenbach, Froriep, Langenbeck, Robert, Wolff and probably others.

104. Amussat, Baudens, Bonnet, Boyer, Colombat, Dufresse-Chassaigne, Guersent, Jobert, Oré, Petrequin, Petit, Richet, Roux, Sequin, Sichel and Velpeau Phillips, originally from Belgium and a student of Dieffenbach, was operating in Paris. This outstrips Russia with Roustoff, Italy with Malagodi and Sante-Sallani, and America, with Mott, Parker and Post.

105. G. Gordon-Taylor, 'The Life and Times of Sir Charles Bell', *Annals of the Royal College of Surgeons of England*, 18 (1956), 1-24. Liston is said to have amputated a limb and deposited it in the sawdust within a minute; Lizars to have ligated the innominate artery for aneurysm.

106. Lucas (1841a), p. 12.

107. Sir D'Arcy Power, rev., *Plarr's Lives of the Fellows of the Royal College of Surgeons of England* (1930), vol. 1, p. 736.

108. Dieffenbach, *Provincial Medical and Surgical Journal*, 1, p. 402. Cf. *Memoir*, p. 12 and above p. 104. In 1830 Schulthess likened stuttering to both photophobia and hydrophobia and proposed *phonophobia* and *lalophobia* as alternative terms for the complaint (Appelt, p. 7; Kussmaul, p. 836n). This may have been the source of Dieffenbach's suggestion.

109. Dieffenbach, p. 10. Cf. above pp. 114-15.

110. Ibid., pp. 14, 17, 26.
111. Ibid., pp. 9, 18-22.
112. 'On the Operations for the Cure of Stammering', *Medico-Chirurgical Review*, 36 n.s. (1841-2), p. 212 (212-3); Lebrun and Bayle, pp. 82, 83.
113. William Brockbank, 'Partial Glossectomy as a Cure of Stuttering', *British Medical Journal*, 2 (1937), 1239-40.
114. Dieffenbach, p. 25.
115. Ibid., pp. 26-7.
116. Academy of Sciences, Paris, p. 366.
117. Amussat (1841), pp. 293-4.
118. Amussat (1841-2), pp. 39-40.
119. Academy of Sciences, Paris, May 5, 'Stammering', *Provincial Medical and Surgical Journal*, 2 (1841), p. 157.
120. 'M. Velpeau . . . ', pp. 196-7.
121. Hunt (1870), pp. 129-30.
122. Review of four recent publications . . ., pp. 211-13. For Colombat's priority claim to this operation see Phillips, pp. 376-7.
123. Academy of Sciences, Paris, March 22, 'Treatment of Stuttering by Division of the Genio-Glossi Muscles', *Provincial Medical and Surgical Journal*, 2 (1841), p. 35.
124. Lizars, pp. 766-7. Letter to *Lancet* reprinted in *Dublin Medical Press*, 6 (1841), p. 127.
125. See above p. 104.
126. Cull (1833), pp. 28-9.
127. M. Phillips, 'Stammering. Section of the Sub-Lingual Nerve', *Dublin Medical Press*, 6 (1841), p. 228; 'On the Section of Lingual Nerves for the Cure of Stammering', *London and Edinburgh Monthly Journal of Medical Science*, 2 (1842), p. 196.
128. Review, *Lancet*, 2 (1840-1), p. 21.
129. Medical Society of London (1840-1b), p. 75.
130. Yearsley, *Statement*, p. 3n.
131. 'Squint-Cutting, and Tongue-Mutilation Rewarded', *London and Edinburgh Monthly Journal of Medical Science*, 1 (1841), p. 769.
132. Physician, p. 39; Review of four recent publications . . . , p. 211n.
133. Franz (1840-1a), pp. 923-4.
134. Lucas (1841b), pp. 109-12.
135. Braid (1841), p. 361.
136. Met. Free Hosp., *Provincial Medical and Surgical Journal*, 2, p. 91.
137. Lucas (1841c), p. 248.
138. P. Bennett Lucas, letter to Yearsley in *Yearsley's Letters*, p. 7.
139. Yearsley (1841), p. 8. Cf. Yearsley's letters to: *Lancet*, 1 (1840-1), 884-5; *London Medical Gazette*, 1 n.s. (1840-1), 919-20 reprinted in *Medico-Chirurgical Review*, 34 n.s. (1840-1), 551-2.
140. Ibid., p. 20.
141. Ibid., pp. 21-2.
142. Yearsley (1843-4), pp. 291-2.
143. Yearsley (1841), p. 20.
144. Ibid., p. 18.
145. Yearsley (1843-4), p. 292. Cf. ibid., p. 289.
146. See for example: M. Malagodi, 'On the Cause of the Frequent Return of Stammering after Division of the Genio-Glossi Muscles, and a new mode of preventing it', *Medical Times*, 6 (1842), 14-15; below, p. 230n37.
147. Westminster Medical Society (1840-1b), p. 81.
148. Yearsley, *Statement*, p. 5.
149. Correspondent, p. 899.

150. Royal Academy of Medicine, Paris, April 27, 'M. Louvrier's Operation for Anchylosis', *Dublin Medical Press*, 5 (1841), p. 294 (293-4).

151. 'On the Operations . . . ', *Medico-Chirurgical Review*, 36 n.s. (1841-2), p. 212.

152. A Hater of Quackery and Falsehood, 'The Stammering Quackery – A new plan of cheating the public', *Lancet*, 2 (1840-1), p. 287.

153. Symonds, *Lancet*, 2 (1840-1), p. 594.

154. Dieffenbach, p. 25; Franz (1840-1b), p. 815.

155. MM. Velpeau and Bonnet, 'Results of Operations for Stammering in France', *British and Foreign Medical Review*, 12 (1841), p. 555 (554-5). For Amussat's problems with abscesses see Hunt (1870), p. 136.

156. Dieffenbach, p. 22.

157. Lucas (1840-1), p. 389.

158. Baudens, p. 165.

159. 'Stammering', *Provincial Medical and Surgical Journal*, 4 (1842), p. 407.

160. Wright (1843), p. 25; Phillips, pp. 392-4.

161. Dieffenbach, pp. 23, 26.

162. Franz (1840-1b), p. 817; 'Death after an Operation for Stammering', *Provincial Medical and Surgical Journal*, 2 (1841), p. 140.

163. M. Guersent, 'Operation for Stuttering followed by Obstinate Haemorrhage', *Dublin Medical Press*, 5 (1841), p. 295; Lee, pp. 58-9.

164. M. Guersent, 'Great Hemorrhage after Division of the Genio-Glossi Muscles for Stammering', *British and Foreign Medical Review*, 12 (1841), p. 252.

165. 'Fatal Hemorrhage following Dieffenbach's Operations for the Cure of Stammering', *London and Edinburgh Monthly Journal of Medical Science*, 1 (1841), p. 678; Phillips, p. 388.

166. Braid (1841), p. 362.

167. Bartlett, pp. 47-9.

168. von Horn, *Lancet*, 2 (1840-1), 15-16.

169. John Harrison Curtis, 'New Operations – Squinting and Stammering', letter to *Lancet*, 2 (1840-1), 229 (228-9).

170. Editorial, 'Spirit of Modern Surgery', *London Medical Gazette*, 1 n.s. (1841-2), p. 154 (153-5).

171. Ed. – L.G., footnote to a report on G. Fowler's *Three Years in Persia* (1841), *Literary Gazette*, no. 1270 (1841), p. 326 (326-8). See above p. 114.

172. Review, *Lancet*, 2 (1840-1), p. 21.

173. Review of four recent publications . . . , p. 209.

174. Review of Dieffenbach's *Memoir*, p. 372.

175. Medical Society of London (1840-1b), p. 77. Cf. Hater of Quackery, *Lancet*, 2 (1840-1), 287.

176. Review of Dieffenbach's *Memoir*, p. 375.

177. Correspondent, p. 900.

178. Medical Society of London (1840-1b), pp. 76-7.

179. Wright (1843), p. 28.

180. Review of four recent publications . . . , p. 213n.

181. Report of J.E. Petrequin's *Traité d'Anatomie Medico-Chirurgicale et Topographique* (1844), *British and Foreign Medical Review*, 20 (1845), p. 135 (133-40).

182. Report of J.F. Dieffenbach's *Die Operative Chirurgie* (1845, 1), *British and Foreign Medical Review*, 21 (1846), p. 331 (285-333).

183. Ibid.

184. Velpeau and Bonnet, *British and Foreign Medical Review*, 12 (1841), pp. 554-5; M. Bonnet, 'Results of Forty-Two Operations for the Cure of Stammering', *Provincial Medical and Surgical Journal*, 2 (1841), p. 425.

185. Review of four recent publications . . ., p. 212; Hunt (1870), p. 136.

186. Lee, p. 44.
187. Braid (1841), p. 361.
188. Yearsley, *Lancet*, 2 (1840-1), p. 589.
189. Lucas (1841a), p. 13.
190. Iatros, 'Of Quacks and Empirics', *Medical and Physical Journal*, 40 (1804), 554-6.
191. Yearsley (1841), p. 21.
192. Lucas (1840-1), p. 389.
193. Dieffenbach, p. 14.
194. Review of Dieffenbach's *Memoir*, p. 373n.
195. Review, *British and Foreign Medical Review*, 11 (1841), p. 198 (194-8).
196. Notice, *Literary Gazette*, no. 1260 (1841), p. 172; Weekly Gossip, *Athenaeum*, no. 699 (20 March 1841), p. 227.
197. 'New Operation for Stammering', *Medical Times*, 3 (1841), p. 298.
198. Yearsley (1841), p. 18n.
199. Correspondent, *The Times*, 5 March 1841, p. 5. The next day, the *Literary Gazette* (p. 158) interpreted the Correspondent as saying 'that Mr. Yearsley has discovered that stammering is cured by cutting the patients' throats and not their tongues, as is done with starlings and magpies, and on the Continent'.
200. *Athenaeum*, nos. 698 & 699 (1841), pp. 211, 227.
201. Medical Society of London (1840-1a), p. 27.
202. Lee, pp. 65-6; *Athenaeum*, no. 699, p. 227.
203. 'On the Cure of Stammering . . . ', p. 590.
204. G. Butler, letter to Yearsley, ibid., also cited in Yearsley's *Statement*, p. 5.
205. See the United States' National Union Catalogue. I have been unable to trace a copy in the United Kingdom.
206. Correspondent, p. 899.
207. Lee, *London Medical Gazette*, 2 n.s. (1840-1), p. 38.
208. Review, *Lancet*, 2 (1840-1), p. 20.
209. Westminster Medical Society, 'Humbug Operations for Stammering. – New Bath. – Defective Vision', *Lancet*, 2 (1840-1), p. 203.
210. James Yearsley, letter to *Lancet*, 2 (1840-1), 413-14.
211. Editorial comment, *Lancet*, 1 (1840-1), p. 885.
212. Yearsley, *Statement*, pp. 2-3. The reviewer of *Traité de Médicine Operatoire* . . . (Paris, 1853, 1855) erroneously suggests that Yearsley's operations were for deafness and not as the author, Dr C. Sédillot, states for stuttering, see *Lancet*, 2 (1855), 583-4.
213. Yearsley, *Lancet*, 2 (1840-1), p. 588.
214. Yearsley, *Statement*, p. 9.
215. Thomas Hunt, letter to *Lancet*, 2 (1840-1), 494-5.
216. James Yearsley, letter in 'Operations for Stammering', *Lancet*, 2 (1840-1), p. 638.
217. Yearsley, *Statement*, p. 9.
218. *Yearsley's Letters*, pp. 1-8.
219. Westminster Medical Society (1840-1a), pp. 24-5.
220. Marshall Hall, letter to Yearsley in *Yearsley's Letters*, p. 6.
221. Physician, pp. i-ii.
222. W. Tyler Smith, letter to Yearsley in *Yearsley's Letters*, p. 7.
223. Editorial (1846b), p. 663.
224. Donnison, pp. 57, 91.
225. Editorial (1846a), p. 558.
226. *Unspeakable*, p. 107.
227. Review of Lee's *On Stammering & c.*, *Athenaeum*, no. 717 (1841), p. 552.

228. 'The Lancet and Mr. Hunt', *Medical Times*, 14 (1846), p. 261.
229. Medical Society of London (1840-1a), pp. 25-7; Bishop (1846), pp. 25-8, abstracted in *Medico-Chirurgical Review*, 3 n.s. (1846), 322-4; see above p. 114.
230. *Unspeakable*, p. 138.
231. Alexander Bell, *The Tongue* (London, W.J. Cleaver, 1846), pp. 63-5.
232. Wyllie, p. 26.
233. Henry Bigelow, *Orthopaedic Surgery and other Medical Papers* (Boston, Little Brown & Co., 1900), pp. 37-53.
234. L. Stevenson, p. 553.
235. Lebrun and Bayle, p. 89.
236. Bristowe [1882], p. 1514.

8 DIDACTIC TECHNIQUES AND REMEDIAL AIDS

Demosthenes provided Victorians with a perfect archetype of the elocutionary ideals to which they aspired, and few treatises on stuttering failed to commend his example. Though defective in speech, he was inspired to greatness by the oratory of Callistratus. He also wisely attended to the counsel of Satyrus, the actor, but personal effort underlay his success. For months he practised daily: diligently monitoring his actions before a mirror; strengthening his frail voice as he pitted it against the waves; conquering shortness of breath by repeating his orations uphill; and developing articulatory precision by speaking with pebbles in his mouth.[1] These practices were given diverse interpretations, the latter providing a precedent for the use of gadgets in stuttering therapy. Indeed, the variety of his practices meant that he held something for everyone and the protagonists of differing systems could each call upon his authority. But his ultimate aim was clear. When asked what was the most important part of oratory, Demosthenes replied three times – delivery.

Delivery was the business of elocutionists. Aside from gesture, it concerned the manner of speaking, the clarity of articulation and the pitch, intonation, sonority and rhythm of voice; in short, the audibility, fluency and energy of utterance. As delivery became detached from rhetoric with the new elocutionary movement, there was a corresponding diminution of its intellectual status and a rise in its popular appeal:

> Like the English renaissance in design and decoration under William Morris, elocution was more than a fad of the era; it amounted to a social movement. Melville Bell was its prophet. On two continents, foreheads were clasped in despair and hands flung wide in supplication in accord with Bell's directions for the delivery of dramatic speech and soliloquies.[2]

The treatment of stutterers was one facet of this groundswell.

Many of the practitioners loosely called elocutionists, obviously considered themselves masters of the art: Thelwall, the Bells, Wright, Foster and Beasley amongst them. Of the doctors treating stutterers, only Shuldham claimed to have made a study of elocution, and he conceded that it was this, not his medical knowledge, which enabled him to help them.[3] But for most of his colleagues, an understanding of vocal physiology was thought to suffice. With this the elocutionists had no quarrel and, indeed, preoccupation with articulatory phonetics gave the treatment to both groups a mechanical orientation. For elocutionists, it reflected not only their linguistic background, but served as a defence against the charge of empiricism, by showing that their treatment was based upon sound principles rather than chance.[4] In other words, their measures were justified by being 'scientific' and thus Melville Bell could distain Demosthenes' pebbles, while using gadgets himself.

There was ample evidence of 'the inefficacy of the knife to *excise a habit*'[5] and a general consensus that this must be altered by contrary associations. The danger of resorting to opposite modes of speech, however, was that these might also be faulty.[6] Whereas moral treatment could rectify anxiety and untoward mental associations, oral retraining could do much to establish the neuro-muscular concord that Charles Bell emphasised was lacking, and enable the stutterer's organs to respond selectively:

> The power of confining the voluntary excitement of the nervous principle to distinct groups of fibres is increased much by exercise, and the more frequently certain groups of fibres are excited into action by the influence of the will, the more capable do they become of isolated action; this is exemplified in performers on the piano-forte, &c.[7]

The analogy with musicians acquiring dexterity on their instruments was popular, and applied to stutterers, meant the systematic correction of obstructive sounds and the establishment of continuity in speech, through rhythmic exercises. Most practitioners introduced breathing and articulatory drills into their programme, but their techniques and emphasis varied, as did their use of mechanical aids.

Breathing, Gadgets and Vocal Gymnastics

If, as Cazalet maintained, stuttering always began with 'a disordered act of respiration',[8] then the therapeutic needs were obvious. Good breathing underlay health, as well as the strength and fluidity of voice, and measures directed towards developing these were commonplace. Advice ranged from McCormac's injunction to speak on a strong exhalation,

Table 8.1: Breathing Exercises

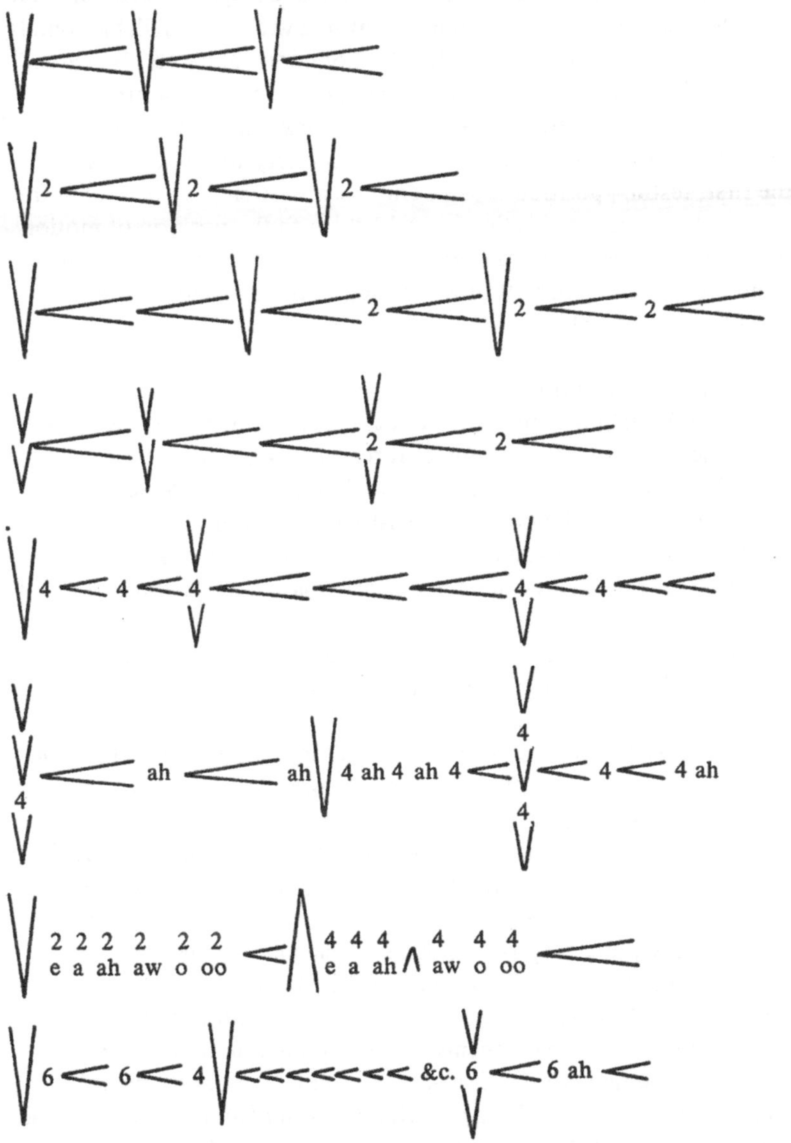

Note: V indicates inhalation through the mouth, inverted V inhalation through the nose, lateral V exhalation, and numbers, the time in seconds.

Source: F. Helmore, *Speakers, Singers and Stammerers*, p. 68.

after filling the lungs completely,[9] to Helmore's systematic exercises (Table 8.1). These, reflecting his profession as a singing instructor, were to be followed by drills combining breathing with monosyllabic sounds, vocal intonation following the direction of curved lines on his charts.[10]

All Helmore's exercises were to be done in front of a mirror, a practice recommended by others including Alexander Bell, who claimed to have discovered the two oral stances necessary for good speech. In the first, resting, position the lips and teeth were slightly parted; in the second their combined action brought them to the position of motion that should precede all articulation.[11] Alexander Melville was even more precise about correct oral postures, as his instructions for articulating N reveal:

> Let him, with a mirror before him, open his mouth as widely as he can, and retain it at its greatest opening, while he places the tongue on the palate, as for D. Here let it rest steady for some time: – it is in the position for either T, D, or N. Let him now produce a continuous sound, without the slightest motion in any visible part of the mouth. This sound – if the tongue has been obstructively placed on the palate – must necessarily pass through the nose . . .[12]

The whole exercise would improve vocal quality and respiratory steadiness. Wright's use of a mirror was rather more general, for he recommended scrutiny of the whole bodily stance,[13] and thought it provided a useful stepping stone from solitary practice to that in front of small groups.[14] Possibly also directed towards mirror-work was Butterfield's Alphabetic Speculum, designed for the prevention and cure of stuttering, manufactured by Weiss and Son, and marketed for one guinea.[15] Unfortunately, it was not described in any publication, but the *Lancet* learned enough from advertisements to deride its merit,[16] only publishing Butterfield's article under protest.[17]

The rationale for mirror-work and what Melville Bell called 'analytic pronunciation' was that patients needed to know how to speak and correct unconscious mannerisms; it was not unnatural but 'merely cautious creeping before walking, wary walking before running'.[18] Since they wanted to talk, they suffered neither from weakness of will nor imagination, but from knowledge,[19] which could explain 99 per cent of their difficulties.[20] Arnott's 'Physiological Alphabet' (Table 2.1, p. 54) was considered useful and such a chart was even recommended in trivial writings like *The Popular Encyclopaedia* (1841). Arnott suggested it should guide the stutterer, as a score directs a musician:

> an analysis and scale of articulate sounds, with minute description of the organic actions required to produce them, like the scale which we possess for music, in the *gamut* and rules for fingering, should give nearly the same assistance to the speaker, which the gamut gives to the player.[21]

Thelwall made use of graphic illustrations,[22] and Wright recommended the teaching methods of Signor G. Lanza. This noted Italian singing master had attached pictures of oral postures to each of the notes of the Solfeggio,[23] probably much like the pictures employed by educators of the deaf. Physicians were particularly inclined to believe that a stutterer's cure had begun once he understood the anatomy and physiology of speech.[24] Sketches such as Figure 2.1 (p. 55) were considered helpful, but to demonstrate how the speech organs were adapted from their biological use, Poett turned to models and preparations of the human larynx.[25]

To Melville Bell it was not theoretical anatomy but 'practical knowledge' of muscular action that was important and the fact that stutterers could speak normally did not seem to enter his reckoning. They were instructed in Visible Speech and analytic pronunciation, aided by mechanical means if necessary. Something similar in size to a paper-cutter was Bell's answer to the locked or misplaced jaw, so often the basis of lingual malaction. For certain sounds, the teeth needed to be slightly parted and for others greater separation was required, always allowing for individual anatomical idiosyncracies. The thin edge of the blade could be employed for sibilant practice, whereas the breadth of the paper-cutter would serve to gauge the correct jaw position for tongue tip and gutteral sounds. A number of therapists had recourse to finger or pencil, Bell considering the latter preferable since it could be held horizontally, its upward or downward displacement revealing any advance or retraction of the jaws.[26] Similar views about opening the jaws were held by Charles Kingsley, who recommended a cork,[27] and about the teeth by Gordon Holmes, who recommended a 'small wedge'.[28] The lips were another source of error and Melville Bell issued precise directions. Their vertical movement should be confined to articulation and horizontal movement to emotional expression. The stutterer, whose extraneous muscular actions were so disfiguring, was enjoined to control the lips and 'prevent their officious meddling with sounds over which they possess no legitimate influence'. One way was to harness them so that enough of the teeth were revealed to avoid a simpering expression but not so much as to simulate a grin. Properly, the upper lip should not move, all enunciatory action being made by the lower jaw. This was hardly easy, even for the most fluent speaker, but the stutterer was not abandoned without help. Labial sounds could be practised with small objects between the teeth and should the lips run riot, a pair of silver hooks could be inserted over their edges and secured with a rubber band behind the head. Alternatively, a slim pencil or ivory knitting needle might serve to keep them correctly retracted.[29] Although Melville Bell thought these gadgets should soon be discarded, it is surprising he advocated them at all, in view of his father's wry comment about tongue bridles made of gold: though this metal could prompt politicians into speech or silence, it had remarkably little effect upon the speech of stutterers.[30]

Mechanical aids were popular in Europe and leading practitioners were numbered amongst their champions: Chégoin lowered the dental arches by a silver 'cintre',[31] Colombat employed a tongue bridle or retractor,[32] Klencke had wooden plates shaped to the lower jaw, Merkel fixed a whalebone clasp to the lower molar,[33] and, in 1829, Wutzer had introduced his glossonochon,[34] also called a glossomochlian or tongue lever.[35] This thin plate was fastened to a lower tooth, giving it a similarity with Merkel's device. However, it was reputedly a modification of Itard's fork, the most widely publicised of all the instruments. The fork, measuring one inch, was designed to lie horizontally and one of Itard's patients became so dextrous he could retain it in his mouth during meals.[36] Later, Malagodi found a surgical use for such devices, which could serve to keep the severed edges of wounds apart and hence prevent a return of stuttering.[37]

The most notorious mechanical treatment was that of an English woman living in New York, the widow Leigh. Her system evidently excited 'more attention than ever given before or since to anything of the kind'.[38] She counteracted any tendency of the tongue to root itself in the floor of the mouth by placing rolls of linen beneath it during the night. In waking hours, the patient's will should suffice and he was enjoined to keep the tip raised to the palate, so that his speech could set off from this point 'as from a spring'.[39] Uncertainty surrounds the origin of this treatment which, though known as the American Method, may have originated in Edinburgh, where a poor man reputedly divulged it to Broster, who is said to have practised it secretly before it appeared in New York.[40] Another version was that Mrs Leigh's husband stuttered and, after nine or nineteen years' observation, she pinpointed his difficulties.[41] It was also ascribed to her experiences with a young 'lady friend',[42] and attributed to Dr Yates, whose daughter it helped. He then informed her governess, Mrs Leigh. Possibly the doctor doubted its orthodoxy, and by passing it on to her he avoided tarnishing his own reputation.[43] Secrecy ensured constant speculation and interest. Malebouche, of Brussels, went to New York, had financial dealings with Mrs Leigh,[44] and subsequently introduced the method into Europe, with his own elocutionary modifications.[45] The most detailed account of these events in English came from James Hunt. Always thorough, he also wished to refute suggestions in foreign publications that his father was associated with the system.[46]

Neither the British government nor the medical profession endeavoured to acquaint themselves with the American method. McCormac, however, during a trip to New York in 1826, was impressed with the testimonials from respectable physicians that Mrs Leigh possessed and this prompted his own conjectures, by reversing his previous conviction that stuttering was incurable.[47] Contrarily, as with surgery, Continentals reacted enthusiastically, the method being hailed as one of 'the most important and useful discoveries' of the century which, once developed, would bring 'great revolutions in medicine and psychology'.[48] Both Crown and State put their weight behind the plight of stuttering citizens: the King of the Netherlands arranged that the poor should be treated free,[49] the Belgian government bought the secret for £10,000,[50] privileges were extended to those practising the method, and Prussian teachers in training received instruction equipping them to handle stuttereres in the classroom.[51] The French likewise interested themselves in the discovery, with no less a figure than Magendie presenting it to the French Academy in 1828.[52] Time soon revealed the gullibility of all concerned and history vindicated the British reserve, though this probably stemmed from indifference rather than perspicacity.

Mrs Leigh is said to have cured 150 people in her establishment between 1828-30 and Malebouche was credited with even greater success.[53] However, Voisin personally gained no lasting benefit from the Leigh system. His solution was to hold the lower jaw half open with the hand.[54] Perhaps to forestall the hanging jaw which Catlin deplored, Tupper was required to wear a crutch under his chin – a 'sort of gag on the rebellious tongue'.[55] Other advice was that the teeth should be kept close together while speaking.[56] Where teeth were damaged, Yearsley believed dentures would benefit speech,[57] and someone, purportedly a 'dental surgeon to all the great orators in the kingdom' recommended that perfectly good teeth be extracted and replaced by artificial ones – a treatment the patient declined.[58] Yet some of these remedies were tried. Almost every sufferer sought relief in pebbles, often on advice from the family physician,[59] and Borthwick admits that as a schoolboy he had been helped by placing a marble or small coin in his mouth.[60] Though not in the same league as mishaps following surgery, accidents inevitably happened. One patient, after swallowing the greater part of his pebbles mercifully 's-p-pat the r-e-e-est' out;[61] another developed an attack of *colica pictonum* following the use of a bullet;[62] and though an 'infallible remedy', the plate of a third slipped back and nearly choked him.[63]

Once again, the distinction between quackery and orthodoxy was blurred, but those devices peddled as a sole and universal cure could be put in the first category. This was probably the case with Schirmann's wooden balls, sold in Paris during 1829,[64] and with the American report of the leaden ball, intended to lodge in the depression above the breastbone when worn round the neck.[65] The latter must have borne a superficial resemblance to the larynx-compressor, one of three appliances devised by the stuttering Mr Bates. These gained respectability by their apparently scientific basis, each being designed to alleviate a specific form of the complaint. They clearly impressed some influential men, for Bates was awarded 'premiums' by an investigative Committee of the Franklin Institute in Philadelphia,[66] and a medal both by the Metropolitan Mechanics Institute (Figure 8.1), and an impressively constituted jury at the International Exhibition held in London during 1862.[67] His contrivances also formed part of the American dental contribution to the Paris Exhibition of 1867, along with the latest in artificial limbs and sanitary supplies.[68] However, the British response had by then cooled, if we are to judge from one medical correspondent's report. The instrument intended for those in difficulty with gutterals was the larynx-compressor, comprising a leather neck-band that could be tightened by a buckle and screw, thereby submitting the wearer to a 'permanent process of strangulation'.[69] The gold and silver tube attached to the upper incisors by means of a strip of wire or rubber, supposedly to obviate dental stuttering, was not a feature of the Paris Exhibition, but seems to have been replaced by a plate perforated at the centre to fit between the teeth as an antidote for lingual stuttering. This particular appliance sounds similar to one used by the august Colombat, whose contributions to the alleviation of stuttering won him the Monthyon prize from the French Academy.[70] Lastly, labial stuttering was to be relieved by a

Figure 8.1: Bates' Advertisement

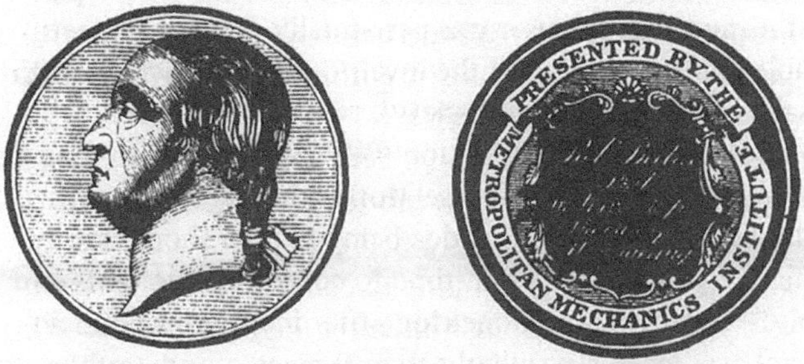

APPLIANCES FOR THE CURE OF

STAMMERING;

INVENTED AND PATENTED BY

ROBERT BATES,

And successfully introduced throughout the United States of America.

Pamphlets containing a description of the appliances, &c. can be had gratis by applying to the Inventor, who will remain in London during the Exhibition, and will be happy to see those who are afflicted with Stammering to test the merits of his invention.

ROBERT BATES,

9, ***Great Castle Street*, *Cavendish Square. W*.**

Can be consulted from 8 to 10 in the morning, and 6 to 8 in the evening, or at his stand in the American Department of the Exhibition during the day.

Ladies and Gentlemen who are desirous of testing the appliances *at their own Residence*, will please send their Address as above, which will be punctually attended to, between the hours of 10 a.m. and 6 p.m.

Note: Birkbeck College have no record of any such award, nor of the Metropolitan Mechanics Institute, which was possibly an American organisation.

Source: John Johnson Collection, New Bodleian Library, Oxford.

device shaped like a flattened bed-pan, the handle projecting between the teeth. In the Exhibition, this projection was concealed in a quill, giving the impression that the user was perpetually picking his teeth, a most desirable habit according to the inventor and 'one which ought to be universally adopted in polite society'.

Foreign bodies also featured in fiction. Pebbles were put to dramatic effect in *Le Voyage en Chine*.[71] George Morley, having failed with these, was advised to use a pipe, the idea being that he should speak between puffs, the pauses giving him time to collect his thoughts and breathe deeply.[72] And William Monckton, after ineptly pronouncing 'cauchouc' [*sic*] was given a peculiarly shaped piece of india rubber to wear beneath his tongue. Monckton's attempts to persevere with this were short-lived since, after 'gobbling about the house like a turkey' for six hours, his guardian could stand it no longer.[73]

Gadgetry might be combined with medical-type treatment, according to a young Mancunian's account of his dealings with one stutter-doctor:

> I went in the morning at about eleven o'clock, and he had two pieces of stick, and thrust them under my tongue; then I held some liquid in my mouth, which burnt the skin off the roof of my mouth: then I had a vapour bath. I held my face over a basin of hot water, with some herbs in it, for half an hour, till my face was as red as it really could be; after that, I had a piece of India-rubber in my mouth under the tongue, and that was the whole of the operation, and I am not any better now.[74]

The rubber was probably caoutchouc, a substance discovered by some French Academicians whilst visiting South America during 1735. Its commercial potential was developed during the nineteenth century, especially for waterproofing and insulation, as was gutta-percha, the latex of certain Malaysian trees. Samples of the latter were sent to London from Singapore in 1843 and its plastic qualities were exploited so quickly that by the time of the Great Exhibition its applications ranged from lifeboats to hats and medical appliances. Predictably, gutta-percha balls also found their way into the mouths of stutterers.[75] The dental profession was especially interested in its use. Obturators for cleft palate speakers were developed, particularly in America,[76] and when a highly vaulted palate was held responsible in one instance of stuttering, the dental department of St Clement's Hospital, Leamington, made a corrective plate, three-eighths in. thick. This particular appliance was secured by suction and made of vulcanite.[77]

As well as being comparable to a musical instrument, the principles under which articulate speech operates could be likened to a machine: the power and resistance to be overcome must be in equilibrium.[78] Taking the analogy of a watch, Melville Bell believed the curative process involved patients in taking their speech apart and examining all its parts, before replacing them in the natural order.[79] Speech, however, subject to the vicissitudes of subjective states, differed from a watch, which had an automatic momentum.[80] Nevertheless, Wright thought there was a comparison between the mainspring and hairspring of a watch:

> if the muscular power upon which the action of the cartilages which constitute the organ of voice, be too weak . . . speech must be impeded; if the lungs be not regularly and systematically inflated and discharged . . . the voice will falter . . . and, though the glottis itself be open, the speech will be impeded; . . . if the resistance made at the organs of enunciation to articulate, (which must, of necessity, even in accurate speaking, transiently impede the breath and voice,) be greater than the power which is given to separate the organs of enunciation, and produce a passage for the utterance of a vowel, – the *breath* and *voice* will be *impeded altogether* and *stopped*, a word or syllable cannot be spoken.[81]

Thus, while Melville Bell's analytic pronunciation aimed to show how the phonetic elements fitted together, Wright seems to have used instruments as an extrinsic counterbalance to disruptive spasms. His array included a silver or ivory device similar to a paper-cutter, for prising tongue from palate, plus a hook and strap, and springs, variously situated, one clipping the nostrils to prevent the nasal escape subsequent upon faulty palatal action.[82]

On the Continent, gadgets were used by doctors and possibly Dr Poett's lip and tongue separators[83] derived from his travels. In England, however, they were generally used by laymen. One of the objects of surgery was the mechanical positioning of the tongue, and phonetic aids may be looked upon as their elocutionary counterpart. It is therefore ironical that the principal gadget-men should come from the ranks of those most critical of surgery: Kingsley, Wright, Melville Bell and the younger Poett.

In fairness, their gadgets were only a remedial sideline, assisting moral treatment[84] and elocution proper. The latter extended to those exercises designed to increase the strength and skill of the speech muscles, which were often called 'vocal gymnastics', words entitling Urling's book. Poett, however, who saw his own writings in Urling's, objected to the name, suggesting 'disciplinitic' as more appropriate, since it was the mind that was in need of training.[85] But Urling was following a well trodden path, Cull having spoken of 'vocal', 'enunciatory' and 'myologic' gymnastics 20 years before.[86] They remained in vogue till the end of the century: Wyllie approved of such exercises, if conducted by a 'well-educated specialist'.[87] So times had changed, for it was on account of this treatment that the *Lancet* had labelled Thomas Hunt 'a mere vocal posture-master'.

An important feature of oral gymnastics was the practice of various sound sequences in nonsense syllables, words and sentences, grouped according to sounds. These sentences comprised 15 pages of Helmore's book. For example:

> Λ Marlborough managed* in a most magnificent manner* to mar by military manoeuvres* the mischievous machinations* of a marvellous multitude* of malicious mounted Mamelukes,* mercurially and malevolently menacing* his merry merry men.[88]

The inverted V (Λ) represents a deep breath and the asterisk a short one. Such 'alliterative exercises' found approval with Tyler Smith,[89] and were employed throughout the century, whether or not the practitioner ascribed stuttering to muscular weakness. Applications varied, however, with Thelwall having isolated sounds articulated in common and triple time,[90] whereas Wyllie put tongue-twisters to diagnostic purpose.

Vocal gymnastics and gadgets raise the question of attention. For those advocating greater conscious control, they were valued for their moderating action. Like the surgically wounded tongue, foreign languages and singing, they necessitated deliberation. The obstacle they provided spurred mental effort, leading to the development of the attention, will, memory and powers of imitation.[91] They also heightened nervous stimulation to the parts.[92] Alternatively, they could be seen as deflecting attention from morbid self-consciousness and thus creating conditions suitable to spontaneity. In fact, almost any device would serve this end, including the metronome and Poett's stammering trumpet, into which the voice was thrown to distract the mind 'from its wild pronunciatory efforts'.[93]

Generally speaking, psychiatric writings maintained that semiautomatic functions were liable to be disrupted by surveillance of the will. Allusions to stuttering were made where this principle was discussed,[94] but only Monro gave the matter serious thought. With 'intermittent stammerers', he believed that mental emotion could be minimised by abstracting the mind from the thought 'I stammer',[95] and, contrary to Melville Bell, he recommended patients to engross themselves in the matter, not manner, of speech. There were various ways this might be done. Though he never recommended silence, a remedy popular on the Continent,[96] he did suggest avoiding speech where failure seemed likely. He also thought it justifiable to resort to any artifice that might help break habitual associations.[97]

With the question of dodges, Monro was on contentious ground. One of the very examples he gave – squeezing the back of the chair – was denounced by Abbotts, along with the practice of reading either lying flat on the floor, or with gadgets.[98] Here he was joined by Mason[99] and Ball,[100] who were disparaging about previous remedies, some of which were facile, like teeth clenching and whispering, but others being the therapeutic mainstay of respectable practitioners, for example syllabic speech, tongue-twisters and rhythm. Needless to say, Ball's answer was little better, the stutterer first being trained to speak in a drawling tone, whilst simultaneously raising his head, the reason being that this position was incompatible with swallowing and hence the stuttering.[101]

Opposed to what might be called the 'articulatory' school was the 'vocal' school, though writers defy neat categorisation. Marshall Hall, for instance, while theoretically belonging to the former, found value in free-flowing speech. The vocal school was impressed by stutterers' fluency during singing and their diminished numbers amongst speakers of musical languages. Its most noted protagonist, Neil Arnott, went a stage further by postulating the open state of the glottis during song. When glottal stricture supervened, vocal continuity could be re-established by using the *e* vowel, as in berry. In time, the drawl would become unnecessary, but meanwhile, mental associations could be developed by imagining continuous sounds, like a waterfall.[102] Similar in practice, was Mr Julion's 'making of a voice', which entailed prefixing and dwelling upon the *u*, as in *u*rn:

> U . . . there-is-u-a-vigi-lance u-of-u-observation, and-u-acc-uracy of-u-dist-inction[103]

which amounted to little more than speaking like 'mental stammerers'. Alexander Bell advised much the same, using some form of the *e* vowel.

Thus, 'a bad case' became:

a-eeb-ad-eek-ase

The idea was to begin slowly, as a tyro 'practises the notes in a bar of music' until all 'will be a harmonious, and an unbroken utterance of the most difficult words'.[104] Arnott's remedy soon went the way of most therapeutic discoveries – discarded but never wholly abandoned – and in 1880 a former sufferer was praising its merits, adding his own modifications.[105]

Since the stutterer supposedly failed to 'throw the whole power of his voice upon the vowels',[106] some reversal of this process was logical. As the impediment might arise in mid-word, Müller developed Arnott's treatment by recommending the practice of sentences devoid of explosive consonants,[107] the compilation of which was not easy.[108] Other criticisms were soon voiced, but not by Munro, who saw it as one way of deflecting attention from 'abnoxious' letters, which might be 'slipped over' or wholly omitted. Moreover, though Arnott's *e* was useful, in certain circumstances it was inferior to the doubling of vocalic sounds, whereby the patient would gradually produce 'a monotonous fluent stream of sound something like the chaunting manner of reading prayer'.[109] Delivery of this kind would obviously be more acceptable to the clergy and it seems to have increased the impressiveness of Kingsley's voice, which 'was partly due to the strange, rich, high-pitched, musical monotone in which he prayed and preached'.[110]

Syllabication and Rhythm

Vocalic stress was not the only antidote to 'consonant-clogged' speech.[111] The principal linguistic symptom of stuttering is disruption to the sequential flow of speech – sounds do not follow as they ought, though individual ones may be perfectly pronounced.[112] Thus, the difficulty was with 'syllabication', a word deriving from the Greek *syllaba* meaning to include or combine together.[113] In other words, it was a rhythmic disorder, calling for rhythmic re-education. This contention was supported by the fact that stutterers experienced less difficulty where rhythm was imposed upon them, as in singing and verse speaking, and it was apparently non-existent among the speakers of primitive languages, in which cadential patterns were more marked. Moreover, it was observed that the defect was also unusual amongst the Cochin Chinese, whose language was monosyllabic. Consequently, there was a *prima facie* case for having stutterers regularise their rhythm by speaking in a similar fashion.

In France, this type of speech was called 'equisyllabic pronunciation',[114] and it evidently excited unusual interest when Dr Serre described it to the Academy of Sciences.[115] There is no doubt that in England this was a technique used to stagger onlookers by producing a near miraculous reduction in hesitation. Although Hunt described it as a 'trick' and pointed out that Serre's enthusiasm waned, so important was it to Melville Bell that once in America he produced a pamphlet on the subject, containing many illustrative sentences:

> Pho – ne – tic sy(l)la – bi – ca – tion is the cure for o – ra – to – ri – cal and o – ther de – fects of speech.[116]

Each vowel was assigned a number, which was placed above it so that patients should not confuse spelling with sounds. Similar advice was given by Tyler Smith, who divided phrases into 'vocal and respiratory feet', the latter being indicated by a comma:

> The – pro – per, – stu – dy – of, – man – kind, – is – man

the feet being gradually lengthened:

> The proper – study of, – mankind – is man

until fluency ensued.[117] His close collaborator, Yearsley, also came to advocate rhythm, though he spoke disparagingly of elocutionists, such as the one who combined walking and talking, each step coinciding first with one syllable and then with several.[118]

Tyler Smith's inspiration derived from Colombat, who viewed rhythm as 'one of the first laws of the animal economy'[119] and was judged to have 'found out the royal road to the cure of stammering'.[120] It is not clear from English writings whether this entailed equisyllabic pronunciation, but he did find speech assisted by regular beats and for this purpose devised a muthonome (*lit.* speech governor),[121] similar to Maelzel's device.[122] This itself grew out of the pendulum, which revolutionised clock mechanisms around 1656. From that time, many apparatuses were conceived to beat at regular speeds within the musical range, yet be practical and easily transportable. In 1816, Johann Maelzel patented, widely advertised, and manufactured an instrument.

But his designs were borrowed from others, not least the Dutchman, Winkel, to whom credit for the invention is now given. Since that time the metronome's popularity as a therapeutic aid has fluctuated, an electric device now being available.[123] Victorians recommended starting rates between 60[124] to 84[125] beats per minute, at which pace 'syllabication' was unavoidable. Shuldham proposed the latter speed, pointing out that this was equivalent to 3-time in music and was especially suited to passages such as Hood's *Lay of the Labourer.*

Thelwall advocated time-beating, but not in the manner prescribed above, which was the very negation of rhythm. He believed that the true unit of rhythm was not the monosyllable, but the cadence, which itself was under the laws of pulsation and remission inherent in muscular action. Thelwall aimed to develop his pupils' ear so that they would no longer exhibit 'tuneless cluttering', 'soporific' drawling or that 'vulgar sing-song style'. For him, the larynx was the principal syllabicator or 'metronome of vocal impulse', and as this was a musical instrument, so was the rhythm of language essentially musical. He therefore had pupils, whether stutterers or not, score passages into 'proper bars, with all the regularity of a piece of music'.[126]

It has been said that Thelwall's approach was 'mechanistic', as opposed to 'natural'. The two categories, however, are not necessarily antithetic and even extreme mechanists took 'Nature as their norm and guide'.[127] Thelwall anticipated the charge and, taking an analogy from dancing, asked whether those skilled in the art necessarily walked with an elaborate or stiff gait. He then pointed out that there was such a thing as 'order without formality, and a stiffness without order; such a distinction as proportioned variety, and monotonous irregularity'. In short, his purpose was to produce 'flexure and harmonic variety' and he denied that mannerism was the inevitable consequence of a strict didactic programme.[128]

The question of what was meant by 'natural' is too involved to pursue here, but most elocutionists aligned themselves with some aspect of the concept. To some, equisyllabism was undesirable, yet Melville Bell, believing speech to be an 'artificial process' rather than a 'natural instinct', furthered its use and justified analytic pronunciation on account of its value in clarifying the muscular postures and movements of normal speech, meanwhile pointing to the unnaturalness of droning, singing, the interpolation of vowels and tricks like stamping.[129] Gerdts similarly objected to any new habit which patients would find difficult to practice regularly. The human organism is ruled by 'natural laws', not least in speech, and therefore stutterers must acquire a 'natural way of speaking', that is, re-establish the normal physiological processes, particularly of exhalation and diaphragmatic movement, first in quiet situations.[130] Though differing from Gerdts on the merits of correspondence courses, Mason also stressed the importance of natural laws. However, little was said in his *Practical Guide*, which was designed to whet the appetite for his *Manual of Instruction on the Natural System*.

The natural rhythms of English might be recognisable, but their underlying principles were poorly understood and much controverted. When Thelwall inveighed against the unrelieved flow of heavy syllables, he was objecting to the manner children were taught to read. Had anyone then proposed equisyllabism as a therapeutic technique, he would have been outraged. As it was, he was liberal in his criticism of most theorists of prosody, not least Benjamin Smart.[131] Prosody, however, was not Smart's principal concern and, rather like Bell, his remedial method gradually centred on the teaching of speech sounds, first in isolation, and then through exercises joining consonant to vowel, syllable to syllable, word to word, until phrases were reached – at which point rhythm became important.[132]

This attention to phonetics reflected Smart's interest in orthoepy, which led to *Walker Remodelled*, where his views on the cure of stuttering were restated.[133] It will be recalled that the other disciple of Walker, James Wright, attended particularly to the difficulties which the subtle pitch changes of conversational speech posed for stutterers. He thought vocal inflection could best be practised in sentences where words' initial consonants had been omitted, but if hesitancy persisted once these were replaced, then the vowel *u* should be prefixed to them. On this point, Wright's cure resembled Arnott's, but he also recommended something similar to equisyllabism, in that he had patients divide words into monosyllables and breath between each. Wright said little about rhythm, and in the sentence:

Truth / is the basis / of excellence

the bars merely indicated convenient pauses for breath.[134]

Elocutionists led the pupils step by step, using poetical and literary extracts as a transition from vocal gymnastics to spontaneous speech. Thelwall, the most ambitious, believed Pope's heroic couplets best suited to beginners, the acmé being *Paradise Lost*, where Milton demonstrated his mastery of English metre. Pupils could learn something of the language by trying their own hand at composition. Also elucidating were the Greeks, whose appreciation of metre was unrivalled. Thelwall therefore had students 'translate the classics into their original measures', by which means 'the study of the vernacular and the learned languages may be made to reflect a reciprocal light, one upon the other, and be rendered mutually conducive to the improvement of the harmony and felicity in speech'.[135]

Testimonials

With livings and reputations at stake, Victorian practitioners needed to establish the reliability of their systems and most realised that some objective evidence was required to back up their own effusive assertions. This might be done through demonstration, as when Bishop displayed his patient to the Medical Society of London,[136] or through public showings, like Beasley's Speech Days. Strangely, James Yearsley's table of figures on 204 post-operative cases was the only serious attempt to quantify results.[137] The preferred alternative was testimonials and many treatises concluded with a series of letters from the nobility and other eminent men. The elder Poett, for example, was well pleased with the following unsolicited letter from a colleague unknown to him:

Tuam, 22nd April, 1828.

SIR, I have just visited young Birmingham, of Milbrook, who was a patient of mine for some months previous to his being placed under your care. During my attendance upon him, *so great was the hesitation of his speech*, that he was almost *unintelligible*, so that in fact it was *through the medium of his mother* I could ascertain the nature of his disease.

I was, therefore, highly gratified, indeed I must confess astonished beyond measure, at finding him so completely cured, that he spoke and read for me *distinctly* and *articulately*.

From your success in this case in particular, I look upon the infallibility of your system proved beyond all question – a system which must be considered as one of the greatest discoveries of ancient or modern times, and one which must secure for you (if the discoverer) a place in the ranks of those who, by their genuis, have rendered their names immortal.

You should have had this communication from me sooner, but that whenever Mr. Birmingham brought in his son to me, I was unfortunately away on my professional duties. You are at liberty to make any use you please of this letter, and to add my name to the list of your referees.

I have the honor to be,
Your very humble Servant,
JOHN PRENDERGAST M.D.[138]

Surgeon POETT

It was usual for the names and addresses of referees to be printed, but 'through motives of delicacy' Broster declined to do so in his pamphlet, which amounted to little more than a string of extracts from letters and the press lauding his system. From a modern standpoint, some only cast doubt upon it: 'I came to Mr. Broster the 20th October, and before I had been with him half an hour, I was perfectly cured of a very bad impediment in my speech.'[139] Possibly this was written the day after he left the institution.

James Hunt pointed out that testimonials had always been a *questio vexata*. Anonymous ones were meaningless and the practice was 'equally the resort of truth and honesty, and of falsehood and fraud'. He valued the word of eminent medical men and the fact that Sir John Forbes MD referred patients to his father for 24 years spoke well for his results.[140] Furthermore, Thomas received backing from the *Literary Gazette*[141] during his difficulties with the *Lancet* and he was congratulated by the presiding magistrate at the trial of John Francis, charged with attempted assassination of the Queen. After a fortnight with Hunt, the key witness, George Pearson, was apparently transformed from inarticulateness to verbal spontaneity.[142] Kingsley also supported the family,[143] and it was to him that James' *Manual* was dedicated. James himself received a similar compliment in *The Unspeakable*, which was unstinting in its praise of him – so much so that one suspects collusion.[144]

Yet these favourable reports cannot be accepted uncritically. *The Unspeakable* was essentially a tale of woe and even Hunt's long-term results were not impeccable, for Kingsley[145] and Dodgson[146] stuttered to the end. So the criterion of success was not unerring fluency. Broster's system, for example, was said to be generally 'effective' but not always '*perfective*'.[147] The records of others were similarly blemished. By 1814, Thelwall had reported one failure,[148] but there must have been more, as it is unlikely that this was the patient who subsequently turned to Broster.[149] Bishop expected only a 1 per cent failure rate,[150] and perhaps this was so in his presence, which was 'magnetic', but Shorthouse for one was little improved in other situations.[151]

Although not more than 10 per cent of Hunt's patients regressed,[152] relapses were probably common. Many stutterers might be relieved whilst adhering to the rules that some practitioners laid down,[153] but these were either so irksome or unnatural that they slipped back into old ways. Poett put blame on the patient:

> There is no system, however perfect, but may be at times abused, and so fail in its application . . . there are many, with minds so weak and vacillating, that every effort to make them sensible of the necessity for their setting their own shoulders to the wheel is only so much time and trouble thrown away by the practitioner. With such individuals the merit of my system must in a manner be obscured, not because it is deficient *in se* . . . but because such people can never be brought to apply it to their own cases.[154]

To avoid 'odium' accruing to his character and method, Poett screened his patients, but despite this safeguard, Martin Tupper gained neither from him, nor from other practitioners.

On the positive side, it is probable that many patients improved significantly and had neither the inclination nor money to protract their treatment in hope of a perfect outcome. Certainly some were well enough satisfied to express their gratitude tangibly as well as verbally. Broster's achievements were recorded in *Blackwood's Magazine* through a poem, ending:

> Oh I have feelings few may guess,
> Which words, even words, cannot express,
> Due to him who loosed my voice, and brought
> The light of words to my darken'd thought;
> Not more grateful could Cain have been, I trow,
> Had the curse of Heaven been erased from his brow![155]

Broster's skill was further acknowledged when the principal booksellers of Edinburgh published, at his pupils' request, a portrait after the painting by John Syme.[156] Thomas Hunt was accorded a similar honour when former patients presented him with his bust, in testimony of 22 years' service. This was exhibited at the Royal Academy during 1849.[157] The artist was Joseph Durham, who had also sculptured

Tupper, and been encouraged by him.[158] In addition, Beasley was the recipient of a handsome marble timepiece and illustrated address from grateful pupils.[159] So there were a number of stutterers who, if not reaching the eloquence of Demosthenes or even their peers, had overcome the social and professional barriers that once intimidated them and consequently were no longer, in the words of their favourite poet, 'debarred from man's true attribute, The proper glorious privilege of Speech'.

Notes

1. *Plutarch's Lives* (Loeb edition), vol. 7, 12-19, 26-7.
2. Mackenzie, *Bell*, p. 43. *Bell's Standard Elocutionist* had sold 169 editions by 1893.
3. Shuldham, p. 36.
4. Cull (1835), pp. 5, 8, 14, 21.
5. A.M. Bell (1900), p. 249.
6. Ibid., p. 238.
7. Müller, p. 939.
8. Cazalet, p. 36.
9. McCormac, p. 83. Cf. G. 'Treatment of Stammering', letter to *Lancet*, 1 (1869), p. 520; Haward, p. 112; Shuldham, pp. 46-58; *Mind, Breath*, pp. 22-3; 'On the Cure of Stammering', *Medico-Chirurgical Review*, 41 n.s. (1844), 203-5; Abercrombie, p. 257, where he says that without breath, the patient '*has no voice*', which prompts another remedy, see below notes 102-10.
10. Helmore (1874), pp. 65-73; Frederick Helmore, *Breathers . . . for the Cure of Stammering* . . . (London, J. Masters & Co. [1880]). Cf. Sandlands, pp. 21-33.
11. A. Bell, pp. 19-21.
12. A.M. Bell (1900), p. 212. Other advocates of the mirror: Ball, p. 29; A. Bernard, p. 18; Colman (1895), p. 1421; Colman (1899), p. 453; Gray, p. 24; Kingsley (1901), vol. 3, p. 269; *Unspeakable*, p. 139.
13. Wright (1839), p. 44. Cf. Sandlands, p. 21.
14. Wright (1835), pp. 32, 39-40.
15. I can find this neither in Weiss's catalogue nor the patent lists.
16. I have been unable to trace these.
17. Editorial (1846a), p. 557, reproduced in *Literary Gazette* (1846), p. 508.
18. A.M. Bell (1900), p. 256.
19. Mason (1884), p. 11.
20. McCormac, p. 14.
21. Arnott (1827), p. 588.
22. Thelwall (1812), p. lxv.
23. Wright (1835), pp. 44-5.
24. Bartlett, p. 41.
25. Poett jnr, pp. v-vii, 18, 26. During these expositions, Poett claims to have coined the verb 'to vocalize', for 'vibrating air in the larynx', but in 1669 Holder had used it for the sound given to breath during its passage through the larynx.
26. A.M. Bell (1900), pp. 239, 246-7.
27. *Charles Kingsley* (1901), vol. 3, p. 268.
28. Holmes, p. 96.
29. A.M. Bell (1900), pp. 244-6.

30. A. Bell, p. 46.
31. Hunt (1861), p. 82.
32. 'Bride-langue' and 'langue-refoule', see Hunt (1870), p. 148. Such a gadget is presumably the 'snaffle-bit' noted in 'The Historical Remedy for Stammering', *British Medical Journal*, 2 (1898), 999-1000. For reproductions of several intra-oral instruments see Wingate, pp. 279-85; Murray Katz, 'Survey of Patented Anti-stuttering devices', *Journal of Communication Disorders*, 10 (1977), 181-206.
33. Kussmaul, pp. 841-2, 852.
34. Caleb, p. 159.
35. Hunt (1870), pp. 92-3.
36. For a description in English see McCormac, pp. 78-9.
37. Malagodi, *Medical Times*, 6 (1842), 14-15. Cf. Physician, pp. 44-5: 'I have heard patients, having undergone an operation, remark that, as long as the parts continued sore, they felt as though a bit and bridle had been applied, which forced them to speak slower, and appeared to render the articulation more manageable.'
38. Potter, p. 46.
39. Yearsley (1843-4), p. 288.
40. 'Wanderungen des Brosterschen Heilverfahrens gegen das Stottern', *Magazin der Ausländischen Literature*, 15 (1828), 93-5.
41. Hunt (1870), p. 72.
42. Caleb, p. 159.
43. Hunt (1870), pp. 69-70.
44. Ibid., p. 72.
45. Lee, p. 30.
46. Hunt (1870), p. 121. Hunt's name was misspelled in these publications. In 1830, Schulthess referred to him as 'Hari' and, in 1833, Rullier's version was 'Hert'. Even further distortions appeared in later writings.
47. McCormac, pp. 30-1.
48. Dr Zitterland, cited by Hunt (1870), p. 73.
49. Hunt (1870), p. 72.
50. Westminster Medical Society, *Provincial Medical and Surgical Journal*, 2 (1841), p. 17. It could be inferred that she negotiated directly with the Belgium government.
51. 'On Stammering and its Cure', *Medical Quarterly Review*, 4 (1835), 261-4.
52. Hunt (1870), p. 74. Cf. Potter, pp. 46, 49, 51.
53. Lee, pp. 29-30.
54. Dr B [*sic*] Voisin, 'New Method for the Cure of Stammering', reported in *British and Foreign Medical Review*, 5 (1838), p. 568.
55. Tupper, *My Life*, p. 72.
56. Correspondent, *Lancet*, 1 (1869), p. 484.
57. Yearsley (1843-4), p. 288.
58. Beasley (1885), p. 11.
59. A.M. Bell (1900), p. 249.
60. Borthwick, p. 49.
61. Wright (1835), p. 37.
62. Physician, pp. 46-7.
63. Abbotts, p. 49.
64. Kussmaul, p. 842.
65. Potter, p. 93.
66. 'Report on Instruments for the Cure of Stammering', *Journal of the Franklin Institute*, 57 (1854), 285-7.
67. *International Exhibition, 1862. Reports by the Juries . . .* (London,

printed for the Society of Arts, 1863), pp. 5, 16.

68. *Reports on the Paris Universal Exhibition, 1867* (London, HMSO, 1868), vol. 2, p. 231.

69. Hunt (1870), p. 303n; Foreign Correspondence, *Medical Times*, 2n.s. (1867), 158-9.

70. Ibid., p. 148.

71. Shuldham, p. 42.

72. Caxton, *What Will He Do With It?*, vol. 1, pp. 318-19. Cf. H. Cuthbert, 'Smoking for Stammerers', letter to *Lancet*, 2 (1895), p. 1673, where it is thought that the purpose was to sedate and improve respiratory power.

73. *Unspeakable*, pp. 78-9.

74. Cited by Hunt (1870), p. 304.

75. Sandlands, p. 44.

76. Wyllie, p. 136. Cf. Wright (1850), pp. 289-90.

77. Williams, p. 396.

78. Wright (1853), p. 32.

79. A.M. Bell (1900), p. 257.

80. Bishop (1851), pp. 78-9; Abbotts, p. 53.

81. Wright (1835), p. 33.

82. Ibid., pp. 31, 42-3; Wright (1839), p. 46; see above p. 119.

83. Poett jnr, p. 29.

84. See above p. 181.

85. Poett jnr, pp. xx-xxii.

86. Cull (1835), pp. 24, 25, 32, 46. Gymnastics seem to have been the basis of Chervin's treatment, which the *Lancet*, 2 (1874, p. 461) implied was '*his* original discovery' according to Alex J.D. D'Orsey's letter to *Lancet*, 2 (1874), p. 505, where he forwards his own claim.

87. Wyllie, p. 26.

88. Helmore, p. 73. Cf. Sandlands, p. 47.

89. Physician, p. 56.

90. *Mr. Thelwall's Lectures on . . . Elocution* (Birmingham, printed by J. Belcher & Son, 1806), pp. 29-34.

91. Lee, p. 37. Cf. Jonathan Osborne, *On some actions performed by voluntary muscles, which by habit become involuntary: with practical applications* (Dublin, University Press, 1860), Pt. 2, pp. 15-16.

92. Review of *Du Bégaiement . . .*, p. 466.

93. Poett jnr, p. 29. This device appears not to have been patented and no description is given.

94. See, for example, Daniel Hack Tuke, *Illustrations on the Influence of the Mind upon the Body*, 2nd edn (London, J. & A. Churchill, 1884), pp. 96-7.

95. Bacc. Med. Oxon., pp. 32, 52-7.

96. Kussmaul, p. 840n; Appelt, p. 35.

97. Bacc. Med. Oxon., pp. 32, 52-7. Cf. 'Stammering', *British Medical Journal*, 1 (1879), 674-5.

98. Abbotts, p. 49.

99. [Mason] (1885), pp. 10-11.

100. Ball, p. 24.

101. Ibid., pp. 27-30. See above pp. 108-9.

102. Arnott (1829), pp. 610-11. The *er* prefix was said to have been the secret remedy of Broster, an auctioneer, who treated stutterers several years before Arnott. For another version of Broster's secret, see Rockey (1979), p. 159.

103. Wright (1835), p. 36.

104. A. Bell, pp. 31, 33. Allied to this is treatment involving singing, intoning, the practice of scales etc. Cf. Notes 107-10, 126 below; A. Bernard, p. 20; Sandlands, pp. 36-7, 52-5; Abercrombie, p. 258 on 'a full and strong current of

voice'; *Mind, Breath*, pp. vi, 17, 25, 26, 27, 46, 48 on keeping up the 'stream of sound'; Wyllie, pp. 3-4 and Colman (1895), p. 1420 on 'vocalizing'. The latter caused Mrs Behnke to press her husband's priority claim and Van Praagh to assert that the method originated on the Continent, see letters to *Lancet*, 1 (1895), pp. 1557, 1620, 1681.

105. 'Hints to Stammerers', *Chambers's Journal*, no. 874 (1880), 635-7.

106. Urling, p. 49; Poett jnr, p. xvii.

107. Müller, p. 1057. This objection was supported by Carpenter, whose views were quoted *in extenso* by the reviewer of the 1842 edition of his *Principles*, *Medico-Chirurgical Review*, 39n.s. (1843), 133-9 (131-43).

108. Physician, pp. 47-8.

109. Bacc. Med. Oxon., pp. 48-9.

110. *Charles Kingsley* (1901), vol. 2, p. 45; vol. 1, p. 235. Cf. Bristowe (1883), p. 846; Abercrombie's (p. 257) church precentor, who 'showed no hestitation when *reading out the line*, as it is called'.

111. Alexander Melville Bell, *Phonetic Syllabication. The Cure for Oratorical and other Defects of Speech* (Washington, Volta Bureau, 1896), p. 17.

112. Müller, p. 1055.

113. Kussmaul, p. 826n.

114. Now called syllable-timed speech.

115. Academy of Sciences, 2 February, 1846, reported in *Medical Times*, 13 (1846), p. 383. Dr Serre d'Uzès is probably the physician usually referred to as Serres d'Alais, the two towns lying close together in the South of France.

116. A.M. Bell, *Syllabication*, p. 24.

117. Physician, pp. 54-7. Cf. Sandlands, pp. 61-8 on word-grouping.

118. Yearsley (1843-4), p. 248.

119. Academy of Medicine, Paris, 7 October 1843, 'Influence of Rhythm', *Medical Times*, 9 (1843), p. 92.

120. Note, *Lancet*, 2 (1842-3), p. 605.

121. For a recent illustration, see Wingate, p. 155. It was one of several time-keepers. An 'isochrome' was used in Europe during 1837 and an 'orthophone' in America, see Perkins, 'Physiological Studies' in Sheehan (ed.), p. 217.

122. Report of Colombat's memoir, *Lancet*, 2 (1842-3), 747.

123. For further information on anti-stuttering devices see Franklin Silverman and William Trotter, 'Bibliography: Literature Related to Use of Instrumental Aids in Stuttering Therapy', *Perceptual and Motor Skills*, 36 (1973), 247-51 and a similarly entitled 'Supplement', ibid., 38 (1974), 1329-30.

124. Bishop (1851), p. 60.

125. Shuldham, p. 34.

126. Thelwall (1812), pp. vii, xxi, xxv, xxx. To denote the light and heavy stresses in his scansions, Thelwall used the terms *arsis* and *thesis*, which, for the ancients, signified the lifting up and down of the hand or foot in time-beating. See also Henry Innes. *The Rhetorical Class Book* (London, John Limbard, 1834), p. 39n.

127. W.M. Parrish, 'The Concept of "Naturalness" ', *Quarterly Journal of Speech*, 37 (1951), p. 448 (448-54).

128. Thelwall (1812), pp. xxv-xxvi.

129. A.M. Bell [1853], pp. 26, 41.

130. Gerdts, pp. 7, 8, 9 and *passim*.

131. Rockey (1979), pp. 158-9.

132. B.H. Smart, *A Grammar of English Sounds . . . To which is prefixed an Introductory Essay, comprising . . . the Cure of Stammering, and the removal of other Defects and Impediments of Speech* (London, printed for John Richardson, 1812), pp. xxx-xliii. Cf. B.H. Smart, *A Practical Grammar of English Pronunciation . . . together with directions to persons who Stammer*. (London,

printed for John Richardson, 1810), pp. xiv, 41-4, 339-97.

133. Smart (1836), pp. xliii-xliv.

134. Wright (1835), pp. 44-51.

135. Thelwall (1812), pp. xviii-xx. Cf. [John Thelwall], *The Poetical Recreations of the Champion* (London, Champion Press, 1822), p. 243.

136. Medical Society of London, *Lancet*, 1 (1846), pp. 304, 553.

137. Yearsley (1841), p. 30.

138. Poett snr (1828), pp. 32-3.

139. Broster, p. 22.

140. Hunt (1861), p. 172.

141. In addition to references cited above, see 'The Cure of Stammering', *Literary Gazette*, no. 1262 (1841), 201-2; ibid., no. 1515 (1846), p. 112.

142. *DNB*, vol. 10, p. 280.

143. Hunt (1861), pp. 173-4.

144. I have been unable to trace any biographical information on James Malcolm Rymer, the author of other books.

145. Tupper, *My Life*, p. 74.

146. Hudson, *Lewis Carroll*, p. 106.

147. Pupil, *London Magazine Review*, 2 n.s. (1825), p. 534.

148. John Thelwall, *Results of Experience in the Treatment of Cases of Defective Utterance* (London, printed by M. M'Creery, 1814), Appendix, p. 4. It is not clear whether this patient was a stutterer.

149. See above p. 177.

150. Medical Society of London (1840-1a), p. 26.

151. *Life . . . of . . . Shorthouse*, vol. 1, p. 15.

152. Hunt (1861), p. 151.

153. A. Bernard, pp. 14-20; Borthwick, p. 37; M'Minn, p. 31; Poett jnr, pp. 27, 28, 33; Wright (1835), p. 35; Bartlett, pp. 43, 67-72. For brief comments on Bartlett's rules see a review of his book, *Medico-Chirurgical Review*, 30 n.s. (1838-9), p. 509 (507-9).

154. Poett snr (1828), pp. 54-5.

155. E.D., *(Blackwood's) Edinburgh Monthly Magazine*, 18 (1825), 730-1.

156. Broster, p. 7. This supposedly came from 'Notice respecting . . .', *(Blackwood's) Edinburgh Monthly Magazine*, 17 (1825), p. 47, but was added later.

157. Royal Academy Catalogue (1849), Item 1336.

158. Tupper, *My Life*, pp. 357-9.

159. B. Beasley, *Stammering: Its Treatment*, 11th edn (Birmingham, Hudson & Son, 1889), inside back cover.

CONCLUSION

The discords and vagaries traced by this book signal the first faltering steps of an ill-defined occupation. Stuttering was the battleground on which it was determined whether speech correction should become another medical specialty or the object of a new profession. That it became the latter is perhaps ironical, for physicians began relinquishing their claims when elocution was academically weak and without its most vigorous champions. From this impoverished beginning speech therapy ultimately grew. In the broader analysis, elocutionists triggered the same medical reflex that other supposed competitors and trespassers initiated. During the process of increasing its authority and dominance, the profession of medicine became engaged in skirmishes on several fronts and many occupational groups found themselves struggling for survival, independence or the right to registration, with varying degrees of success – chemists, dentists, veterinarians, herbalists, bone-setters, masseuses, corn-cutters, oculists, midwives,[1] and those laymen assisting the mentally ill. Basically at issue were power, status and financial reward. Victorian elocutionists achieved nothing tangible in the way of professional structure or state backing, nor were they sufficiently organised even to envisage or desire this, but they did hold the fort, and contemporary speech therapists are their heirs, though the conduct and professional relationships of the two groups differ, and direct continuity between them is tenuous. They find a point of contact, however, in the Behnkes, whose work continued well into this century, and whose close co-operation with doctors, and position in hospitals, is now commonplace. What is novel is the breadth of this professional harmony, which has not been without its price: physicians have surrendered therapy into the hands of laymen, who themselves have sacrificed much of the autonomy they once enjoyed. Langwill, a student of Wyllie, was perhaps the first to put this trend into words. Writing for *The Practitioner* during 1903, he urged, in the spirit of Victorians, that stuttering was a nervous rather than an educational problem, but he also admitted that it was impractical for medicine to claim total jurisdiction over it. Instead, he thought that physicians should supervise treatment after the fashion that orthopaedic surgeons prescribe remedial gymnastics. This suggestion was in line with the control doctors were then trying to establish over the midwives they had failed to oust.[2] Speech therapists, however, have resisted auxiliary status,[3] and the clinical independence they have managed to retain gives them some communion with their forebears.

The discipline as well as the profession was taking shape during the nineteenth century, from roots that had been laid down in the previous decades. The modern era in speech pathology, however embryonic, is recognisable in its symptomatology, aetiology, nosology and the more systematic approach to treatment, which was characterised by a proliferation and variety of methods. Previously, the rhetorical and medical traditions were distinct, but a more eclectic approach developed, especially amongst doctors, who began to blend the respective techniques. While limited to its phonetic and gross respiratory characteristics, the first comprehensive descriptions of stuttering began to appear, but little attention was paid to its development. Also new, were questions relating to its incidence and distribution. Fact gathering, albeit haphazard, conferred a measure of objectivity upon speculations, but the science that investigators craved was confounded by methodological and statistical naivety, together with a paucity of tests capable of probing beneath the manifest physiological and psychological symptoms. In sharp contrast is the situation now; indeed, it is the investigative method, rather than hypotheses or practices, that most distinguish the Victorian from our own approach. Accordingly, serious nineteenth century British treatises lacked rigor and savour more of today's popular writings, characteristics no doubt fostered by the limited academic audience and the relative importance of commercial ends.

Impressions are not always reliable, but in the absence of other information, it is worth noting that there appear to have been more writers of substance on the Continent and consequently more influence from that direction than vice versa. Certainly there was no British medical equivalent to Guillaume's article 'Bégaiement' in *Dictionnaire Encyclopédique des Sciences Médicales* (1868). Though far from widespread and uniform throughout their respective countries, the initiative of French and German writers is evident in their statistics, school clinics, free treatment centres, teacher training programmes, investigative committees and moves towards establishing professional bodies. The extent to which this was correlated with the fact that many were doctors or deaf educators can only be conjectured. Before drawing any firm conclusions more attention must be given to their work, to the European equivalent of the elocutionary movement, to the social significance of speech, and to the position of education and science in their countries.

British stutterers and practitioners acted out their roles in the wings of the Victorian stage. Though some were famous, most were bit-part players remaining out of the limelight and seeing little of whatever welfare was available. Certainly moves towards the systematic management of stuttering did faintly echo developments in mental health services and special education, but unlike other handicapped individuals, speech defectives prompted no government action. Nor did they, even as a group, inspire philanthropy. True the stutterer's plight aroused sympathy, not least amongst those therapists with first-hand experience, but their humanitarian motives were mixed with financial considerations as, having overcome their own problem, they endeavoured to derive from this knowledge a means of livelihood.

Nevertheless, nineteenth century speech correction was Victorian in essence. It was fashioned largely by current ideas in oro-vocal physiology, phonetics, phrenology, neurology and association psychology, which readily lent themselves to interpretations of speech breakdown. Furthermore, practices were typical of the times, often being family affairs kept afloat (one suspects precariously) by the enthusiasm of entrepreneurial proprietors, whose dynamic effect upon patients cannot be underestimated. This fact was recognised by Alexander Bell, who, cutting across all talk about the merits of individual systems, and overlooking his disagreement with aspects of his sons' book, said: 'That which is best administered is best.' What was, in fact, administered was frequently repetitive drills, themselves a reflection of the mechanical outlook of the age. But such routines could be mitigated by another contemporary influence – moral treatment, the curative properties of which were probably as great as any didactic system.

The Victorian ideals of self-help, self-improvement and excellence accorded well with the stutterer's situation, as did the popular classes in elocution, public performances of prose and verse, penny reading groups, and the like. Consequently, perhaps contrary to his position on the Continent, or today within the hospital clinic, the stutterer was more pupil than patient. In seeking the services of an elocutionist, he was not joining the sparce ranks of the pathologically inarticulate, but moving with the tide of a highly popular fashion. Though often withdrawn from society, he was not a social outcast. From the relatively little we know of him, however, it seems that his situation was ironical, since despite the variety of remedies at his disposal, for which extravagant claims were made, he frequently remained uncured, disillusioned and out of pocket. Such paradoxes were typical of his disorder, fascinating to many but understood by few, occasioning optimism in the midst of failure, open to numerous interpretations and antidotes, yet strangely elusive to all.

In part, this situation stemmed from lack of intellectual and professional cohesion amongst practitioners, which fostered dissension in a subject already disposed to arouse controversy by its complexity and obscurity. But instead of key issues being isolated and their implications explored, unproductive polemics were often substituted, with hyperbole replacing the measured language of science. Further, knowledge became a partisan affair, with some physicians giving consideration to the views only of eminent colleagues.

Many arguments centred on the issue of quackery, the definition of which was far from clear, and could be extended to include imprudent physicians, all non-medical men, well-meaning amateurs, sharp practitioners and outright tricksters, who seem to have been in the minority, if they entered the arena at all. In actuality, the therapeutic techniques used by reputable persons and those deemed charlatans differed little, respectability being conferred upon them by the spirit in which they were used. Socially acceptable practitioners were those for whom financial considerations were supposedly secondary, and who evidently acted in good faith for their patients' benefit. Frequently, their remedies were legitimised by being made 'scientific', that is, some apparently logical reason was found for them, often retrospectively. This phenomenon, of course, is still with us. Empiricism continues to flourish under the camouflage of science. Consequently, with poorly understood disorders, the dividing line between untrained practitioners and professionals may be fainter than the latter care to admit. One of the more fashionable stuttering treatments of late, for instance, well-known to Victorians, derived from an unorthodox source, hastily forgotten, while the remedy was garlanded in statistics and other scientific paraphernalia.

Contemporary mystification over the empirical nature of many modern remedies extends well beyond speech therapy and is related to professionalisation, a specialist's status being intimately bound up with his claim to operate through reason rather than chance. This appeal to reason results in an overriding attention to quantifiable facts and a conviction that a knowledge of causes is the key to fruitful treatment. Experiment, aetiology and theory assume great importance and become the edifice whereby orthodoxy raises itself above quackery. Thus, for example, endeavours to improve breathing are justified, not because they (may) work, but because they supposedly flow logically from the cause, say, a paucity of breath. Such reasoning reflects an ingrained belief within the professional mind that the cure is entailed in the causal proposition, sometimes expressed in the diagnosis. This question, fundamental to any philosophical analysis of treatment,[4] has several aspects, none of which can be explored here in detail. Suffice it to recall the difficulties inherent within the concept of cause touched on in Chapter 3. The most proper cause, taken philosophically, is the proximate, yet if this is indistinguishable from the complaint itself any theoretical appeal to causality begs the question. Aside from the ever present possibility of faulty aetiological inferences, the situation is further complicated by the variety of so-called causes and the level of their operation, both of which enable practitioners to administer differing and perhaps contradictory treatments with impunity. Hence, a patient whose tongue sticks fast will be given lingual gymnastics by one, while another, attributing this symptom to undue speech consciousness, will deplore mechanical rehabilitation and substitute a moral remedy. Each may justify his activities by an appeal to logic and causality, and it is pretty much a lottery what treatment a patient actually receives. Even when benefit does flow, it may not be for the reasons supposed: spontaneous cures, for example, though uncommon in stuttering, are always possible, and hence a happy outcome proves neither the correctness of the aetiological assumptions nor the logical basis of the treatment. Rather than concentrating on causes, it may be helpful to examine the natural history of a complaint, so that more can be learned of the conditions necessary to the production of a symptom. It then becomes tempting to suppose that by interfering with these conditions the problem will disappear, as indeed may happen but of which there can be no logical certainty. Syllogistic conclusions reveal only what is already known implicitly within the premiss, and this does not encompass the multiplicity of physiological, neurological and psychological reactions possible for any individual at any given time and place. The amount of information necessary to make a truly logical therapeutic inference is immense and years of research must be expected before the full causal story of some disorders is known.

Meanwhile, the best course is to recognise the situation, to see that there may be many paths to one goal, and that cures can happen as if by fluke. Prayer may well have been beneficial to a man of Martin Tupper's inclinations. Should a pill or some elocutionary exercise work with others, all well and good. If a particular technique helps many sufferers, so much the better. And if a valid explanation can be found, better still. The pejorative connotations of empiricism should not be allowed to conceal its existence or value. The inspired therapist often operates intuitively and need not apologise, nor be disdained, if reasons for a patient's new-found fluency are lacking. There is little justification for the belief that a body of scientific knowledge is, or need be, the only basis for effective treatment in the medical and allied specialties – psychiatry, for example, has proceeded accidentally for years, and in the matter of stuttering, speech therapy is in a similar position. Fortunately, the profession's reputation does not rest with this one complaint.

There are risks in failing to acknowledge the worth or presence of empiricism. For a start, the scientific drive may lead to a patient being taken apart rather than reintegrated. And despite it being a therapeutic cliché that everyone be treated as an individual, some clinics unremittingly subject their patients to one technique as experimenters set about controlling all variables for fact-gathering purposes, ambitious theorists with reputations to establish seek to keep some idea aloft at least long enough to publish a string of papers, whilst humbler clinicians are liable to follow trustingly the impressively decked out findings of their more illustrious colleagues. When the inherent limitations of this idea can no longer be overlooked, there follows a critique or refutation, which is presented as profound insight or new step forward. Thus 'progress' comes to involve the discarding of remedies already discounted by our predecessors. This practice is not peculiar to speech therapy, nor to Britain, where the scope for establishing logopaedic fashions is limited. Yet it is still apparent and predictable. Recently, for example, the tide has turned again as a 'multi-factorial' and pragmatic approach finds favour over the single technique.

Another danger is the self-confidence and sense of impunity practitioners may gain if convinced they are guided by logic and science. A possible consequence is that, with double standards operating, patients may be prepared to undergo and doctors experiment with treatments of dubious theoretical merit and distressing effects, which in the hands of quacks would be considered outrageous. The surgery of stuttering provides a rather extreme illustration, but time will doubtless reveal that some current medical practices are similarly misguided. Stuttering surgery demonstrates how patients are not necessarily best served by experts apparently at the frontiers of knowledge, since such patients are liable to become unsuspecting guinea pigs. In 1841, the stutterer was better off amongst the less imaginative British, than on the Continent, where the drive to help him seems to have been greater. The episode also shows how professional curiosity and competitiveness can distort therapeutic judgement and obscure the patient's real needs. One of the handicaps of contemporary British speech pathology is its lack of funding for research, difficulties in penetrating university circles, and relatively poor academic position. These may not be unconnected with its therapeutic strength, taken in relation to the totality of disorders. *Vis-à-vis* North America, the profession in Britain is most poorly placed, but its patients, with certain exceptions, are not.

It was in desire, rather than fact, that Victorian pathologists of stuttering embraced science, their motives being partly sociological, as indeed are those of their descendants, at least in Britain, science being one of the ways for an occupation to become professionalised, increase its status and command greater financial support. That speech pathologists should seek firm foundations for their discipline is most necessary, but speech correction, like the practice of medicine and agriculture, is essentially a servile art, co-operating with nature and thereby drawing out her best. To those convinced that science is the key to all ills, who believe in the linearity of progress and the distance between ourselves and the past, who are anxious to divest themselves of any taint of empiricism, and who wish to aggrandise their profession, this may be unwelcome. But with maturity should come the ability to delineate areas of ignorance, the patience to await the results of diligent research and the confidence to accept its limitations openly. There are signs that professional sensibilities are becoming less tender, for it is currently said that a realistic aim for stuttering treatment is the patient's acquisition of control over his symptom – cure being a medical concept applicable only to disease, which gives a new twist to the medico-elocutionary debate. The niceties of such verbal distinctions may well be lost on the hapless patient, desiring only to be rid of his complaint. Yet once again he is beset by paradox, since within the contention is a tactic admission that he must learn to live with his stuttering because current techniques are unlikely to be wholly effective. Thus, he cannot count on finding relief from the profession designed to help him. What, then, can he do? One may recall Sir Benjamin Brodie's words on quackery, written over a century ago when any hint of charlatarism raised a hue and cry. Reminding his colleagues that they were not infallible, he said that where medicine had no answer to an ailment it should not frown upon those who seek relief for their suffering elsewhere.[5]

To conclude: hindsight, bitter experience and unproductive enquiries have now demonstrated the intricacies of the problem. Stuttering remains an enigma. Theory does not, as two writers recently admit, 'reflect the kind of progressive change and refinement which one might have expected from a developing science'.[6] Yet advances have been made. Experimental findings, though largely negative, are none the less useful and have contributed towards the more coherent formulation of theories which, even if they remain unsatisfactory as explicatory models, subject the issues to more penetrating analysis. Cures, contrarily, have had a cyclical life, for current therapeutic fashions are often little more than discarded remedies given a new lease of life by the enthusiasm of therapists not yet tempered by failure. Creditably, contemporary social changes have made treatment freely available to all, which has minimised financial and other malpractices. But this alone is no cause for complacency, since there is no certainty that stuttering has been correspondingly reduced. At present, clinics replace the private homes or relaxing institutions of Huntingdon, Swanage and Hastings; and for most patients, weekly visits substitute for the intensive and extended supervision formerly given. Services may now be more widespread, but it is questionable whether they rival the best Victorians had to offer.

Notes

1. Donnison, pp. 44, 60-1, 88, 90, 116-17, 159, 165, 176, 180.
2. Ibid., pp. 161, 164-70, 175.
3. Department of Education and Science, pp. 12-13; Rockey (1979), p. 157.
4. For one article touching on this important, but much neglected subject see B.A. Farrell, 'Mental illness: a conceptual analysis', *Psychological Medicine*, 9 (1979), 21-35.
5. Review of books, *Quarterly Review*, 71 (1842-3), p. 105 (83-106).
6. Beech and Fransella, p. 55. Cf. ibid., p. 79.

BIBLIOGRAPHY

Abbotts, W. (1894), *Stammering, Stuttering and other Speech Affections* (London, Savoy Press)

Abercrombie, Dr (1843), 'Observations on the Impediment of Speech commonly called Stammering', *London & Edinburgh Monthly Journal of Medical Science*, 3, 257-8

Academy of Medicine, Paris, 16 February 1841 (1841), 'Treatment of Stuttering by Division of the Muscles of the Tongue', *Dublin Medical Press*, 5, 135-6

—— 26 February 1841 (1840-1), 'Cure of Stammering', *Provincial Medical and Surgical Journal*, 1, p. 381

Academy of Sciences, Paris, 15 February 1841 (1840-1), 'Operation for the Cure of Stuttering', *Provincial Medical and Surgical Journal*, 1, p. 366

Amussat, M. (1841), 'Cases of Section of the Muscles of the Tongue as a Cure for Stuttering', *Edinburgh Medical and Surgical Journal*, 56, 293-4

—— (1841-2), 'Clinical Observations on Stammering', *Provincial Medical and Surgical Journal*, 3, 39-40

Appelt, A. (1911), *The Real Cause of Stammering and its Permanent Cure* (London, Methuen)

Arnott, N. (1827), *Elements of Physics*, 2nd edn (London, printed Thomas & George Underwood)

—— (1829), *Elements of Physics*, 4th edn (London, Longman), vol. 1

Ashburner, J. (1843), *On Dentition, and some Coincident Disorders* (London, Longman)

Bacc. Medicinel Oxon. (1850), *On Stammering, and its Treatment* (London, John Churchill)

Ball, J.C. (1890), *The New Theory and Practice for the Cure of Stammering, Stuttering, and all other Defects of Speech* (London, Bretano's)

Bartlett, T. (1839), *Stammering Practically Considered* (London, Sherwood, Gilbert & Piper)

Bastian, H.C. (1898), *A Treatise on Aphasia and other Speech Defects* (London, H.K. Lewis), pp. 55-60

Baudens, M. (1841), 'On the Operations for Stuttering', *Dublin Medical*

Press, 5, 164-5

Beasley, B. (1885), *Stammering: its Treatment*, 8th edn (Birmingham, W.G. Moore & Co., printers)

—— (1905), *Stammering: its Treatment; and Reminiscences of a Stammerer*, 21st edn (Birmingham, Hudson & Son)

Beech, H.R. and Fransella, F. (1968) *Research and Experiment in Stuttering* (Oxford, Pergamon Press)

'Emile Behnke on the Nature and Treatment of Stammering' (1891), *Journal of Laryngology and Rhinology*, 5, 257-60

Behnke, E. [1893], *Stammering. Its Nature and Treatment. With Appendix on Voice Production in Speaking*, 4th edn (London, T. Fisher Unwin)

Behnke, R. [*sic*] (1897), 'Cure of Stammering', *Guy's Hospital Gazette*, 11 n.s., p. 324

Bell, A. (1849), *Stammering, and other Impediments of Speech*, 2nd edn (London, T. Hookam)

Bell, A.M. [1853], *Observations on Speech; the Causes and the Cure of Stammering, Mal-articulations and Defects* (Edinburgh, W.P. Kennedy)

—— (1900), *Principles of Speech and Dictionary of Sounds* (Washington, Volta Bureau)

Bell, C. (1832), 'Of the Organs of the Human Voice', *Philosophical Transactions of The Royal Society of London*, 122, 299-320

Bernard, A.G. (1889), *On the Causes, Treatment, and Cure of Stammering* (London, J. & A. Churchill)

Bernard, C. (1949 reprint of 1927 edn), *An Introduction to the Study of Experimental Medicine*, trans. Henry Copley Green (n.p. Henry Schuman)

Bishop, J. (1846), 'Observations on the Cause and Treatment of Stammering, and on the pathology and therapeutics of some of the less aggravated forms of Aphonia', *Transactions of the Medical Society of London*, 1 n.s., 25-37

—— (1851), *On Articulate Sounds; and on the Causes and Cure of Impediments of Speech* (London, Samuel Highley)

Blake, E. (1890), *Lip Chorea and Paresis of the External Pterygoid Muscles, commonly called "Stammering"* (London, Harrison & Son)

Blathwayt, R. (April 1900), 'A Talk with Mr. Beasley of Brampton Park', *Cassell's Magazine*, pp. 574-8

Bloodstein, O. (1969), *A Handbook on Stuttering* (Chicago, Nat. Easter Seal Co. for Crippled Children & Adults)

Bluemel, C.S. (1913), *Stammering and Cognate Defects of Speech*

(New York, Stechert & Co.), Vols. 1 and 2

Borthwick, T. (1836), *Remarks on the Elements of Language, and the Physiology of Respiration, as the means of producing Voice and Speech, illustrative chiefly of the nature of Stammering* (Edinburgh, The Edinburgh Printing Co.)

Bostock, J. (1830), 'History of a Case of Stammering, successfully treated by the long continued use of cathartics', *Medico-Chirurgical Transactions*, 16, 72-7

Braid, J. (1840-1), 'Cure of Stammering', *London Medical Gazette*, 2 n.s., 116-18

—— (1841), 'Observations on Talipes, Strabismus, Stammering, and Spinal Contortion, and the best methods of removing them', *Edinburgh Medical and Surgical Journal*, 56, 338-64

Bristowe, J.S. (1880), *The Physiological and Pathological Relations of Voice and Speech being the Lumleian Lectures, 1879* (London, David Bogue). These lectures first appeared in the *Lancet* during 1879

—— [1882], 'Stammering' in *A Dictionary of Medicine*, ed. Richárd Quain (London, Longmans, Green & Co.), Pt. 2, pp. 1512-14

—— (1883), 'The Throat, Voice, and Speech' in *The Book of Health*, ed. Malcolm Morris (London, Cassel), pp. 811-52

—— (1892), 'Stammering' in *A Dictionary of Psychological Medicine*, ed. D. Hack Tuke (London, J. & A. Churchill), 2, 1191-3

Broster, J. (1826), *Progress of the System for the Effectual Removal of Impediments in Speech* (London, C. Roworth)

Browne, L. and Behnke, E. (1883), *Voice, Song, and Speech: A Practical Guide for Singers and Speakers* (London, Sampson Low)

Burdin, G. (1940), 'The Surgical Treatment of Stammering: 1840-42', *Journal of Speech Disorders*, 5, 43-64

Butterfield, H. (1846), 'On the Immediate Cause of Stammering, and the Means of Cure', *Lancet*, 1, 336-7

Bynum, W. (1974), 'Rationales for Therapy in British Psychiatry: 1780-1835', *Medical History*, 18, 317-34

Caleb, C.C. (1883), 'On Stammering', *The Students' Journal and Hospital Gazette*, 11, 135-6, 147-9, 158-60

Carpenter, W.B. (1844), *Principles of Human Physiology*, 2nd edn (London, J. Churchill), ch. 6

Cazalet, W.W. (1873), *Stammering: the Cause and Cure; and on Defective Utterance* 5th edn (London, Henry Renshaw)

Colman, W.S. (1895), 'A Lecture on Stammering and other Impediments of Speech, and their treatment on physiological principles',

Lancet, 1, 1419-21
—— (1899), 'Impediments of Speech' in *A System of Medicine*, ed. Thomas Allbutt (London, Macmillan & Co.), 7, 448-56
Combe, A. (1852), *The Principles of Physiology applied to the Preservation of Health, and to the Improvement of Physical and Mental Education*, ed. James Coxe, 14th edn (Edinburgh, MacLachlan & Stewart), ch. 12
Coote, H. (1868), 'Notes of a Clinical Lecture on Stuttering and Stammering', *British Medical Journal*, 2, pp. 611-12
Copland, J. (1858), 'Voice and Speech' in *A Dictionary of Practical Medicine* (London, Longman), 3, Pt. 2, pp. 1360-6
Correspondent (1840-1), 'Stammering versus Squinting', *Lancet*, 1, 899-900
Crichton, A. (1798), *An Inquiry into the Nature and Origin of Mental Derangement* (London, printed for T. Cadell junior & W. Davies), 2, 72-82
Cull, R. (1833), *Observations on Impediments of Speech*, 2nd edn (London, Renshaw & Rush)
—— (1835), *Stammering, considered with reference to its Cure by the Application of those Laws which Regulate Utterance* (London, Henry Renshaw)
Darwin, E. (1794), *Zoonomia; or, the Laws of Organic Life* (London, printed for J. Johnson), Vol. 1, pp. 185-97, Vol. 2, p. 505
Department of Education and Science (1972), *Speech Therapy Services* (London, HMSO)
Dieffenbach, J.F. (1841), *Memoir on the Radical Cure of Stuttering by a Surgical Operation*, trans. Joseph Travers (London, Samuel Highley)
Donnison, J. (1977), *Midwives and Medical Men* (London, Heinemann)
Editorial (1846a), *Lancet*, 1, 557-8
—— (1846b), *Lancet*, 1, 663-4
Eldridge, M. (1968), *History of the Treatment of Speech Disorders* (Edinburgh, Livingstone)
Firth, J.R. (1957), 'The English School of Phonetics' in *Papers in Linguistics 1934-1951* (London, Oxford UP), pp. 92-120
Forshaw, C.F. (1887), *The Cause and Cure of Stammering* (Stanningley, J.W. Birdsall printers)
Foster, J.E. [1885], *Impediments of Speech. The Cause and Cure* (London, Simpkin & Marshall)
—— [1900], *Defects in Speech: Their Cause and Cure*, 4th edn (London, Simpkin)
Franz, A. (1840-1a), 'An Account of Dieffenbach's New Operation

for the Cure of Stuttering. With Case', *London Medical Gazette*, 1 n.s., 920-4

Franz, A. (1840-1b), 'Final Result of a Case in which Dieffenbach's Operation for Stammering was Performed: with Observations', *London Medical Gazette*, 2 n.s., 814-17

Freidson, E. (1970), *Profession of Medicine. A Study of the Sociology of Applied Knowledge* (New York, Dodd, Mead & Co.)

Gerdts, A.E. (1883), *The Impediments of Speech and their Cure*, enl. edn (Bingen-on-Rhine)

Good, J.M. (1829), *The Study of Medicine*, ed. Samuel Cooper, 3rd edn (London, Thomas & George Underwood), Vol. 1, pp. xxx, 565-8

Graves, R.J. (1884), *Clinical Lectures on the Practice of Medicine* reprinted from 2nd edn (London, New Sydenham Soc.), Vol. 1, 652-60

Gray, W.R. (1862), *The Tongue and its Training* (London, William Knight & Co.)

Gutzmann, H. (1891), 'Defects in Speech among School Children', *Physique*, 1, 141-3

Hall, M. (1825), 'Some Observations on the Physiology of Speech read to a Literary Society, at Nottingham, on January the 3rd, 1825', *Quarterly Journal of Science, Literature and the Arts*, 19, 8-16

—— (1831), 'Some Observations on Dr. Arnott's explanation of the nature of Stammering', *Journal of the Royal Institution*, 12, 253-61

—— (1841), 'Stammering; Chorea' in *On the Diseases and Derangements of the Nervous System* (London, H. Baillière), ch. 5

Harms, E. (1957), 'Modern Psychotherapy – 150 Years Ago', *Journal of Mental Science*, 103, 806-9

Hartley, A.M. (1833), *Observations on the different kinds of Impediments of Speech, particularly Spasmodic Stammering; with instructions how to remove them* (London, Simpkin & Marshall)

Hartley, D. (1749), *Observations of Man, his Frame, his Duty and his Expectations* (London, printed by S. Richardson), Vol. 1, ch. 2

Hartwell, E.M. (1895), 'Stuttering and Stammering', *Werner's Magazine*, 17, 17-22

Haward, W. (1887), 'Clinical Lecture on some forms of Defective Speech', *Lancet*, 1, 111-12

Helmore, R. (1874), *Speakers, Singers, and Stammerers* (London, Joseph Masters & Co.)

Holmes, G. (1884), *The Science of Voice Production and Voice Preservation*, new edn (London, Chatto & Windus)

Hunt, J. (1854), *A Treatise on the Cure of Stammering etc.* (London, Longman)

Hunt, J. (1858), *A Few Words on Impediments of Speech etc*, 2nd edn (Hastings)
—— (1859), *A Manual of the Philosophy of Voice and Speech* (London, Longman)
—— (1861), *Stammering and Stuttering, their Nature and Treatment* (London, Longman). Facsimile edition, New York & London, Hafner Pub. Co., 1967
—— (1863), *Stammering and Stuttering, their Nature and Treatment*, 5th edn (London, Longman)
—— (1870), *Stammering and Stuttering, their Nature and Treatment*, ed. H.F. Rivers, 7th edn (London, Longmans)
H–T, J. (1860), 'Stammering', *Encyclopaedia Britannica*, 8th edn (Edinburgh, Adam & Charles Black), Vol. 20, 533-5
Hunt, T. (1846), Letter in *Literary Gazette*, no. 1532, 503-4
Hunter, R. and Macalpine, A. (1963), *Three Hundred Years of Psychiatry, 1535-1860* (London, Oxford UP)
Jones, K. (1972), *A History of the Mental Health Services* (London, Routledge & Kegan Paul)
Charles Kingsley; His letters and memories of his life (1901), ed. by his wife (London, Macmillan & Co.), Vol. 1, pp. 22-3, 234-5; Vol. 2, pp. 44-5; Vol. 3, pp. 18, 267-9
Kussmaul, A. (1878), 'Disturbances of Speech', in *Cyclopaedia of the Practice of Medicine*, ed. H. von Ziemssen, trans. E. Buchanan Baxter *et al.* (London, Sampson Low), Vol. 14, 581-865
Lebrun, Y. and Bayle, M. (1973), 'Surgery in the Treatment of Stuttering', *Neurolinguistic Approaches to Stuttering*, ed. Y. Lebrun and R. Hoops (The Hague, Mouton), pp. 81-9
Lee, E. (1841), *On Stammering, Squinting, and on the Methods for their Removal* (London, John Churchill)
Lizars, A.J. (1840-1), 'Division of the Genio-Hyo-Glossi Muscles, for Stammering', *Lancet*, 2, 766-7
Lucas, P.B. (1840-1), 'On Division of the Genio-Glossi Muscles, for the Cure of Stammering', *Provincial Medical and Surgical Journal*, 1, 389-90
—— (1841a), 'On the Treatment of Stammer by Surgical Operation', *Provincial Medical and Surgical Journal*, 2, 12-15
—— (1841b), 'Case of Stammering, in which Professor Dieffenbach's Operation was Performed', *Provincial Medical and Surgical Journal*, 2, 109-12
—— (1841c), 'Remarks on the New Attempts to Cure or Relieve Stammer, and other Impediments in Speech, by Surgical Operation',

Provincial Medical and Surgical Journal, 2, 247-9
Mason, N.H. (1884), *A Practical Guide to the Cure of Stammering* (London, Wyman & Sons)
[——] (1882), 'Notes on Stammering', *Elocutionist*, 1, 90-1
[——] (1883), ibid., 1, 152-3
[——] (1885), ibid., 3, no. 33, p. 13, no. 34, 10-11
McCormac, H. (1828), *A Treatise on the Cause and Cure of Hesitation Speech, or Stammering* (London, Longman)
M'Minn, T. (1897), *Stammering: its Cause and Cure, considered in the light of modern medical science* (Belfast, Marcus Ward & Co.)
Medical Society of London (1840-1a), 'Is an Operation Necessary for the Cure of Stammering?', *Lancet*, 2, 25-7
—— (1840-1b), 'Stammering a Purely Functional Affection. – Influence of Mental Impressions on its Cure', *Lancet*, 2, 75-7
The Mind, the Breath, and Speech; or Practical Remarks on Stammering (1848), (London, James Madden)
A Minute Philosopher (1859), 'The Irrationale of Speech', *Fraser's Magazine*, 60, 1-14
Müller, J. (1842), *Elements of Physiology*, trans. William Baly (London, printed for Taylor & Walton), Vol. 2, pp. 939, 1054-8
'On the Cure of Stammering, by the Removal of the Uvula and Tonsils', (1840-1), *Lancet*, 2, 587-94
Paget, J. (1868), 'Remarks on Stammering with other Organs than those of Speech', *British Medical Journal*, 2, p. 437-8
Palmer, S. (1829), *Popular Illustrations of Medicine* (London, Baldwin & Cradock), pp. 63-75
Pershing, H.T. (1897), 'The Disorders of Speech' in *Twentieth Century Practice, an International Encyclopedia of Modern Medical Science*, ed. Thomas Stedman (London, Sampson, Low, Marston & Co.), Vol. 10, 777-805
Phillips, C. (1841), *De La Ténotomie &c.* (Paris, Baillière), ch. 13
A Physician Incognita (1843), *A Treatise on the Nature and Causes of Stammering* (London, Samuel Highley)
Plumptre, C.J. (1883), *King's College Lectures on Elocution*, 4th edn (London, Trübner & Co.)
Poett, J. snr (1828), *Observations on Psellismus, or Stammering, with accompanying cases of Cure* (Dublin, Joseph Blundell printers)
—— (1833), *A Practical Treatise on Stammering, and Nervous Affections of Speech*, 4th edn (London, S. Highley, booksellers)
—— (1840-1), 'Operations for Stammering', *Lancet*, 2, 414-16

Poett, J.H.A. jnr (1858), *A Practical Treatise on Stammering, its Pathology, Predisposing, Exciting, and Proximate Causes, and its most successful mode of Cure, scientifically explained* (London, John Churchill)
Potter, S.O.L. (1882), *Speech and Its Defects* (Philadelphia, B. Blakiston, Son & Co.)
Pritchard, D.G. (1963), *Education and the Handicapped 1760-1960* (London, Routledge & Kegan Paul)
'Psellism' in *Household Words* (1856), 14, 464-9
Review of *Du Bégaiement, ses Causes, &c., et Moyens Thérapeutiques pour Prévenir, Modifier, ou Guérir, cette Infirmité*; par M. Felix Voisin in *Phrenological Journal and Miscellany* (1826-7), 4, 458-67. Reprinted in *Journal of Communication Disorders* (1977), 10, 146-52
Review of Dieffenbach's *Memoir, London and Edinburgh Monthly Journal of Medical Science* (1841), 1, 372-5
Review of four recent publications on stuttering surgery, *British and Foreign Medical Review* (1841), 12, 209-14
Richerand, A. (1807), *Elements of Physiology*, trans. Robert Kerrison, 2nd edn (London, printed for John Callow)
Rockey, D. (1977), 'The Logopaedic Thought of John Thelwall, 1764-1834: First British Speech Therapist', *British Journal of Disorders of Communication*, 12, 83-95
—— (1979), 'John Thelwall and the Origins of British Speech Therapy', *Medical History*, 23, 156-75
Romberg, M.H. (1853), *A Manual of the Nervous Diseases of Man*, trans. and ed. Edward Sieveking (London, Sydenham Soc.), Vol. 1, 362-6
Rosenthal, M. (1881), *A Clinical Treatise on the Diseases of the Nervous System*, trans. L. Putzel (London, Sampson Low), Vol. 2, 131-5
Sandlands, J.P. (1886), *How to Develop General Vocal Power and Cure Stammering and Defective Speech* (London, Sampson Low)
Schoolfield, L.D. (1938), 'The Development of Speech Correction in America in the 19th Century', *Quarterly Journal of Speech*, 24, 101-16
Sheehan, J.G. (ed.) (1970), *Stuttering: Research and Therapy* (New York, Harper Row)
Shuldham, E.B. [1879], *Stammering and its Rational Treatment; with remarks on Canon Kingsley's Elocutionary Rules* (London, Homœopathic Pub. Co.)
Smart, B.H. (ed.) (1836), *Walker Remodelled. A New Critical*

Pronouncing Dictionary (London, printed for T. Cadell), pp. iv-xliv
'Stammering' in *The Penny Cyclopaedia* (London, Charles Knight & Co., 1842), Vol. 22, 429-34
Stevenson, L.G. (1968), 'The Surgery of Stammering: a forgotten enthusiasm of the nineteenth century', *Bulletin of the History of Medicine*, 42, 527-54
Stevenson, R.S. and Guthrie, D. (1949), *A History of Oto-laryngology* (Edinburgh, E. & S. Livingstone)
'Terminology for Speech Pathology', *Speech Pathology and Therapy* (1960), 3, 35-9
Thelwall, J. (1810), *A Letter to Henry Cline Esq.* (London, printed by Richard Taylor & Co)
—— (1812), *Illustrations of English Rhythmus* (London, printed by J.M. 'Creery)
The Unspeakable; or, the Life and Adventures of a Stammerer (1855) (London, Clarke & Beeton)
Urling, G.F. (1857), *Vocal Gymnastics; or, a Guide for Stammerers, and for Public Speakers and Others* (London, John Churchill)
Van Riper, C. (1971), *The Nature of Stuttering* (Englewood Cliffs, Prentice-Hall)
'M. Velpeau – Surgical Treatment of Stuttering' (1841), *Dublin Medical Press*, 5, 196-7
Walk, A. (1954), 'Some Aspects of the "Moral Treatment" of the Insane up to 1854', *Journal of Mental Science*, 100, 807-37
Wallace, W. (1974), *Causality and Scientific Explanation* (Ann Arbor, University of Michigan Press), Vol. 2, 76-160
Westminster Medical Society (1840-1a), 'Stammering, its Causes and Treatment', *Lancet*, 2, 23-5
—— (1840-1b), 'The Nature, Causes, and Treatment of Stammering by Operation, and Otherwise', *Lancet*, 2, 77-81
Williams, W.C. (1872), 'Stuttering Relieved by an Artificial Palate', *British Journal of Dental Science*, 15, p. 396
Wingate, M.E. (1976), *Stuttering. Theory and Treatment* (New York, Irvington)
Wright, J. (1835), *A Treatise on the Causes and Cure of Stuttering, with reference to certain modern theories* (London, Whittaker & Co.)
—— (1839), *Impediments of Speech. Three Letters to Sir Charles Bell, K.G.H. F.R.S.L. & E. on the Causes and Cure of Stuttering* (London, Whittaker & Co.)
—— (1843), *The Stutterer's Friend*, 2nd edn (London, printed for

Sherwood, Gilbert, & Piper)

Wright, J. (1850), 'A Lecture on the Mental and Mechanical Obstacles Present in the Defects of Speech, termed Stammering and Stuttering', *Lancet*, 2, 287-91

Wyllie, J. [1894], *The Disorders of Speech* (Edinburgh, Oliver & Boyd)

XYZ (1852), *A Few Words on Stammering* (London, W. Brickhill)

Yearsley, J. (1841), *Stammering, and other Imperfections of Speech, treated by Surgical Operations on the Throat* (London, Churchill)

—— (n.d.), *Statement of facts relative to some new Operations lately proposed for the relief of Stammering: in refutation of false and interested counter-statements recently published in the Lancet* (n.p.)

—— (n.d.), *Mr. Yearsley's Letters to the President and Council of the Royal College of Surgeons in London, on the unprofessional conduct of Mr. Liston* (n.p.)

—— (1843-4), 'On Stammering, its Causes, Varieties, and Treatment', *Lancet*, 1, 244-8, 288-93

Yearsley, W.A. (1909), *A Practical Self-Cure of Stammering and Stuttering* (Accrington, Mrs. W.A. Yearsley)

Young, R.M. (1970), *Mind, Brain and Adaptation in the Nineteenth Century* (Oxford, Clarendon Press)

INDEX

For Product Safety Concerns and Information please contact our EU representative GPSR@taylorandfrancis.com Taylor & Francis Verlag GmbH, Kaufingerstraße 24, 80331 München, Germany